A Guide to
Radiological Procedures

A Guide to Radiological Procedures

Third Edition

Edited by

Stephen Chapman
MB BS, MRCS, MRCP, FRCR

Consultant Radiologist
The Children's Hospital, Birmingham,
Senior Clinical Lecturer, University of Birmingham.

Richard Nakielny
MA, BM, BCh, FRCR

Consultant Radiologist (CT Scanning)
Royal Hallamshire Hospital, Sheffield;
Honorary Clinical Lecturer, University of Sheffield

Baillière Tindall
London Philadelphia Toronto Sydney Tokyo

Baillière Tindall	24–28 Oval Road
W. B. Saunders	London NW1 7DX

The Curtis Center
Independence Square West
Philadelphia, PA 19106–3399, USA

55 Horner Avenue
Toronto, Ontario, M8Z 4X6, Canada

Harcourt Brace Jovanovich Group
(Australia) Pty Ltd
30–52 Smidmore Street
Marrickville
NSW 2204, Australia

Harcourt Brace Jovanovich Japan Inc
Ichibancho Central Building,
22–1 Ichibancho
Chiyoda-ku, Tokyo 102, Japan

First published 1981
Second edition 1986
Third edition 1993

A catalogue record for this book is available from the British
Library

ISBN 0-7020-1678-0

Typeset by Colset Private Limited, Singapore
Printed and bound in Great Britain by Mackays of Chatham PLC,
Chatham, Kent

Contents

Contributors

The numbers in brackets following the contributors' names refer to the chapters written or co-written by the contributors.

C.M. Boivin *BSc, MPhil* [1–5,7–12,14,15]
Senior Computer Scientist,
Deputy Head of Nuclear Medicine,
Queen Elizabeth Hospital, Birmingham

T.J. Cleveland *FRCS* [1–3,8]
Senior Registrar in Radiology
Royal Hallamshire Hospital, Sheffield

W.D. Jeans *FRCR* [8,9]
Prof of Radiology
University of Oman

S. Olliff *MRCP, FRCR* [3–6,9,15]
Consultant Radiologist
Queen Elizabeth Hospital, Birmingham
Senior Clinical Lecturer, University of Birmingham

V. Cassar-Pullicino *FRCR* [12]
Consultant Radiologist
Robert Jones and Agnes Hunt Orthopaedic Hospital, Oswestry
Senior Clinical Lecturer, University of Birmingham

M. Collins *FRCR* [4,5]
Consultant Radiologist
Royal Hallamshire Hospital, Sheffield,
Honorary Clinical Lecturer, University of Sheffield

J.F.C. Olliff *MRCP, FRCR* [3–6,9,15]
Consultant Radiologist
Queen Elizabeth Hospital
Senior Clinical Lecturer, University of Birmingham

M.J.W. Sparks *FRCS* [1,7,9–11]
Senior Registrar in Radiology
The Royal Hallamshire Hospital, Sheffield

Foreword to the First Edition

Ten years ago the Royal College of Radiologists (at that time named the Faculty of Radiologists) revised its examination structure and introduced a Part I examination. The syllabus for this was to cover the basic sciences of radiology, and in radiodiagnosis it was to cover physics as applied to radiodiagnosis, radiographic photography, apparatus construction, radiological anatomy and radiological procedures, including the pharmacology of contrast media.

Radiological procedures are defined as being that aspect of our work concerned with the carrying out of investigations on patients and necessitate a knowledge of radiography and a knowledge of how to carry out special procedures in the Department of Radiodiagnosis. All radiologists must be trained to carry out these procedures and all radiographers must know how such procedures are performed, and be able to prepare the scene for and carry out the radiographic aspects of the procedure.

To date, no concise authoritative book has been produced on this subject. It seemed to the two writers, who were recently successful in the examination, that it would be useful if a reference book could be made available covering just this field, and they were encouraged to produce one. The result is this highly practicable book.

The preparation of such a book is bound to be subjective and largely dependent on the practice in the department in which the radiologists concerned are training and practising. No secret is made of the fact that the methods and procedures described in this book are those in use in the Teaching Hospital of the University of Bristol, and no claim is made to establish what is described as being the only way to conduct these examinations. It can, however, be claimed that in Bristol these examinations are carried out successfully and safely by these methods.

The two writers have worked with immense enthusiasm and energy which has been reflected in the constructive criticism of their colleagues and teachers.

Recourse has been made to the literature, and relevant references and suggested further reading is given at logical points in the text. A uniform method of presentation of the procedures has been used throughout, and certain other useful data included.

I believe that this book will come to be regarded as essential reading for all trainee radiologists, and will become a standard reference book in every Department of Radiology throughout the country, and indeed, wherever diagnostic radiology is practised.

I recommend it to all radiologists, to all Schools of Radiography, and to all radiographers working in departments where special procedures are carried out.

I am confident of its success.

April 1981   *Sir Howard Middlemiss*

Preface to the Third edition

Since the second edition of this book there have been significant changes in the Royal College of Radiologists' guidelines for the Part I Fellowship examination. This new edition has taken these into account. There are also substantial additions of ultrasound and radionuclide imaging within the chapters. Basic information on MRI and CT is also included. The increased amount of clinical information in this edition is aimed to facilitate the progression from Part I radiology onto true clinical radiology.

We welcome several new contributors to this edition who have provided not only expertise in their specialist fields but have also helped in maintaining the book as it was originally intended, i.e. as a basic guide for the new trainee in radiology.

Stephen Chapman
Richard Nakielny

Preface to the Second Edition

At the time of writing the first edition the new generation of low-osmolar contrast media were just being introduced and were not available for general clinical usage. Now that they are widely available and their place in diagnostic radiology is more clearly defined, it is time to produce a new edition.

A new chapter on water-soluble contrast media has been included and the text elsewhere updated. Some older procedures such as double-contrast cystography have been omitted, while newer techniques such as percutaneous nephrolithotomy have been introduced. The decision to retain gynaecography and, to a lesser extent, air encephalography was a difficult one. These techniques are now seldom performed but candidates may well be faced with examples of them in the examinations.

We hope that we have complied with most of the changes that have been suggested to us, in particular the need for more illustrations. However, we have again confined ourselves to X-ray techniques only. We could not hope to cover all the imaging modalities and still retain a book of this size.

Finally we must record our thanks to our colleagues who have helped with the preparation of this edition. Our particular thanks go to Bill Jeans and Mike Collins, who have rewritten several sections and to Victor Cassar-Pullicino of the Robert Jones and Agnes Hunt Hospital, Oswestry, who updated the section on lumbar discography. Thanks also to Nicholas Dunton and the others at Baillière Tindall who have maintained their confidence in us and to Susan Sheehan who typed much of the manuscript.

Stephen Chapman
Richard Nakielny

Preface to the First Edition

The impetus for producing this book came from the difficulty experienced by junior radiologists in assembling all the basic information on radiological procedures. We do not deny that the information is available in the many excellent standard works on radiological sub-specialties, but there is at present no work that brings this information together into one book. We have not intended this to be an exhaustive text, but we do believe it contains sufficient information to satisfy the needs of clinical practice and the requirements of the primary Fellowship examination.

Although principally intended for junior doctors at the commencement of their training in radiology, we also believe this book will be useful to radiographers, especially those taking a higher diploma, and serve as an *aide memoire* in the X-ray suite.

Each chapter begins with a list of the different methods by which an organ or system may be imaged. It should be stressed, however, that no attempt has been made to suggest any order of investigation. The modalities of ultrasound, radioisotopes and computerized tomography may well be the first choice in the investigation of a particular clinical problem. Details of these imaging methods have not been included, as to deal with them adequately would have considerably increased the size of the book. Relevant references have been given should the reader require further information, and useful books are included in a further reading list. Detailed radiography has also been omitted, again to reduce the length of the text and because this aspect is comprehensively covered by well-known books on radiography.

Each procedure is laid out in a logical and consistent manner, as suggested by the Royal College of Radiologists in their Part I syllabus. The technique of each procedure is essentially that which is practised in the United Bristol Hospitals and the reader may find that his hospital adopts a slightly different approach. Consequently a wide left-hand margin has been incorporated for the reader to add modifications in technique to suit local practices and also to add information he may acquire during wider reading. We have adopted a note style of writing as we are well aware of the volume of reading that has to be undertaken by today's junior doctors. We would also emphasize that the acquisition of knowledge about practical procedures should be in conjunction with tuition from and supervision by experienced radiologists. Reading is no substitute for practical experience.

Finally, we wish to record our thanks to everyone in the Department of Radiodiagnosis at the Bristol Royal Infirmary who criticized, helped and encouraged.

Stephen Chapman
Richard Nakielny

Abbreviations

Throughout the text the following abbreviations have been used:

AP	anteroposterior
PA	posteroanterior
RAO	right anterior oblique
LAO	left anterior oblique
RPO	right posterior oblique
LPO	left posterior oblique
CT	computerized tomography
MRI	magnetic resonance imaging
LOCM (370)	low-osmolar contrast medium (containing 370 mg ml^{-1} iodine)
HOCM	high-osmolar contrast medium

1 General Notes

Radiology

The procedures are laid out under a number of sub-headings which follow a standard sequence. The general order is outlined below, together with certain points which are omitted from the discussion of each procedure to avoid repetition. Minor deviations from this sequence will be found in the text where this is felt to be more appropriate.

Methods

Indications

Contraindications All radiological procedures carry a risk. The risk incurred from undertaking the procedure must be balanced against the benefit to the patient from the information obtained. Contraindications may, therefore, be relative (the majority) or absolute.

Factors that increase the risk to the patient can be considered under three headings: due to radiation; due to the contrast medium; due to the technique.

Due to radiation Radiation effects on humans may be hereditary, i.e. revealed in the offspring of the exposed individual, or somatic. Somatic injuries fall into two groups: stochastic and non-stochastic. The latter, e.g. skin erythema and cataracts, occur when a critical threshold has been reached and are not relevant to diagnostic radiology. Stochastic effects are 'all or none'.[1] The cancer produced by a small dose is the same as the cancer produced by a large dose but the frequency of its appearance is less with the smaller dose. It is obviously impossible to avoid some radiation exposure to staff and patients and stochastic effects cannot be completely eliminated. There is an excess of cancers following diagnostic levels of irradiation to the fetus[2] and the female breast[3], and trends of increasing rates of cancer are seen in workers in the nuclear power industry exposed to low doses[4]. The total collective population dose from medical X-rays could be responsible for between 200 and 500 of the 160 000 cancer deaths each year in the United Kingdom[5]. A number of principles guide the use of diagnostic radiation:

1. *Justification* that a proposed examination is of net benefit to the patient[6].
2. *ALARA* – doses should be kept As Low As Reasonably Achievable, economic and social factors being taken into account[7].

Justification is particularly important when considering the irradiation of women of reproductive age because of the risks to the developing fetus. In addition to the tumour risk from diagnostic levels of radiation and the risks that have been extrapolated from atomic bomb survivors[8], Otake and Schull[9] have shown that irradiation of the maternal abdomen between 8 and 15 weeks post-conception also results in an increased incidence of arrested forebrain development and mental subnormality. Earlier advice by national and international bodies aimed at confining less urgent radiological examinations of the lower abdomen and pelvis on females of child-bearing age to the 10 days following the start of menstruation – the 'ten-day rule'[10, 11]. This would be a time when there is the least likelihood of harm to any possible developing fetus because conception is unlikely to have occurred. Patients exempted from this rule were:

1. Women who denied recent sexual intercourse.
2. Women who were menstruating at the time.
3. Women who had been taking an oral contraceptive pill for not less than 3 months and were satisfied that it was effective.
4. Women who had an intrauterine contraceptive device for not less than 3 months and had found it effective.
5. Women who had been sterilized.

The arguments against the 'ten-day rule' have been summarized under four headings[12]:

1. *Timing.* Organogenesis occurs during the fourth to eighth week after conception. Thus, irradiation after the tenth day of the menstrual cycle but before the next menstrual cycle will not result in radiation damage to organogenesis.
2. *Irradiation of the unfertilized ovum.* There is no evidence that irradiation of the conceptus is any more dangerous than irradiation of the unfertilized ovum.
3. *Magnitude of the hazard.* The risks are extremely small and are greatly outweighed by the likely benefits to the mother or fetus of an earlier diagnosis. Irradiation of a fetus during the first few weeks of gestation will, if it has any detrimental effect, induce a spontaneous abortion. This is unlikely to be of serious personal or social concern unless the couple is subfertile[13].
4. *Cost-effectiveness.* The cost of implementing the ten-day rule appeared to be 100 times greater than the value of the possible benefit derived from it, assuming a benefit existed.

More recent advice[14] has superseded the earlier ten-day rule recommendation and is based on a statement by the International Commission on Radiological Protection[15] which reads 'During the first ten days following the onset of a menstrual period there can be no risk to any conceptus, since no conception will have occurred. The risk to a child who had previously been irradiated in utero during the remainder of a four week period following the onset of menstruation is likely to be so small that there need be no special limitation on exposures required within these four weeks.'

The chain of responsibility for ensuring that the fetus is not exposed to ionizing radiation is:

1. The patient.
2. The referring clinician.
3. The radiologist.
4. The radiographer.

Clinicians and radiologists should regard any woman as pregnant if her period is overdue or missed unless she is definitely known not to be pregnant. A pregnancy test may be helpful. It may be possible to defer the answer to a clinical question until it is known that she is not pregnant or it may be possible to answer the question using a safer technique such as ultrasonography. If the examination is necessary, a technique that minimizes the number of films and the absorbed dose per film should be utilized. However, the quality of the examination should not be reduced to the level where its diagnostic value is impaired. The risk to the patient of an incorrect diagnosis may be greater than the risk of irradiating the fetus. Radiography of areas remote from the pelvis and abdomen may be safely performed at any time during pregnancy with good collimation and lead protection.

Due to the contrast medium

The following are high risk factors associated with the administration of intravascular contrast medium:

1. *Proven or suspected hypersensitivity to iodine.*
2. *A previous severe adverse reaction to contrast medium.* With HOCM this carries a 20% risk of a similar reaction on a subsequent occasion. The risk is decreased to 5% with LOCM[16]. Radioisotopes, ultrasound, CT or MRI may provide an alternative means of investigation.
3. *Asthma or a significant allergic history.*
4. *Heart disease.* Cardiac failure and arrhythmias can be precipitated. The risk is less with LOCM but if only HOCM are available, meglumine-containing salts are preferable to those containing sodium.
5. *Infants and small children.*
6. *Hepatic failure.*
7. *Moderate to severe impairment of renal function,* especially when associated with diabetes. A deterioration in renal function may follow but can be minimized if the patient is well hydrated.
8. *Myelomatosis.* Bence Jones protein may be precipitated in renal tubules. The risk is diminished by ensuring good hydration.
9. *Poor hydration.*
10. *Sickle-cell anaemia.* The risk of precipitating a sickle-cell crisis is less with LOCM.
11. *Thyrotoxicosis.* The enormous iodine load has a

statistically significant effect on thyroid function tests, but this is of little practical clinical significance[17]. Hyperthyroidism may recur in patients previously treated for Graves' disease.

12. *Pregnancy.* A possible teratogenic risk has not been excluded.

Contraindications to other contrast media, e.g. barium, water-soluble contrast media for the gastro-intestinal tract and biliary contrast media are given in the relevant sections.

For further discussion of contrast media see Chapter 2.

Due to the technique *Skin sepsis* at the needle puncture site.

Specific contraindications to individual techniques are discussed with each procedure.

Contrast medium Volumes given are for a 70 kg man.

Equipment For many procedures this will also include a trolley with a sterile upper shelf and a non-sterile lower shelf. Details of trolley layout are given by Bryan[18]. Emergency drugs and resuscitation equipment should be readily available (see Appendix III).

See pp. 199–203 for introductory notes on angiography equipment and angiography catheters.

If only a simple radiography table and overcouch tube are required, then this information has been omitted from the text.

Patient preparation 1. Will admission to hospital be necessary?

2. If the patient is a woman of child-bearing age, the examination should be performed at a time when the risks to a possible fetus are minimal (see above). Any female presenting for radiography or a nuclear medicine examination at a time when her period is known to be overdue should be considered to be pregnant unless there is information indicating the absence of pregnancy. If her cycle is so irregular that it is difficult to know whether a period has been missed and it is not practicable to defer the examination until menstruation occurs, then a pregnancy test or pelvic US examination

may help to determine whether she is pregnant.

The risk to a fetus irradiated during the first 4 weeks following the onset of the last menstruation is likely to be so small that there need be no special limitation on radiological exposures within these 4 weeks. The 'ten-day rule' should still apply for hysterosalpingography, so that the risks of mechanical trauma to an early pregnancy are reduced[12].

3. The procedure should be explained to the patient and consent obtained when necessary[19]. Following recent case law in the United Kingdom (*Gillick v West Norfolk and Wisbech Area Health Authority*) and the introduction of 'The Children's Act', in which the capacity of children to consent has been linked with the concept of individual ability to understand the implications of medical treatment, there has come into existence a standard known as 'Gillick competence'. Nevertheless, it appears that where there is more than one person or body who could give consent, treatment would be vetoed only where *all those who could consent had refused to do so*. A parent has a right to consent to the treatment of a minor, and this right lasts as long as minority does (i.e. until the age of 18 years)[20].

4. If the procedure has a risk of bleeding and a bleeding disorder is suspected, e.g. liver disease or concurrent administration of warfarin, then that disorder must be investigated and appropriate steps taken to normalize blood clotting[21, 22].

5. Bowel preparation is used:
   (a) prior to investigation of the gastrointestinal tract,
   (b) when considerable faecal loading obscures other intra-abdominal organs,
   (c) when opacification of an organ is likely to be poor, e.g. the gall bladder in oral cholecystography.

   For other radiological investigations of abdominal organs bowel preparation is not always necessary and when given may result in excessive bowel gas. Bowel gas may be reduced if the patient is kept ambulant prior to the examination and those who routinely take laxatives should continue to do so[23].

6. Previous films and notes should be obtained.

7. Premedication will be necessary for painful procedures or where the patient is unlikely to co-operate for any other reason. Suggested premedication for *adults* include:

BENZODIAZEPINES
(a) diazepam, 10 mg orally 2 hours prior to the procedure, or up to 0.3 mg kg^{-1} i.v., or
(b) midazolam, (which has a shorter duration of action than diazepam) up to 0.1 mg kg^{-1} i.v., or i.m., or
(c) temazepam (which also has a shorter action than diazepam and has a more rapid onset) 20–40 mg (elderly 10–20 mg) 1 hour before the procedure, or
(d) lorazepam (which produces more prolonged sedation than temazepam and has greater amnesic properties), 1–5 mg orally 2–6 hours before the procedure.

(Droperidol, 5–10 mg orally, is usefully combined with a benzodiazepine to produce a quieter patient. It should not be used alone.)

OPIOID ANALGESICS
(a) morphine, 10 mg i.m., or ⎱
(b) papaveretum, 20 mg i.m., or ⎬ 1 hour prior to the procedure
(c) pethidine, 50–100 mg i.m., or ⎰
(d) fentanyl, 50–200 μg i.v. or
(e) alfentanil, up to 500 μg i.v. over 30 s.

Useful drugs for *children* are:
(a) up to 10 kg chloral hydrate 50 mg kg^{-1} orally, *or*
(b) over 10 kg temazepam 1 mg kg^{-1}(up to 30 mg) *and* droperidol 0.2 mg kg^{-1} (up to 2.5 mg), *or*
(c) quinalbarbitone 7–10 mg kg^{-1}

Weight (kg)	Dose (mg)
6–7	50
7–10	75
10–15	100
15–17	150
17–20	175
>20	200

Complex procedures on children or very unco-operative patients will be performed under general anaesthesia.
8. The patient should micturate prior to the procedure so that it will not be disrupted. Some procedures are of lengthy duration.

Preliminary films The purpose of these films is:
1. To make any final adjustments in exposure factors, centring, collimation and patient's position for which the film should always be taken using the same equipment as will be used for the remainder of the procedure.
2. To exclude prohibitive factors such as residual barium from a previous examination or excessive faecal loading.
3. To demonstrate, identify and localize opacities which may be obscured by contrast medium.
4. To elicit radiological physical signs.

Films should have on them the patient's name, registration number, date and a side marker. The examination can only proceed if satisfactory preliminary films have been obtained.

Technique 1. 1. For aseptic technique the skin is cleaned with chlorhexidine 0.5% in 70% industrial spirit or its equivalent.
2. Local anaesthetic used is lignocaine 1% without adrenaline.
3. Gonad protection is used whenever possible, unless it obscures the region of interest.

Films When films are taken during the procedure rather than at the end of it, they have, for convenience, been described under 'Technique':

Additional techniques
or
Modifications of technique

Aftercare May be considered as:
1. Instructions to the patient.
2. Instructions to the ward.

Complications Complications may be considered under three headings.

Due to the anaesthetic
1. General anaesthesia
2. Local anaesthesia:
   (a) allergic – unusual
   (b) toxic.

The maximum adult dose of lignocaine is 200 mg (0.3 mg kg^{-1}; 20 ml of a 1% solution). Anaesthetic lozenges contribute to the total dose.

Symptoms are of paraesthesia and muscle twitching which may progress to convulsions, cardiac arrhythmias, respiratory depression and death due to cardiac arrest.

Treatment is symptomatic and includes adequate oxygenation

Due to the contrast medium
BILIARY CONTRAST MEDIA See pp. 105–108.

BARIUM See p. 46.

WATER-SOLUBLE CONTRAST MEDIA
i.e. urographic/angiographic agents.

The overall incidence of side-effects is in the range 4–13% for HOCM and 1–4% for LOCM[24-26]. Mortality rates for HOCM are 1:100 000 compared with 1:200 000 for LOCM but, because the actual numbers of fatalities are so small, comparison of this end point is difficult. A meta-analysis of several large studies has shown no statistical difference between mortality rates for HOCM and LOCM[27].

Excluding death, adverse reactions can be classified in terms of severity as:
1. Major reactions, i.e. those that interfere with the examination and require treatment.
2. Minor reactions, i.e. those that interfere with the examination but do not require treatment.
3. Trivial reactions, i.e. those that do not interfere with the examination and require only firm assurance.

The adverse effects of water-soluble contrast media are discussed more fully in Chapter 2.

PROPHYLAXIS FOR ADVERSE REACTIONS

1. *Pre-testing.* Involves applying contrast medium to the cornea or injecting a 1 ml test dose intravenously a few minutes prior to the full intravenous injection. However, a negative result does not preclude a major reaction when the full dose is given and a severe reaction may result from the test dose itself. The technique has, therefore, fallen into disfavour.

2. *Pre-treatment with steroids.* Those who have had a previous severe adverse reaction or who are 'at risk' may benefit from pre-treatment with steroids[28]. A suggested regime is methyl prednisolone 32 mg orally 12 and 2 hours prior to injection of contrast medium[29]. However, the reduction in the incidence of adverse reactions using oral steroids is not as great as that achieved by the use of LOCM[30].

3. *Pre-treatment with antihistamines.* Prophylactic chlorpheniramine (Piriton) is of no benefit and, when given, is associated with a three-fold increase in the incidence of flushing[31].

4. *Change of contrast medium* to a LOCM.

5. *Reduction of patient anxiety and apprehension*[32].

Due to the technique   Specific details are given with the individual procedures and may be conveniently classified as:
1. Local.
2. Distant or generalized.

References

1. Russell, J.G.B. (1984) How dangerous are diagnostic x-rays? *Clin. Radiol.* **35**, 347–351.
2. MacMahon, B. (1962) Prenatal x-ray exposure and childhood cancer. *J. Natl. Cancer Inst.* **28**, 1 173–1191.
3. Boice, J.D., Rosenstein, M. & Trout, E.D. (1978) Estimation of breast doses and breast cancer risk associated with repeated fluoroscopic chest examinations of women with tuberculosis. *Radiat. Res.* **73**, 373–390.
4. Kendall, G.M., Muirhead, C.R., MacGibbon, B.T., et al. (1992) Mortality and occupational exposure to radiation: first analysis of the National Registry of Radiation Workers. *BMJ* **304**, 220–225.
5. Field, S. (1992) Just how harmful are diagnostic x-rays? – the college response. *Clin. Radiol.* **46**, 295.
6. International Commission on Radiological Protection (1982) *Protection Against Ionising Radiation from*

External Sources used in Medicine. Publication 33. Oxford: Pergamon Press.

7. International Commission on Radiological Protection (1973) *Implication of Commission Recommendation that Doses be Kept as Low as Readily Achievable.* ICRP Publication 22. Oxford: Pergamon Press.

8. United Nations Scientific Committee on the Effects of Atomic Radiation (1972) *Ionising Radiation: Levels and Effects.* New York: United Nations.

9. Otake, M. & Schull, V.J. (1984) In utero exposure to A bomb radiation and mental retardation: a reassessment. *Br. J. Radiol.* **57**, 409–414.

10. International Commission on Radiological Protection (1970) *Protection of the Patient in X-Ray Diagnosis.* Oxford: Pergamon Press.

11. Department of Health and Social Security (1972) *Code of Practice for the Protection of Persons Against Ionising Radiations Arising from Medical and Dental Use.* London: Her Majesty's Stationery Office.

12. Russell, J.G.B. (1986) The rise and fall of the ten-day rule. *Br. J. Radiol.* **59**, 3–6.

13. Mole, R.H. (1979) Radiation effects on pre-natal development and their radiological significance. *Br. J. Radiol.* **52**, 89–101.

14. National Radiological Protection Board (1985) *Exposure to Ionising Radiation of Pregnant Women: Advice on the Diagnostic Exposure of Women who are, or who may be, Pregnant ASP8.* London: Her Majesty's Stationery Office.

15. International Commission on Radiological Protection (1984) *Statement from the Washington Meeting of the ICRP.* Oxford: Pergamon Press.

16. Fischer, H. (1991) Personal communication. In: McClennan B.L. & Stolberg H.O. Intravascular contrast media. Ionic versus nonionic: current status. *Radiol. Clin. N. Am.* **29**, 437–454.

17. Jaffiol, C., Baldet, L., Bada, M. & Vierne, Y. (1982) The influence on thyroid function of two iodine containing radiological contrast media. *Br. J. Radiol.* **55**, 263–265.

18. Bryan, G.J. (1987) *Diagnostic Radiography. A Concise Practical Manual,* 4th edn. Edinburgh: Churchill Livingstone.

19. Craig, J.O.M.C. (1988) Editorial. Consent in diagnostic radiology. *Clin. Radiol.* **39**, 1.

20. Smith, A.McC. (1992) Consent to treatment in childhood. *Arch. Dis. Child.* **67**, 1247–1248.

21. Silverman, S.G., Mueller, P.R. & Pfister, R.C. (1990) Hemostatic evaluation before abdominal interventions: an overview and proposal. *AJR* **154**, 233–238.

22. Rapaport, S.I. (1990) Assessing hemostatic function before abdominal interventions. *AJR* **154**, 239–240.
23. Payne-Jeremiah, W.D. (1977) Pre-radiographic bowel preparation: a comprehensive reappraisal of factors. *Radiography* **43**, 3–14.
24. Katayama, H., Yamaguchi, K., Kozuka, T., Takashima, T., Seez, P. & Matsuura, K. (1990) Adverse reactions to ionic and nonionic contrast media. A report from the Japanese Committee on the safety of contrast media. *Radiology* **175**, 621–628.
25. Palmer, F.J. (1988) The R.A.C.R. survey of intravenous contrast media reactions: Final report. *Australas. Radiol.* **32**, 426–428.
26. Wolf, G.L., Arenson, R.L. & Cross, A.P. (1989) A prospective trial of ionic vs nonionic contrast agents in routine clinical practice: comparison of adverse effects. *AJR* **152**, 939–944.
27. Conseil d'Evaluation des Technologies de la Santé du Québec (1990) Evaluation of low vs high osmolar contrast media: 1) Principal report. 2) Technical document. Feb 16, 1990, Quebec.
28. Lasser, E.C., Lang, J., Sovak, M., Kollo, W., Lyon, S. & Hamlin, A.E. (1977) Steroids: theoretical and experimental basis for utilization in prevention of contrast media reactions. *Radiology* **125**, 1–9.
29. Lasser, E.C., Berry, C.C., Talner, L.B., et al. (1987) Pretreatment with corticosteroids to alleviate reactions to intravenous contrast material. *N. Engl. J. Med.* **317**, 845–849.
30. Wolf, G.L., Mishkin, M.M., Roux, S.G., et al. (1991) Comparison of the rates of adverse drug reactions: ionic contrast agents, ionic agents combined with steroids, and nonionic agents. *Invest. Radiol.* **26**, 404–410.
31. Davies, P., Roberts, M.B. & Roylance, J. (1975) Acute reactions to urographic contrast media. *BMJ* **ii**, 434–437.
32. Lalli, A.F. (1980) Contrast media reactions: data analysis and hypothesis. *Radiology* **134**, 1–12.

Further reading   Craig, O. (1985) The radiologist and the courts. *Clin. Radiol.* **36**, 475–478.

Radionuclide Imaging

Radiopharmaceuticals Radionuclides are shown in symbolic notation, the most frequently used in nuclear medicine being ^{99m}Tc, a 140 keV gamma-emitting radioisotope of the element technetium with $T_{1/2} = 6.0$ hours.

Activity administered The maximum activity values quoted in the text are those currently recommended in the Guidance Notes of the Administration of Radioactive Substances Advisory Committee[1] (ARSAC) who advise the health ministers on the Medicines (Administration of Radioactive Substances) Regulations 1978 (MARS). Using the ALARA principle, centres will frequently be able to administer lesser activities depending upon the capabilities of their equipment and local protocols. Typical figures are given where they differ from the recommended maximum values. In exceptional circumstances, a clinical director (ARSAC licence holder) is permitted to give activity higher than the recommended maximum to a named patient.

ARSAC recommends that activities administered for paediatric investigations should be reduced in proportion to body weight[1], subject to the minimum practicable activity for each procedure and local techniques and facilities. As a general guide:

$$\text{Paediatric dose} = \text{Adult dose} \times \frac{Wt}{70}$$

where Wt is body weight (kg) and the minimum dose is $0.1 \times$ adult dose.

Radioactive injections Administration of radioactive substances can only be carried out by an individual who has received training to physically direct an exposure, and it must be carried out under the supervision of someone trained to clinically direct an exposure, as specified in the Ionising Radiation Regulations 1988 (commonly known as POPUMET)[2].

Technique

Patient positioning   The resolution of gamma camera images is critically dependent on the distance of the collimator surface from the patient, falling off approximately linearly with distance. Every effort should therefore be made to position the camera as close to the patient as possible. For example, in posterior imaging with the patient supine, the thickness of the bed separates the patient from the camera, as well as interposing an attenuating medium. In this case, imaging with the patient sitting or standing directly against the camera is preferable.

Patient immobilization is very important for the duration of image acquisition. If a patient is uncomfortable or awkwardly positioned, they will have a tendency to move gradually and perhaps imperceptibly, which can have a severe blurring effect on the image. Point marker sources attached to the patient away from areas being examined can help to monitor and possibly permit correction for movement artefact.

'Oldendorf' bolus injection[3]   For some investigations the Oldendorf technique is recommended to provide an abrupt bolus:
1. Place a butterfly needle (20G or larger) in the antecubital vein.
2. Attach to a three-way tap connected to two syringes, one containing 10 ml saline and the other the radiopharmaceutical in a small volume (< 1 ml).
3. Place a blood pressure cuff on the arm and inflate to below diastolic pressure for about 1 min to suffuse veins.
4. Inflate above systolic pressure for 1–2 min to provoke reactive hyperaemia when cuff is released.
5. Inject radionuclide.
6. Release cuff and flush with saline.

Images   The image acquisition times quoted in the text should only be considered an approximate guide, since the appropriate time for a particular department and patient will depend upon such factors as the sensitivity of the available equipment, the amount of activity injected and the size of the patient.

An acceptable time will always be a compromise between the time available and the counts required for a diagnostic image.

Aftercare

Radiation safety Special instructions should be given to patients who are breast feeding regarding expression of milk and interruption of feeding[1]. Precautions may have to be taken with patients leaving hospital or returning to wards, depending upon the radionuclide and activity administered. Details are given in the Guidance Notes for the Ionisation Radiation Regulations 1985[4].

Complications With few exceptions (noted in the text), the amount of active substance injected with radionuclide investigations is at trace levels and very rarely causes any systemic reactions. Those that may occasionally cause problems are labelled blood products, antibodies and substances of a particulate nature.

References 1. Administration of Radioactive Substances Advisory Committee (1993) *Notes for Guidance on the Administration of Radioactive Substances to Persons for Purposes of Diagnosis, Treatment or Research.* London: HMSO.
2. *The Ionising Radiation (Protection of Persons Undergoing Medical Examination or Treatment) Regulations* (1988) London: HMSO.
3. Oldendorf, W.H., Kitano, M. & Shimizy, F. (1965) Evaluation of a simple technique for abrupt intravenous injection of radionuclide. *J. Nucl. Med. 6*, 205–209.
4. National Radiological Protection Board. *Guidance Notes for the Protection of Persons Against Ionising Radiations Arising from Medical and Dental Use* (1988) London: HMSO.

Computerized Tomography

Patient preparation

Many CT examinations require little physical preparation. An explanation of the procedure, the time it is likely to take, the necessity for immobility and the necessity for breath holding whilst scanning chest and abdomen should be given. Waiting times should be kept to a minimum as this tends to increase anxiety. The patient should be as pain-free as is practical but too heavy sedation or analgesia may be counter-productive — patient co-operation is often required. Children under the age of 4 years will usually need sedation; a suitable regime is given on p. 7. Children should also have an i.v. cannula inserted at the time sedation is administered or local anaesthetic cream (e.g. Emla, Astra Pharmaceuticals) applied to two sites if i.v. contrast is needed. If these simple steps are taken the number of aborted scans will be reduced and the resultant image quality be improved.

Intravenous contrast medium

Many CT examinations will require i.v. contrast medium. Allergy and atopy should be excluded. If present, follow the relevant guidelines regarding the use of steroid prophylaxis and use LOCM. An explanation of the need for contrast enhancement should be given to the patient.

The dose will depend on the area examined: head — 50 ml; abdomen — 100 ml, given initially as a bolus of 20 ml followed by 2 ml s^{-1} during scanning. In children a maximum dose of 2 ml kg^{-1} body weight (300 mg I ml^{-1}) should be observed.

Oral contrast medium

For examinations of the abdomen, opacifying the bowel satisfactorily can be problematic. Water-soluble contrast medium [2–3% Urografin flavoured to disguise the taste (15–20 ml Urografin 150 diluted in 1 litre of orange squash] or low-density barium suspensions (2% w/v) can be used. Timing of administration is given in Table 1.1. Doses of contrast media in children depend on age.

Pelvic scanning

Rarely it may be necessary to opacify the rectum using direct instillation of contrast medium or air via catheter. The concentration of contrast medium should be the same as for oral administration. 150 ml is adequate. Vaginal tampons may also be used. The air trapped by the tampon produces good negative contrast.

Table 1.1 Timing and volume for oral contrast medium in CT.

	Volume (ml)	Time before scan (min)
ADULT		
Full abdomen and pelvis	1000	gradually over hour before scanning
Upper abdomen, e.g. pancreas	500	gradually over ½ hour before scanning
CHILD		
Newborn	60–90	full dose 1 hour before scanning and a further half dose immediately prior to the scan
1 month to 1 year	120–240	
1 year to 5 years	240–360	
5 years to 10 years	360–480	
Over 10 years	as for adult	
	If the large bowel needs to be opacified then give the contrast medium the night before or 3–4 hours before scanning	

Ultrasonography

Patient preparation
For many US examinations no preparation is required. This includes examination of tissue such as thyroid, breast, testes, musculoskeletal, vascular and cardiac. In certain situations simple preparatory measures are required.

Abdomen
For optimal examination of the gallbladder it should be dilated. This requires fasting for 6–8 hours before scanning.

Pelvis
To optimally visualize the pelvic contents bowel gas must be displaced. This is easily accomplished by filling the urinary bladder to capacity. This then acts as a transonic 'window'. The patient should be instructed to drink 1–2 pints of water during the hour prior to scanning and not to empty their bladder.

In practice, both abdominal and pelvic scanning are often performed at the same attendance. Oral intake of clear fluids will not provoke gallbladder emptying and so the two preparations can be combined.

Endoscopic
Endoscopic examination of rectum or vagina requires no physical preparation but an explanation of the procedure in a sympathetic manner is needed.

Examination of the oesophagus or transoesophageal echocardiography require preparation similar to upper gastrointestinal endoscopy. The patient should be starved for 4 hours prior to the procedure to minimize the risk of vomiting, reflux and aspiration. Anaesthesia and sedation are partly a matter of personal preference of the operator. Local anaesthesia of the pharynx can be obtained using 10% lignocaine spray. Care to avoid overdose is essential as lignocaine is rapidly absorbed via this route. The maximum dose of lignocaine should not exceed 200 mg; the xylocaine spray metered dose applicator delivers 10 mg per dose. Intravenous sedation using benzodiazepines such as Diazemuls 10 mg or midazolam 2–5 mg may also be necessary. If local anaesthetic has been used then the patient must be instructed to avoid hot food or drink until the effect has worn off (1–2 hours).

Children   Ultrasound examination in children can, in most cases, be performed with no preparation apart from explanation and reassurance to both child and parent. In some cases where the child is excessively frightened or where immobility is required then sedation may be necessary. With echocardiography in infants sedation is essential to obtain optimal recordings. The sedation regimes described on p. 7 may be used.

2 Intravascular Contrast Media

The first report of opacification of the urinary tract by renal excretion rather than by retrograde introduction of a contrast agent appeared in 1923 when Osborne et al. took advantage of the fact that intravenously injected 10% sodium iodide solution, which was used in the treatment of syphilis, was excreted in the urine[1]. In an effort to detoxify the iodine, Binz and Rath in Berlin synthesized a number of pyridine rings containing iodine. One of these, selectan-neutral, was excreted in the urine but the images were poor and there was anxiety about the side effects. Swick suggested some modifications to the molecule and in 1928 and 1929 the first intravenous urograms with the compound uroselectan (Iopax) were performed[2-4]. This mono-iodinated compound was developed further into the di-iodinated compounds, uroselectan-B (Neoiopax) and diodone (Diodrast, Umbradil), and in 1952 the first tri-iodinated compound, sodium acetrizoate (Urokon), was introduced into clinical radiology.

Uroselectan

Diodone (Diodrast, Umbradil)

Sodium acetrizoate (Urokon)

Sodium acetrizoate was based on a 6-carbon ring structure, tri-iodo benzoic acid, and was the precursor of all modern water-soluble contrast media.

In 1955 a much safer derivative became available — diatrizoate (Urografin, Hypaque). This was a fully substituted benzoic acid derivative with an acetamido group at the previously unsubstituted position 5. Isomerization of diatrizoate and substitution at position 5 of N-methyl carbamyl produced the iothalamate ion (Conray) in 1962. Modern HOCM are distinguished by differences at position 5 of the anion and by the cations sodium and/or meglumine.

Diatrizoate
(side chains at positions
3 and 5 are identical)

Iothalamate
(side chains at positions
3 and 5 differ)

All conventional ionic water-soluble contrast media or high-osmolar contrast media (HOCM) are hypertonic with osmolalities of 1200–2000 mosmol kg^{-1} water, 4–7 × the osmolarity of blood. Almén first postulated that many of the adverse effects of contrast media were the result of high osmolality and that by eliminating the cation, which does not contribute to diagnostic information but is responsible for up to 50% of the osmotic effect, it would be possible to reduce the toxicity of contrast media[5, 6].

Table 2.1 Schematic illustration of the development of contrast media.

Name	Chemical structure	No. of iodine atoms/ions (A)	No. of particles in solution (B)	Ratio of A/B	Osmolality of a 280 mg I ml[1] solution
Sodium iodide	Na⁺ I	1	2	0.5	
Diodone	Na⁺ (RCOO-pyridine ring structure, O)	2	2	1	
Diatrizoate Iothalamate Metrizoate Iodamide	Na⁺ / Meg⁺ (COO, R, R ring) monomeric – monoacidic	3	2	1.5	1500
Iocarmate	Meg⁺ Meg⁺ (COO⁻ COO⁻ dimeric ring, R—R) dimeric – diacidic	6	3	2	1040
Ioxaglate	Na⁺ Meg⁺ (R COO⁻ dimeric ring, R—R) dimeric – monoacidic	6	2	3	490
Iopamidol Iohexol Iopramide Iopentol Ioversol	(R, R, R ring) monomeric – non-ionic	3	1	3	470
Iotrolan	ROH ROH HOR—(R)—ROH dimeric – non-ionic	6	1	6	

Meg = meglumine
R = an unspecified side-chain

In order to decrease the osmolality without changing the iodine concentration the ratio between the number of iodine atoms and the number of dissolved particles must be increased. Conventional ionic contrast media have a ratio of three iodine atoms per molecule to two particles in solution, i.e. a ratio of 3:2 or 1.5 (Table 2.1). In 1972 a new agent was introduced for radiculography. This was produced by linking two iothalamate molecules to form a dimer — iocarmate (Dimer X). This has since been withdrawn for toxicological reasons, but the iodine/particle ratio was increased to two and the osmolality decreased (Table 2.1).

Further development has proceeded along two separate paths. The first was, again, to combine two tri-iodinated benzene rings to produce an anion with six iodine atoms. Replacement of one of the carboxylic acid groups with a non-ionizing radical means that only one cation is necessary for each molecule. This anion, ioxaglate, is marketed as a mixed sodium and meglumine salt (Hexabrix). The alternative approach was to produce a compound that does not ionize in solution and so does not provide radiologically useless cations. Contrast media of this type include metrizamide (Amipaque), iopamidol (Niopam), iohexol (Omnipaque), iopramide (Ultravist) and ioversol (Optiray).

For both types of contrast media the ratio of iodine atoms in the molecule to the number of particles in solution is 3:1. Compared with conventional HOCM, the new LOCM show a theoretical halving of osmolality for equi-iodine solutions. However, because of aggregation of molecules in solution the measured reduction is approximately one-third[7] (Figure 2.1).

A further development of LOCM has been non-ionic dimers. These have a ratio of six iodine atoms for each molecule in solution and satisfactory iodine concentrations can now be obtained at iso-osmolality. In addition to the increased financial cost these compounds also have the problem of high viscosity at room temperature[9]. With development having reached the stage of iso-osmolality, further development has been targetted on decreasing the

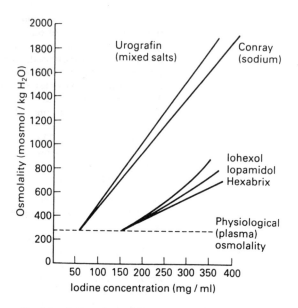

Fig. 2.1 A plot of osmolality against iodine concentration for new and conventional contrast media. From Dawson and Howel[8]. (Reproduced by courtesy of the editor of *Clinical Radiology*.)

chemotoxicity of the molecule. Increased hydrophilicity due to an increased number of hydroxyl groups provides a high affinity for water and shelters the toxic iodine atoms from the human body.

It should be noted that the terms 'low-osmolar' and 'non-ionic' are not synonymous. Iopamidol, iohexol, iotrolan, iopramide, ioversol and ioxaglate are all low osmolar but the latter is not non-ionic. The major clinical difference between the two groups is that ionic contrast media cannot be used in the subarachnoid space.

Adverse effects of contrast media

The manifestations of adverse reactions to intravenous contrast medium are:

1. *Mucocutaneous reactions* — flushing, pallor, rhinorrhoea, urticaria and, in the most severe cases, angioneurotic oedema. Onset may be immediate or delayed up to 3 days.

2. *Nausea and vomiting.*
3. *Headache.*
4. *Sneezing.*
5. *Arm pain* – locally, due to perivenous injection or extending further up the arm and due to stasis of the contrast medium in the vein. Less common with LOCM.
6. *Thrombophlebitis and venous thrombosis.*
7. *Abdominal pain.*
8. *Rigors.*
9. *Bronchospasm* – predisposed to by a history of asthma and concurrent therapy with β-blockers[10]. In most patients the bronchospasm is subclinical.
10. *Hypotension* – usually accompanied by tachycardia but in some patients there is vagal overreaction with bradycardia[11, 12]. The latter is rapidly reversed by atropine 0.6–2 mg i.v. Hypotension is usually mild and is treatable by a change of posture. Rarely it is severe and may be accompanied by pulmonary oedema[13].
11. *Haematological changes* – blood micro-viscosity is increased and is due to increased rigidity of the red cell wall. If this results in blockage of pulmonary arterial capillaries then pulmonary hypertension may be exacerbated.
    Sickle-cell crisis may be provoked.
12. *Sloughing of skin* – secondary to extravasation of contrast medium. Less common with LOCM.
13. *Convulsions* – especially in patients with an epileptic tendency and in patients with cerebral tumours undergoing CT[14, 15] This is probably secondary to contrast medium leaking across the blood–brain barrier. Convulsions may also occur secondary to the cerebral hypoxia caused by hypotension ± cardiac arrest.
14. *Cardiac arrest* – due to (a) arrhythmia, (b) ischaemia secondary to hypotension or (c) coronary artery spasm during an anaphylactoid reaction.

Mechanisms of contrast medium reactions

Mechanisms of contrast medium reactions can be classified as follows:
1. Overdose.
2. Anaphylaxis.
3. Complement/histamine/kallikreins.

4. Chemotoxicity.
5. Cardiovascular — both cardiac and vascular.
6. Anxiety.

Overdose Some kinds of patients may be overdosed with contrast medium. Small infants having multiple injections during angiocardiography and adults with cardiac, renal or hepatic failure may be given an excessive osmotic or sodium load. Acute lethal dose (LD_{50}) studies in mice have shown that the LOCM have less toxicity than HOCM (Table 2.2). Because of the difficulty of extrapolating from animals to man, only major differences are significant.

Table 2.2 LD_{50} data for some commonly used contrast media.

	LD_{50} (mouse i.v. gl kg^{-1})
Urografin 370	7.6
Conray 420	8.0
Ioxaglate (Hexabrix)	12.5
Iopamidol (Niopam)	21.8
Iohexol (Omnipaque)	24.2

Data from manufacturers' references.

Anaphylaxis All drugs may provoke an anaphylactic response and this is also true of contrast media. Anaphylactic (following previous sensitization) or anaphylactoid (without previous sensitization) reactions are manifested by bronchospasm, glottic oedema, circulatory collapse, abdominal cramps and diarrhoea. The patient may die unless immediate resuscitative steps are taken. There is probably no difference in the incidence of acute anaphylaxis between LOCM and HOCM. The possible mechanisms of contrast medium-induced anaphylaxis have been reviewed by Preger[16] and include generation of anaphylatoxins (C3a and C5a) by complement activation, and direct release of histamine and kallikreins. The great majority of adverse reactions are not mediated this way[17].

Histamine release Contrast media do cause the release of histamine from mast cells and basophils and this could provide a mechanism for the phenomena of flushing, urticaria, metallic taste, hypotension, collapse and angioneurotic oedema. While hyperosmolality is a factor, isosmolar concentrations of contrast media will also stimulate histamine release. The basophils of allergic individuals do release more histamine than those of normal individuals[18]. The histamine-releasing properties of contrast media differ, with LOCM causing less histamine release than HOCM. Meglumine salts have a greater effect than sodium salts and this is reflected in the $4 \times$ increase in the incidence of bronchospasm when the former is compared with the latter. Bronchospasm may be due to the effect of contrast medium on pulmonary-bed mast cells and dysrhythmias from the effect on cardiac mast cells.

Endothelial damage Endothelial cells can be damaged by both the direct chemotoxicity of contrast media and as a result of their hyperosmolality. Contrast medium-induced thrombophlebitis and venous thrombosis are particular complications of lower limb venography with a four-fold increase with HOCM compared to LOCM.

Activation systems Lasser et al[19] have hypothesized that damage to vascular endothelium stimulates a complex of activation systems resulting in the formation of kinins, thrombus, fibrinogen degradation products, histamine release and haemolysis. A number of inhibitors limit the extent to which these systems function. One such inhibitor, Cl-inhibitor, has been shown to be lower in those exhibiting contrast medium-induced reactions than in non-reactors and the variability of severity of reactions, both between patients and in any individual on different occasions, may be related to variable inhibitor levels. As LOCM cause less endothelial damage than HOCM it is to be expected that activation systems will be less important with the new contrast media.

Chemotoxicity In addition to the toxicity of the contrast medium because of its intrinsic structure, the electrical charge on the particles of the HOCM and of Hexabrix (sodium/meglumine ioxaglate) is of particular importance in intracoronary and intrathecal use. The cations are clinically more toxic than the anions and sodium is more toxic than meglumine to brain (increased incidence of convulsions in patients with altered blood–brain barrier) and myocardium (increased incidence of arrhythmias). The toxicity of intracoronary ionic agents is partly related to their greater propensity to bind calcium[20]. The high incidence of adverse reactions when LOCM or sodium/meglumine ioxaglate is introduced into the subarachnoid space is almost certainly related to the electrical charge on the particles.

Although the major adverse effect on erythrocytes is due to hyperosmolality, even contrast medium which is iso-osmolar with plasma produces changes in red blood cell morphology which reveal the intrinsic chemotoxicity of contrast medium molecules[21].

Protein binding and enzyme inhibition
Contrast media are weakly protein bound and the degree of protein binding correlates well with their ability to inhibit the enzyme acetylcholinesterase[22]. Contrast medium side-effects such as vasodilatation, bradycardia, hypotension, bronchospasm and urticaria are all recognized cholinergic effects and may be related more to cholinesterase inhibition than osmolality. LOCM are less effective enzyme inhibitors as well as having lower osmolality, whilst the biliary contrast agent, meglumine ioglycamide, is the most strongly protein-bound contrast agent and the most toxic.

The chemoreceptor trigger zone is situated in the lateral walls of the fourth ventricle and is unprotected by the blood–brain barrier. There is a cholinergic link between the chemoreceptor trigger zone and the emesis centre, and the greater capacity of some contrast media to stimulate vomiting is probably a result of their greater ability to inhibit acetylcholinesterase. Of the newer contrast media, ioxaglate has the greatest ability to inhibit cholinesterase activity and is associated with the highest incidence of nausea and vomiting[23].

The anticholinesterase activity of sodium iothalamate is almost identical to sodium iodide but both are less than iohexol[24]. This finding suggests that it may be the 'available' iodine which matters in this phenomenon. In both sodium iodide and simple molecules, like iothalamate, which have short side chains the iodine is 'exposed'. More complicated molecules, such as the non-ionics, have long side chains which 'hide' the iodine. Their large hydrophilic side chains, which increase their solubility and compensate for the loss of the carboxyl group common to the ionic agents, have a steric hindrance effect. As the size and complexity of the hydroxyl-carrying side chains increases in the new non-ionics (to increase solubility) the effect is to produce compounds with lower protein binding and greater steric hindrance. (Ioxaglate retains a carboxyl group and, as expected, behaves like iothalamate leaving its iodines 'available'.)

Calcium binding HOCM are weak binders of ionic calcium[25]. Significant reductions in ionic calcium are caused by diatrizoate compounds because of the addition of the chelating agent sodium citrate as a stabilizing agent. The effects are obviously of greatest significance with direct intracoronary injection.

Other hyperosmolality effects 1. HAEMODYNAMIC AND SYSTEMIC EFFECTS
The injection of a hypertonic contrast medium causes significant fluid and ion shifts. Immediately after injection there is a significant increase in serum osmolality. This causes an influx of water from the interstitial space into the vascular compartment, an increase in blood volume and an increase in cardiac output. These effects are particularly important in young children and those with cardiac impairment.

Injection of a HOCM produces a significant, transient decrease in systemic arterial pressure, a decrease in peripheral vascular resistance, peripheral vasodilatation and tachycardia and an increase in pulmonary arterial blood pressure. This is accompanied by clinical perception of heat and, with intra-arterial injections, there is often pain. LOCM produce significantly less fluid shifts, changes in measurable parameters, heat and pain.

2. CARDIAC EFFECTS
Coronary arteriography with HOCM has adverse inotropic and chronotropic effects on the heart.

There is a decrease in peak left ventricular systolic pressure, an increase in left ventricular end diastolic pressure, a biphasic decrease then increase in coronary artery blood flow, and bradycardia. LOCM have less effect on these parameters, although ioxaglate produces more depression of left ventricular contraction during coronary arteriography than the other LOCM, probably because of its ionic nature. LOCM also produce fewer electrocardiographic changes, including ventricular fibrillation.

3. RED CELL EFFECTS

When red blood cells are placed in a hypertonic contrast medium, water leaves the interior of the cells by osmosis and they become more rigid. Red cell rigidity or deformability is, thus, dependent on osmolality and isosmolar solutions have no effect on red cell deformability[21]. Red cells that deform less easily are less able to pass through capillaries and may occlude them. This is the explanation for the transient rise in pulmonary arterial pressure during pulmonary arteriography[26] and the reason why LOCM should be used when there is any likelihood of pre-existing pulmonary hypertension. It may also be a factor in the deterioration of renal function that is occasionally encountered after contrast administration[27].

Increasing concentrations of contrast media have an increasing sickling effect on red cells in sickle-cell anaemia. LOCM have a lesser effect and their use is indicated in this disease[28].

Haemolysis and coagulation

In the presence of a high concentration of contrast medium, such as withdrawal of blood into a syringe of contrast medium, damage to red cell walls occur and haemolysis follows. Haemolysis and haemoglobinuria have been reported following angiocardiography with diatrizoate and acute renal failure may supervene. It is advisable not to re-inject blood that has been mixed with contrast medium.

Two further effects of contrast media on red cells are red cell aggregation and coagulation. In the presence of highly concentrated contrast medium, e.g. 350 mg I/ml, red cells show irregular and disorganized aggregation. However, disaggregation occurs easily and this is not likely to be of any clinical significance[29].

All contrast agents have inhibitory effects on coagulation, LOCM being less 'anticoagulant'[30]. Thrombus formation does occur and is more common when blood is mixed with LOCM. However, the role of the syringe is also significant and thrombus formation is maximal when blood is slowly withdrawn into a syringe so that it layers on top of the contrast medium, against the wall of the syringe. Activation of coagulation by the tube material (worse with styrene acrylonitrile) probably plays a significant role.

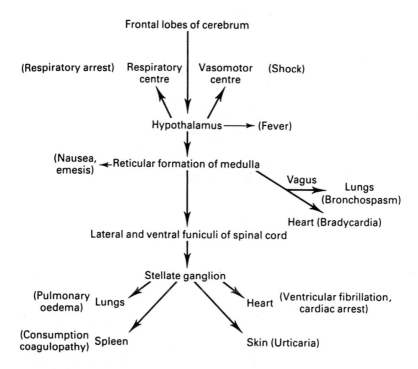

Fig. 2.2 Central nervous system and contrast media reactions. From Lalli (1980). (Reproduced by courtesy of the editor of *Radiology*.)

Anxiety Lalli[31] has postulated that most, if not all, contrast medium reactions are the result of the patient's fear and apprehension. The high autonomic nervous system activity in an anxious patient will be stimulated further when the patient experiences the administration of contrast medium. Furthermore, contrast medium crossing the blood–brain barrier can stimulate the limbic area and hypothalamus to produce further autonomic activity. This autonomic activity is responsible for contrast medium reactions by the sequence of events illustrated in Figure 2.2.

Support for Lalli's hypothesis is found in the work of Heron et al[32] who showed a significant correlation between ECG changes and more subjective side-effects experienced after contrast injection. When compared with HOCM, LOCM resulted in less frequent ECG abnormalities and subjective side-effects.

Mechanisms of contrast-induced bronchospasm Uncertain but include:
1. Direct histamine release from mast cells and platelets.
2. Cholinesterase inhibition.
3. Vagal overtone.
4. Complement activation.
5. Direct effect of contrast media on bronchi.

Bronchospasm is much less pronounced with LOCM than with HOCM[33].

Mechanisms of contrast-induced nephrotoxicity Recent reviews on the incidence of contrast-induced nephrotoxicity suggest an incidence of approximately 5%[34-36]. For the majority the renal impairment is temporary. There are a number of predisposing factors:
1. Pre-existing impairment of renal function. This is present in 90% of reported cases of contrast medium nephrotoxicity.
2. Diabetes mellitus, which is present in 50% of cases of contrast medium nephrotoxicity. Approximately 75% of patients with juvenile onset diabetes mellitus and renal insufficiency will show deterioration of renal function after HOCM. In as many as 50% of these patients the renal function

will not return to baseline levels.
3. Dehydration.
4. Age — because of the greater incidence of cardio-vascular disease in the elderly.
5. Very large doses of contrast medium.
6. Multiple myeloma.

The mechanisms of contrast medium-induced nephrotoxicity have been reviewed by Dawson and are summarized below[37]:
1. Impaired renal perfusion.
   (a) Adverse cardiotoxic effects
   (b) Increased peripheral vasodilatation
   (c) Renal vascular bed changes (increased blood flow followed by a more prolonged decrease)
   (d) Increased rigidity of red cells
   (e) Pre-dehydration
   (f) Osmotic diuresis.
2. Glomerular injury:
   (a) Impaired perfusion
   (b) Hyperosmolar effects
   (c) Chemotoxic effects.
3. Tubular injury:
   (a) Impaired perfusion ⎤ manifest histologic-
   (b) Hyperosmolar effects ⎬ ally as cytoplasmic
   (c) Chemotoxic effects. ⎦ vacuolation.
4. Obstructive nephropathy:
   (a) Cytoplasmic vacuolation in tubules
   (b) Precipitation of Tamm–Horsfall protein
   (c) Precipitation of Bence Jones protein in multiple myeloma.

Experimental work and theoretical considerations suggest that LOCM are less nephrotoxic. However, the available evidence[38], including a review of 43 clinical trials comparing LOCM and HOCM, concluded that there was no difference[39].

Indications for the use of low-osmolar contrast media

The advantages of LOCM are:
1. More comfortable arteriograms and i.v. injections.
2. Less tissue toxicity.
3. Reduction in adverse reactions.

If it was not for their expense, there would have been a complete switch to LOCM many years ago[40]. The financial implications of using LOCM for all patients and all procedures are so great that a selection process to identify those at risk must be instituted. The following should receive LOCM in preference to HOCM[41]:

1. Those at high risk from the hyperosmolar effects:
   (a) Infants and small children and the elderly
   (b) Those with renal and/or cardiac failure
   (c) Poorly hydrated patients.
   (d) Patients with diabetes, myelomatosis or sickle-cell anaemia
   (e) Patients who have had a previous severe contrast medium reaction with LOCM or those with a strong allergic history.
2. Those who would suffer unnecessarily from the hyperosmolar effects of HOCM e.g. arteriography under local anaesthesia.

References

1. Osborne, E.D., Sutherland, C.G., Scholl, A.J. & Rowntree, L.G. (1923) Roentgenography of the urinary tract during excretion of sodium iodid. *JAMA* **80**, 368–373.
2. Swick, M. (1929) Darstellung der niere und harnwege in roentgenbild durch intravenose einbringung eines neuen kontraststoffes: des uroselectans. *Klin. Wochenschr.* **8**, 2087–2089.
3. Von Lichtenberg, A. & Swick, M. (1929) Klinische prüfung des uroselectans. *Klin. Wochenschr.* **8**, 2089–2091.
4. Swick, M. (1978) Radiographic media in urology. The discovery of excretion urography: Historical and developmental aspects of the organically bound urographic media and their role in the varied diagnostic angiographic areas. *Surg. Clin. N. Am.* **58**, 977–994.
5. Almén, T. (1969) Contrast agent design. Some aspects of synthesis of water-soluble contrast agents of low osmolality. *J. Theor. Biol.* **24**, 216–226.
6. Almén, T. (1985) Development of nonionic contrast media. *Invest. Radiol.* **20 (suppl)**, S2–S9.
7. Grainger, R.G. (1980) Osmolality of intravascular radiological contrast media. *Br. J. Radiol.* **53**, 739–746.
8. Dawson, P., Grainger, R.G. & Pitfield, J. (1983) The new low-osmolar contrast media: a simple guide. *Clin. Radiol.* **34**, 221–226.
9. Dawson, P. & Howel, M. (1986) The non-ionic dimers: a new class of contrast agents. *Br. J. Radiol.* **59**, 987–991.

10. Ansell, G., Tweedie, M.C.K., West, C.R. & Evans, D.A.P. (1982) Risk factors for adverse reactions in intravenous urography. In: Amiel, M. (ed.) *Contrast Media in Radiology*, pp. 7–10. Berlin: Springer-Verlag.
11. Andrews, E.J. (1976) The vagus reaction as a possible cause of severe complications of radiological procedures. *Radiology* 34, 227–230.
12. Stanley, R.J. & Pfister, R.C. (1976) Bradycardia and hypotension following use of intravenous contrast media. *Radiology* 121, 5–7.
13. Chamberlin, W.H., Stockman, G.D. & Wray, N.P. (1979) Shock and noncardiogenic pulmonary edema following meglumine diatrizoate for intravenous pyelography. *Am. J. Med.* 67, 684–686.
14. Scott, W.R. (1980) Seizures, a reaction to contrast media for computed tomography of the brain. *Radiology* 137, 359–361.
15. Fischer, H.W. (1980) Occurrence of seizures during cranial computed tomography. *Radiology* 137, 563–564.
16. Preger, L. (1984) Some drug-induced complications that should be known to the radiologist. In: Steiner, R.E. (ed.) *Recent Advances in Radiology and Medical Imaging*, Vol. 7, Chap. 10, pp. 199–202. Edinburgh: Churchill Livingstone.
17. Carr, D.H. & Walker, A.C. (1984) Contrast media reactions: experimental evidence against the allergy theory. *Br. J. Radiol.* 57, 469–473.
18. Arroyave, C.M. (1980) An in vitro assay for radiographic contrast media idiosyncracy. *Invest. Radiol.* 15, S21–S25.
19. Lasser, E.C., Lang, J.H., Hamblin, A.E., Lyon, S.G. & Howard, M. (1980) Activation systems in contrast idiosyncracy. *Invest. Radiol.* 15, S2–S5.
20. Haywood, R. & Dawson, P. (1984) Contrast agents in angiocardiography. *Br. Heart. J.* 52, 361–368.
21. Dawson, P., Harrison, M.J.G. & Weisblatt, E. (1983) Effect of contrast media on red cell filtrability and morphology. *Br. J. Radiol.* 56, 707–710.
22. Dawson, P. & Edgerton, D. (1983) Contrast media and enzyme inhibition. 1. Cholinesterase. *Br. J. Radiol.* 56, 653–656.
23. Manhire, A.R., Dawson, P. & Dennet, R. (1984) Contrast agent induced emesis. *Clin. Radiol.* 35, 369–370.
24. Howel, M.J. & Dawson, P. (1985) Contrast agents and enzyme inhibition. II. Mechanisms. *Br. J. Radiol.* 58, 845–848.
25. Morris, T.W., Sahler, L.G. & Fisher, H.W. (1982) Calcium binding in radiographic media. *Invest. Radiol.* 17, 501–505.

26. Effros, R.M. (1972) Impairment of red cell transit through the canine lungs following injections of hypertonic fluids. *Circ. Res.* **31**, 590–601. ˜
27. Golman, K. & Holtas, S. (1980) Proteinuria produced by urographic contrast media. *Invest. Radiol.* **15**, S61–S66.
28. Rao, V.M., Rao, A.K., Steiner, R.M., Burka, E.R., Grainger, R.G. & Ballas, S.K. (1982) The effect of ionic and nonionic contrast media on the sickling phenomenon. *Radiology* **144**, 291–293.
29. Dawson, P., McCarthy, P., Allison, D.J., Garvey, B. & Bradshaw, A. (1988) Non-ionic contrast agents, red cell aggregation and coagulation. *Br. J. Radiol.* **61**, 963– 965.
30. Dawson, P., Hewitt, M.R., Mackie, I.J., Machin, S.J., Amis, S. & Bradshaw, A. (1986) Contrast, coagulation and fibrinolysis. *Invest. Radiol.* **21**, 248–252.
31. Lalli, A.F. (1974) Urographic contrast media reactions and anxiety. *Radiology* **112**, 267–271.
32. Heron, C.W., Underwood, S.R. & Dawson, P. (1984) Electrocardiographic changes during intravenous urography: a study with sodium iothalamate and iohexol. *Clin. Radiol.* **35**, 137–141.
33. Dawson, P., Pitfield, J. & Britton, J. (1983) Contrast media and bronchospasm: a study with iopamidol. *Clin. Radiol.* **34**, 227–230.
34. Gomes, A.S., Lois, J.F., Baker, J.D., McGlade, C.T., Bunnell, D.H. & Hartzman, S. (1989) Acute renal dysfunction in high risk patients after angiography: Comparison of ionic and nonionic contrast media. *Radiology* **170**, 65–68.
35. Parfrey, P.S., Griffiths, S.M., Barrett, B.J., et al. (1989) Contrast material induced renal failure in patients with diabetes mellitus, renal insufficiency or both: a prospective controlled study. *N. Engl. J. Med.* **320**, 143–149.
36. Schwab, S.J., Hlatky, M.A., Pieper, K.S., et al. (1989) Contrast nephrotoxicity: a randomized control trial of nonionic and ionic radiographic contrast agent. *N. Engl. J. Med.* **320**, 149–153.
37. Dawson, P. (1985) Contrast agent nephrotoxicity. *Br. J. Radiol.* **58**, 121–124.
38. Schwab, S.J., Hlatky, M.A., Piepers, K.S., et al. (1989) Contrast nephrotoxicity. A randomised controlled trial of a non-ionic (iopamidol) and an ionic radiographic contrast agent (diatrizoate). *N. Engl. J. Med.* **320**, 149–153.
39. Kinnison, M.L., Powe, N.R. & Steinberg, E.P. (1989) Results of radiologic controlled trials of low vs high osmolality contrast media. *Radiology* **170**, 381–389.

40. Grainger, R.G. (1987) Annotation: radiological contrast media. *Clin. Radiol.* **38**, 3–5.
41. Grainger, R.G. (1984) The clinical and financial implications of the low-osmolar contrast media. *Clin. Radiol.* **35**, 251–252.

Further reading   Ansell, G. & Wilkins, R.A. (1987) *Complications in Diagnostic Imaging.* Oxford: Blackwell Scientific Publications.

Carr, D.H. (1988) *Contrast Media.* Edinburgh: Churchill Livingstone.

Grainger, R.G. (1982) Intravascular contrast media – the past, the present and the future. *Br. J. Radiol.* **55**, 1–18.

Grainger, R.G. & Dawson, P. (1990) Editorial. Low osmolar contrast media: an appraisal. *Clin. Radiol.* **42**, 1–5.

McClennan, B.L. & Stolberg, H.O. (1991) Intravascular contrast media. Ionic versus nonionic: current status. *Radiol. Clin. N. Am.* **29**(3), 437–454.

Contrast Agents in MRI

Mechanism of action

To enhance the inherent contrast between tissues, MRI contrast agents must alter the rate of relaxation of the protons within the tissues. The changes in relaxation must vary for different tissues in order to produce differential enhancement of the signal (see Figures 2.3 and 2.4). These show that, for a given time t, if the T1 relaxation is more rapid then a larger signal is obtained (brighter images), but the opposite is true for T2 relaxation where more rapid relaxation produces reduced signal intensity (darker images).

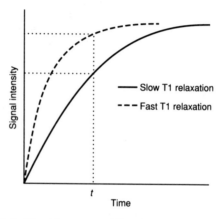

Fig. 2.3 Signal intensity and T1 relaxation time.

MRI contrast agents must exert a large magnetic field density (a property imparted by their unpaired electrons) to interact with the magnetic moments of the protons in the tissues and so shorten their T1 relaxation time which will produce an increase in signal intensity (see Figure 2.3). The electron magnetic moments also cause local changes in the magnetic field which promotes more rapid proton dephasing and so shortens the T2 relaxation time. Agents with unpaired electron spins are therefore potential contrast agents in MRI. These may be classified into three groups:

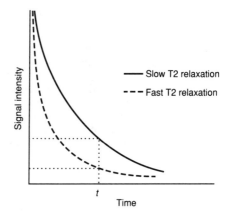

Fig. 2.4 Signal intensity and T2 relaxation time.

1. *Ferromagnetic.* These have magnetic moments which align with the scanner's applied field. They will maintain their alignment even when the applied field is removed. This retained magnetism may cause particle aggregation and interfere with cell function, making them unsafe as MR contrast agents.

2. *Paramagnetic* — e.g. gadolinium (see below). These agents have magnetic moments which align to the applied field, but once the gradient field is turned off, thermal energy within the tissue is enough to overcome the alignment. They may be made soluble by chelation and can therefore be injected intravenously. Their maximum effect is on protons in the water molecule, shortening the T1 relaxation time and hence producing increased signal intensity (white) on T1 images (Figure 2.3).

3. *Superparamagnetic* — e.g. ferrite. These are aggregates of paramagnetic ions in a crystalline lattice. They cause abrupt changes in the local magnetic field which results in rapid proton dephasing and reduction in the T2 relaxation time, and hence producing decreased signal intensity (black) on T2 images (Figure 2.4). They are less soluble than paramagnetic agents, due to their chemical structure and so are available only as a colloidal suspension.

Both paramagnetic and superparamagnetic substances can be used as gastrointestinal contrast agents (see below).

Gadolinium (Gd)

Chemistry   Gd is chelated to diethylenetriaminepenta-acetic acid (DTPA). The official generic name is dimeglumine gadopentate (Magnevist, Schering).

Indications   1. CNS tumours — particularly small acoustic neuromas and spinal seedlings from posterior fossa tumours.
2. Demyelinating diseases — for differentiating acute from chronic plaques.
3. More accurate delineation of tumour margins from oedema.
4. Discrimination of tumour recurrence from post-therapy fibrosis (although fibrosis may enhance even several years after therapy, particularly if due to radiation).
5. Discrimination of recurrent intervertebral disc prolapse from postoperative fibrosis. Images must be obtained within 30 min of the injection as fibrosis enhances immediately but disc material may enhance approximately 20 min after injection.
6. Cardiac/aortic imaging.

Contraindications   No absolute contraindications are known, but roughly they are contraindicated in similar situations to iodinated contrast media. There is little experience with any form of MRI during pregnancy and even less with the use of contrast agents, particularly in the first trimester.

Dose   0.1 mmol kg^{-1} body weight (e.g. 0.2 ml of Magnevist kg^{-1}); up to 0.2 mmol kg^{-1} when used in low field magnets.

Administration should be by relatively slow intravenous injection (60 s for a 40 kg individual, up to 120 s for a 100 kg person) to reduce side-effects.

Side-effects   Few are described and include:
1. Warmth.
2. Pain at injection site.

3. Seizure.
4. Strange taste.
5. Nausea.
6. Headache.
7. Dizziness.
8. Anaphylactoid reactions may occur (at the present time seven episodes have been reported to Schering worldwide) and so medical cover should be readily available, as should resuscitation equipment.

Of these the first two are the most common, but in all they add up to only about 3% of injections (Schering Technical Brochure).

Gastrointestinal contrast agents These are used to distinguish bowel from adjacent soft tissue masses. As with CT, all bowel contrast agents need to mix readily with the bowel contents to ensure even distribution. They must also be palatable. They can be divided into two groups:

Positive agents e.g. fatty oils and gadolinium.
Act by T1-shortening effects.
Appear white on T1 images.

DISADVANTAGES
1. The high signal increases the effect of bowel motion artefact.
2. The effect varies with the pulse sequence and the contrast concentration within the bowel. This can produce non-uniformity in the signal which may cause confusion.
3. Expensive.

Negative agents e.g. ferrite and barium sulphate (60–70% w/w).
Act by T2-shortening.
Appear black on T2 images.

DISADVANTAGES
1. High concentrations result in image distortion and blurring of adjacent structures.
2. The required dose of ferrite is a potentially lethal dose and so enteric preparations need to be chelated to reduce the absorption of iron.
3. Rather unpalatable.

Other aids to abdominal MRI

1. Prone position of the patient results in reduced respiratory artefact.
2. Smooth muscle relaxants help reduce motion artefact due to bowel peristalsis.
3. Saturation pulses reduce motion artefact due to diaphragmatic movement.
4. Breath holding.
5. FLASH sequences. This is a rapid method of acquiring T2-weighted images by using a low flip angle (FLASH = Fast Low Angle SHot).
6. Corsets.

3 Gastrointestinal Tract

Methods of imaging the gastrointestinal tract

1. Plain film.
2. Barium swallow.
3. Barium meal.
4. Barium follow-through.
5. Small bowel enema.
6. Barium enema.
7. Ultrasound
   - transcutaneous
   - endosonography.
8. Radionuclide imaging
   - Gastro-oesophageal reflux
   - Gastric emptying
   - Bile reflux study
   - Meckel's scan
   - Gastrointestinal bleeding.
9. Angiography.
10. CT.

Further reading

Balthazar, E.J. (1989) CT of the gastrointestinal tract: principles and interpretation. *Am. J. Roentg.* **156**, 23–32.

Davies, E.R. (1990) Review. Radionuclides and the gut. *Clin. Radiol.* **42**, 80–84.

Gore, R.M. (ed.) (1989) CT of the gastrointestinal tract. *Radiol. Clin. N. Am.* **27**(4).

Joseph, A.E.A. & Macvicar, D. (1990) Editorial. Ultrasound in the diagnosis of abdominal abscesses. *Clin. Radiol.* **42**, 154–156.

Kaufman, R.A. (1989) Technical aspects of abdominal CT in infants and children. *Am. J. Roentg.* **153**, 549.

Kelvin, F.M. (ed.) (1992) Radiology of the alimentary tract. *Radiol. Clin. N. Am.* **20**(4).

Introduction to Contrast Media

WATER-SOLUBLE CONTRAST MEDIA

e.g. Gastromiro, Gastrografin.

Proprietary name	Chemical name	Iodine concentration (mg ml^{-1})
Gastromiro	iopamidol 61% w/v	300
Gastrografin	{ meglumine diatrizoate 66% w/v / sodium diatrizoate 10% w/v }	370

Indications
1. Suspected perforation.
2. Meconium ileus.
3. To distinguish bowel from other structures on CT. A dilute solution of water soluble contrast medium (e.g. 15 ml of Gastrografin in 1 litre of flavoured drink) is used so that minimal artefact 'shadow' is produced.
4. LOCM is used if aspiration is a possibility.

Complications
1. Pulmonary oedema if aspirated (not LOCM).
2. Hypovolaemia in children — due to the hyperosmolality of the contrast media drawing fluid into the bowel (not with LOCM).
3. Allergic reactions — due to absorbed contrast media.
4. May precipitate in hyperchlorhydric gastric acid (i.e. 0.1 N HCl) — not non-ionics.
5. Ileus — may occur in 4% of patients examined in the postoperative phase.

Use in the gastro-intestinal tract of neonates and infants

The use of LOCM in neonates and infants has been reviewed Cohen[1]

Advantages
1. Isotonic at iodine concentrations which are satisfactory for good images of the bowel. There is no effect on the infant's haematocrit or serum osmolality.
2. Isosmolar concentrations are not diluted with time.

3. Rapid absorption of LOCM that enters the peritoneal cavity.
4. No damage to bowel mucosa or peritoneal mesothelium.
5. Very slow absorption from the gut, resulting in good bowel visualization many days after the administration of contrast medium.
6. Stable in bowel secretions.
7. No adverse effects on the lungs when used in isosmolar concentrations.

Disadvantages
1. Cost
2. Slightly inferior image quality because LOCM are still less dense than barium sulphate[2].
3. Diarrhoea may be more common[2].

Recommendations for use
1. When contrast medium is likely to enter the lungs, e.g. swallowing disorders, tracheo-oesophageal fistula and CNS impairment. *In most cases barium is still the contrast medium of choice.*
2. Possible leakage of contrast medium from the gastrointestinal tract.
3. Suspected necrotizing enterocolitis.
4. The gasless abdomen.

References
1. Cohen, M.D. (1987) Choosing contrast media for the evaluation of the gastrointestinal tract of neonates and infants. *Radiology* **162**, 447–456.
2. Cohen, M.D., Towbin, R., Baker, S., et al. (1991) Comparison of iohexol with barium in gastrointestinal studies of infants and children. *Am. J. Roentg.* **156**, 345–350.

BARIUM

Barium suspension is made up from pure barium sulphate. (Barium carbonate is poisonous.) The particles of barium must be small (0.1–3 μm), since this makes them more stable in suspension. A nonionic suspension medium is used, for otherwise the barium particles would aggregate into clumps. The resulting solution has a pH of 5.3, which makes it stable in gastric acid.

There are many varieties of barium suspension in use. Exact formulations are secret. In most situations the preparation may be diluted with water to give a lower density.

Proprietary name	Density
Baritop 100	100% w/v
Baritop G powder	150% w/v
EPI-C	150% w/v
E-Z Paque	170% w/v
E-Z HD	250% w/v
Micropaque liquid	100% w/v
Micropaque powder	76% w/v
Micropaque DC	100% w/v
Polibar	125% w/v

Examinations of different parts of the gastrointestinal tract require barium preparations with differing properties.

1. *Barium swallow*, e.g. Baritop G 150% w/v. 100 ml (or more, as required).
2. *Barium meal*, e.g. E-Z HD 250% w/v. 135 ml. A high-density, low-viscosity barium is required for a double-contrast barium meal to give a good thin coating that is still sufficiently dense to give satisfactory opacification. E-Z HD fulfils these requirements. It also contains simethicone (an anti-foaming and coating agent) and sorbitol (a coating agent)[1].
3. *Barium follow-through*, e.g. Baritop G 100% w/v. 300 ml (150 ml if performed after a barium meal). This preparation is partially resistant to flocculation.
4. *Small bowel enema*, e.g. two tubs of E-Z Paque made up to 1500 ml. N.B. As the transit time through the small bowel is relatively short in this investigation, there is a reduced chance of flocculation. This enables the use of barium preparations which are not flocculation-resistant. Some advocate the addition of Gastrografin to the mixture as this may help reduce the transit time still further.
5. *Barium enema*, e.g. Polibar 125% w/v. 500 ml (or more, as required).

Complications
1. *Perforation*. The escape of barium into the peritoneal cavity is extremely serious, and will produce pain and severe hypovolaemic shock. Despite treatment, which should consist of i.v. fluids, steroids, and antibiotics, there is still a 50% mortality rate. Of those that survive, 30% will develop peritoneal adhesions and granulomata. Intramediastinal barium also has a significant mortality rate.

   It is therefore imperative that a water-soluble contrast medium is used for any investigation in which there is a risk of perforation, or in which perforation is already suspected.
2. *Aspiration*. Barium, if aspirated, is relatively harmless. The only treatment required is physiotherapy, which should be arranged for the patient before he leaves hospital (the same applies to aspirated LOCM).

For further complications of the use of barium, see the specific procedure involved.

Reference
Lintott, D.J., Simpkins, K.C., de Dombal, F.T. & Noakes, M.J. (1978) Assessment of double contrast barium meal: method and application. *Clin. Radiol.* **29**, 313–321.

Introduction to Pharmacological Agents

Hyoscine-N-butyl bromide (Buscopan)

Adult dose 20 mg i.v.

Advantages
1. Reduced bowel peristalsis during the examination, owing to the smooth muscle relaxant action.
2. Immediate onset of action.
3. Short duration of action (approx. 15 min).

Disadvantage Anticholinergic side-effects, e.g. blurring of vision, dry mouth, tachycardia, urinary retention, acute gastric dilatation. Its use is contraindicated in glaucoma and cardiovascular disease — glucagon may be used in these circumstances.

N.B. Buscopan has replaced propantheline as the smooth muscle relaxant of choice. The latter has an unnecessarily long duration of action (3 hours or more).

Glucagon

Adult dose 0.3 mg i.v. for barium meal[1].
1.0 mg i.v. for barium enema.

Paediatric dose 0.5–1.0 μg kg^{-1} for barium meal.
0.8–1.25 μg kg^{-1} for barium enema[2].
(A smooth muscle relaxant is seldom needed in paediatric practice.)

N.B. Glucagon is available in vials which contain either 1 unit or 10 units. Both sizes are supplied with a diluent, but if the 10-unit vials are reconstituted they contain a bacteriocide which enables them to be stored in a refrigerator for up to 1 week provided the temperature of the refrigerator is 4°C.

Advantages
1. It is a more potent smooth muscle relaxant than Buscopan.
2. Onset of action within 1 min.
3. Short duration of action (approx. 15 min).
4. It does not interfere with the small bowel transit time.

Disadvantages
1. Hypersensitivity reactions are possible, as it is a protein molecule.
2. Phaeochromocytoma and insulinoma are contra-indications.
3. It is expensive.

Metoclopramide (Maxolon)

Adult dose 20 mg oral or i.v.

Advantage Increased gastric peristalsis enhances the transit of barium during a follow-through examination.

Disadvantage Extrapyramidal side-effects may occur if the dose exceeds 0.5 mg kg^{-1}. This is more likely to occur in children.

References
1. Kreel, L. (1975) Review article. Pharmaco-radiology in barium examinations with special reference to glucagon. *Br. J. Radiol.* **48**, 691–703.
2. Ratcliffe, J.F. (1980) Glucagon in barium examinations in infants and children: special reference to dosage. *Br. J. Radiol.* **53**, 860–862.

Further reading Lintott, D.J., Simpkins, K.C., de Dombal, F.T. & Noakes, M.J. (1978) Assessment of the double contrast barium meal: method and application. *Clin. Radiol.* **29**, 313–321.

General Points

A tilting table, and a fluoroscopic unit with a spot film device are standard equipment for all barium investigations. The need for these will not be mentioned further in the text. In all barium work a high-kV technique is used (90–110 kV). As in all radiological procedures, the ALARA (As Low As Reasonably Achievable) principle is adhered to.

Barium Swallow

Barium is used unless there are indications to do otherwise, because of the superior contrast qualities.

Indications
1. Dysphagia.
2. Pain.
3. Assessment of tracheo-oesophageal fistula in children — a non-ionic agent is preferable.
4. Assessment of the site of perforation — it is essential that a water soluble contrast medium is used, e.g. Gastrografin or LOCM.

Contraindications   None.

Contrast medium
1. Baritop G 150% w/v. 100 ml (or more, as required).
2. Gastrografin
3. LOCM (approx. 350 mg I ml^{-1}).

N.B. LOCM or barium may be used for the investigation of a tracheo-oesophageal fistula.

Equipment   Rapid serial radiography (6 frames per s) or video recording may be required for assessment of the laryngopharynx and upper oesophagus during deglutition.

Patient preparation   None. (But as for barium meal if the stomach is also to be examined — see p. 53.)

Preliminary films   None.

Technique
1. The patient is in the erect RAO position to throw the oesophagus clear of the spine. An ample mouthful of barium is swallowed, and spot films of the upper and lower oesophagus are taken. Oesophageal varices are better seen in the prone RPO position, as they will be more distended.
2. If rapid serial radiography is required, it may be performed in the right lateral, RAO, and PA positions.

Modification of technique   *To demonstrate a tracheo-oesophageal fistula in infants*, a nasogastric tube is introduced to the level of the mid-oesophagus, and the contrast agent (barium or LOCM) is syringed in to distend the oesophagus. This will force the contrast medium through any small fistula which may be present. It is important to take radiographs in the lateral projection during simultaneous injection of the contrast medium and withdrawal of the tube. Although some authors recommend that the infant be examined in the prone position whilst lying on the foot step of a vertical tilting table, satisfactory results are possible with the child on his side on a horizontal table.

The contrast medium is introduced through a nasogastric tube because infants may aspirate into the trachea during swallowing from a bottle. It would then not be possible to determine whether contrast in the bronchi was due to a small fistula, which was difficult to see, or due to aspiration.

Aftercare   None.

Complications   1. Leakage of barium from an unsuspected perforation.
2. Aspiration.

Barium Meal

Methods
1. *Double contrast* — the method of choice to demonstrate mucosal pattern.
2. *Single contrast* — uses:
   (a) children — since it usually is not necessary to demonstrate mucosal pattern
   (b) very ill adults — to demonstrate gross pathology only.

Indications
1. Dyspepsia.
2. Weight loss.
3. Upper abdominal mass.
4. Gastrointestinal haemorrhage (or unexplained iron deficiency anaemia).
5. Partial obstruction.
6. Assessment of site of perforation — it is essential that a water-soluble contrast medium, e.g. Gastrografin or LOCM, is used.

Contraindications
Complete large bowel obstruction.

Contrast medium
E-Z HD 250% w/v. 135 ml.

Patient preparation
1. Nil orally for 6 hours prior to the examination.
2. The patient must not smoke on the day of the examination, as this causes increased gastric motility.
3. It should be ensured that there are no contraindications to the pharmacological agents used.

Preliminary films
None.

Technique
The double contrast method (Figure 3.1)
1. A gas-producing agent is swallowed. The requirement of these agents are as follows[1]:
   (a) production of an adequate volume of gas — 200–400 ml
   (b) non-interference with barium coating
   (c) no bubble production
   (d) rapid dissolution, leaving no residue
   (e) easily swallowed
   (f) low cost.

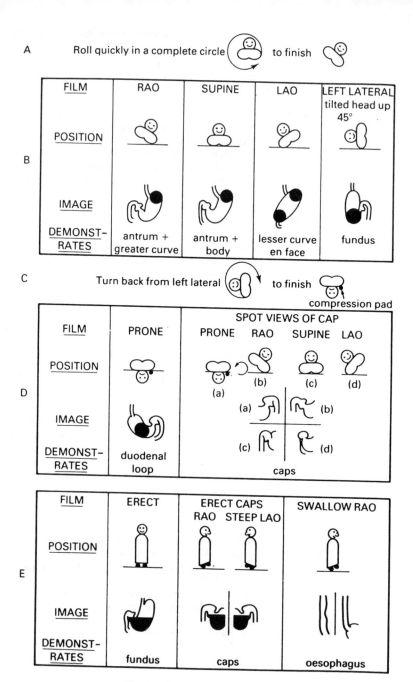

Fig. 3.1 Barium meal sequence.

Carbex granules and fluid satisfy most of these requirements, but have the disadvantage of being relatively costly.

2. The patient then drinks the barium while lying on his left side, supported by his elbow. This position prevents the barium from reaching the duodenum too quickly and so obscuring the greater curve of the stomach.

3. The patient then lies supine and slightly on his right side, to bring the barium up against the gastro-oesophageal junction. This manoeuvre is screened to check for reflux, which may be revealed by asking the patient to cough or to swallow water while in this position. The significance of reflux produced by tipping the patient's head down is debatable, as this is an unphysiological position. If reflux is observed, spot films are taken to record the level to which it ascends.

4. An i.v. injection of a smooth muscle relaxant (Buscopan 20 mg or glucagon 0.3 mg) is given. The administration of Buscopan has been shown not to effect the detection of gastro-oesophageal reflux or hiatus hernia[2].

5. The patient is asked to roll onto his right side and then quickly over in a complete circle, to finish in an RAO position. This roll is performed to coat the gastric mucosa with barium. Good coating has been achieved if the areae gastricae in the antrum are visible.

Films There is a great variation in views recommended, and the following is only the scheme used in our departments. In some departments fewer films are taken to reduce the cost and radiation dose.

1. Spot films of the stomach (lying):
   (a) RAO — to demonstrate the antrum and greater curve
   (b) supine — to demonstrate the antrum and body
   (c) LAO — to demonstrate the lesser curve *en face*
   (d) left lateral tilted, head up 45° — to demonstrate the fundus.

From the left lateral position the patient returns to a supine position and then rolls onto his left side and over into a prone position. This sequence of movement is required to avoid barium flooding into the duodenal loop, which would occur if the patient were to roll onto his right side to achieve a prone position.

2. Spot film of the duodenal loop (lying):
   (a) prone — the patient lies on a compression pad to prevent barium from flooding into the duodenum.

   An additional view to demonstrate the anterior wall of the duodenal loop may be taken in an RAO position.

3. Spot films of the duodenal cap (lying):
   (a) prone
   (b) RAO — the patient attains this position from the prone position by rolling first onto the left side, for the reasons mentioned above
   (c) supine
   (d) LAO.

4. Additional views of the fundus in an erect position may be taken at this stage, if there is suspicion of a fundal lesion.

5. Spot films of the oesophagus are taken, while barium is being swallowed, to complete the examination.

Modification of technique for young children

The main indication will be to identify a cause for vomiting. The examination is modified to identify the three major causes of vomiting — gastro-oesophageal reflux, pyloric obstruction and mal-rotation.

1. Single contrast technique using 100% w/v barium sulphate and no paralytic agent.

2. A relatively small volume of barium — enough to just fill the fundus — is given to the infant in the supine position. A film of the distended oesophagus is exposed.

3. The child is turned semi-prone into a LPO or RAO position. A film is exposed as barium passes through the pylorus. The pylorus is shown to even better advantage if 20–40° caudocranial angulation can be employed with an overhead screening unit. Gastric emptying is prolonged if

the child is upset. A dummy coated with glycerin is a useful pacifier.

4. Once barium enters the duodenum, the infant is returned to the supine position, and with the child perfectly straight a second film is exposed as barium passes around the duodenojejunal flexure.

5. Once malrotation has been diagnosed or excluded, a further volume of barium is administered until the stomach is reasonably full. The child is gently rotated through 180° in an attempt to elicit gastro-oesophageal reflux.

Aftercare

1. The patient should be warned that his bowel motions will be white for a few days after the examination, and to keep his bowels open with laxatives to avoid barium impaction, which can be painful.

2. The patient must not leave the department until any blurring of vision produced by the Buscopan has resolved.

Complications

1. Leakage of barium from an unsuspected perforation.

2. Aspiration.

3. Conversion of a partial large bowel obstruction into a complete obstruction by the impaction of barium.

4. Barium appendicitis, if barium impacts in the appendix.

5. Side-effects of the pharmacological agents used.

It must be emphasized that there are many variations in technique, according to individual preference, and that the best way of becoming familiar with the sequence of positioning is actually to perform the procedure oneself.

References

1. de Lacey, G.J. Wignall, B.K. & Bray, C. (1979) Effervescent granules for the barium meal. *Br. J. Radiol.* **52**, 405–408.

2. Rajah, R.R. (1990) Effects of Buscopan on gastro-oesophageal reflux and hiatus hernia. *Clin. Radiol.* **41**, 250–252.

Barium Follow-through

Methods
1. Single contrast.
2. In the investigation of suspected disaccharidase deficiency the examination is performed first without, and then with 25 g of the appropriate sugar added to the barium[1].
3. Enhanced with an effervescent agent[2].
4. Enhanced with a pneumocolon technique[3].

Indications
1. Pain.
2. Diarrhoea.
3. Bleeding.
4. Partial obstruction.
5. Abdominal mass.
6. Failed small bowel enema.

Contraindications
1. Complete obstruction.
2. Suspected perforation (unless a water-soluble contrast medium is used).

Contrast medium
Baritop G 100% w/v. 300 ml (150 ml if performed immediately after a barium meal). The transit time through the small bowel has been shown to be reduced by the addition of 10 ml of Gastrografin to the barium[4]. In children 3–4 ml kg^{-1} is a suitable volume.

Equipment
Overcouch tube in addition to a fluoroscopy unit.

Patient preparation
1. Metoclopramide 20 mg orally 20 min before the examination.

Preliminary film
Plain abdominal film.

Technique
The aim is to deliver a single column of barium into the small bowel. This is achieved by lying the patient on his right side after the barium has been ingested. The metoclopramide enhances the rate of gastric emptying. If the transit time through the small bowel is found to be slow, a dry meal may help to speed it up. If a follow-through examination is combined with a barium meal, glucagon is used for the duodenal cap views rather than Buscopan because it has a short

length of action and does not interfere with the small-bowel transit time.

Films
1. Prone PA films of the abdomen are taken every 20 min during the first hour, and subsequently every 30 min until the colon is reached. The prone position is used because the pressure on the abdomen helps to separate the loops of small bowel.
2. Spot films of the terminal ileum are taken supine. A compression pad is used to displace any overlying loops of small bowel that are obscuring the terminal ileum.

Additional films
1. To separate loops of small bowel:
   (a) obliques
   (b) with X-ray tube angled into the pelvis
   (c) with the patient tilted head down.
2. To demonstrate diverticula:
   (a) erect — this position will reveal any fluid levels caused by contrast medium retained within the diverticula.

Aftercare
As for barium meal.

Complications
As for barium meal.

References
1. Laws, J.W., Spencer, J. & Neale, G. (1967) Radiology in the diagnosis of disaccharidase deficiency. *Br. J. Radiol.* **40**, 594–603.
2. Fraser, G.M. & Preston, P.G. (1983) The small bowel follow-through enhanced with an oral effervescent agent. *Clin. Radiol.* **34**, 673–679.
3. Fitzgerald, E.J., Thompson, G.T., Somers, S.S. & Franic, S.F. (1985) Pneumocolon as an aid to small bowel studies. *Clin. Radiol.* **36**, 633–637.
4. Frazer, G.M. & Adam, R.D. (1988) Modifications to the gas-enhanced small bowel barium follow-through using Gastrografin and compression. *Clin. Radiol.* **39**, 537–541.

Further reading
Garvey, C.J., de Lacey, G. & Wilkins, R.A. (1985) Preliminary colon cleansing for small bowel examinations: results and implications of a prospective study. *Clin. Radiol.* **36**, 503–506.

Small Bowel Enema

Advantage   This procedure gives better visualization of the small bowel than that achieved by a barium follow-through because rapid infusion of a large, continuous column of contrast medium directly into the jejunum avoids segmentation of the barium column and does not allow time for flocculation to occur.

Disadvantage   Intubation may be unpleasant for the patient, and may occasionally prove difficult. It is also time-consuming for the radiologist.

Indications }
Contraindications }   The same as for a barium follow-through. In some departments it is only performed in the case of an equivocal follow-through.

Contrast medium   Micropaque 100% w/v.

This is diluted with tap water to give a volume of 1000 ml with a specific gravity of 1.3. The reduced viscosity produces better mucosal coating, and the reduced density permits the visualization of bowel loops which may otherwise have been obscured by a denser contrast medium in an overlying loop.

An alternative way to gain a double contrast effect is to use a small (100 ml) bolus of Micropaque, followed by a continuous infusion of methyl cellulose (100 ml of Cologel made up to 2 litres with distilled water).

Equipment   A choice of tubes is available.
(a) Bilbao–Dotter tube with a guide-wire (the tube is longer than the wire so that there is reduced risk of perforation when introducing the wire).
(b) Silk tube (E. Merck Ltd). This is a 10F, 140 cm long tube with a tungsten-filled guide-tip. It is made of polyurethane and the stylet and the internal lumen of the tube are coated with a water activated lubricant to facilitate the smooth removal of the stylet after insertion.

Patient preparation   1. A low-residue diet for 2 days prior to the examination.

2. If the patient is taking any antispasmodic drugs, they must be stopped 1 day prior to the examination.
3. Amethocaine lozenge 30 mg, 30 min before the examination.
4. Immediately before the examination the pharynx is anaesthetized with lignocaine spray.

Preliminary film   Plain abdominal film if a small bowel obstruction is suspected.

Technique

1. The patient sits on the edge of the X-ray table. The pharynx is thoroughly anaesthetized with lignocaine spray. If a per nasal approach is planned the patency of the nasal passages is checked by asking the patient to sniff with one nostril occluded. The Silk tube should be passed with the guide-wire pre-luricated and fully within the tube, whereas for the Bilbao–Dotter it may be more comfortable to introduce the guide-wire after the tube tip is in the stomach.
2. The tube is then passed through the nose or the mouth, and brief lateral screening of the neck may be helpful in negotiating the epiglottic region. The patient is asked to swallow as the tube is passed through the pharynx. The tube is then advanced into the gastric antrum.
3. The patient then lies down and the tube is passed into the duodenum. Various manoeuvres may be used alone or in combination, to help this part of the procedure which may be difficult.
   (a) Lie the patient on his left side so that the gastric air bubble rises to the antrum, thus straightening out the stomach.
   (b) Advance the tube whilst applying clockwise rotational motion (as viewed from the head of the patient looking towards the feet).
   (c) In the case of the Bilbao–Dotter tube, introduce the guide-wire.
   (d) In the case of the Silk tube, lie the patient on his right side, as the tube has a Tungsten-weighted guide-tip which will then tend to fall towards the antrum.
   (e) Get the patient to sit up, to try to overcome

the tendency of the tube to coil in the fundus of the stomach.

(f) Metoclopramide (20 mg i.v.) may help.

4. When the tip of the tube has been passed through the pylorus, the guide-wire tip is maintained at the pylorus as the tube is passed over it along the duodenum to the level of the ligament of Treitz. Clockwise torque applied to the tube may again help in getting past the junction of the first and second parts of the duodenum. The tube is passed as far as the duodenojejunal flexure to diminish the risk of aspiration due to reflux of barium into the stomach.

5. Barium is then run in quickly, and spot films are taken of the barium column and its leading edge at the regions of interest, until the colon is reached. If methyl cellulose is used, it is infused continuously, after an initial bolus of 100 ml of barium, until the barium has reached the colon.

6. The tube is then withdrawn, aspirating any residual fluid in the stomach. Again, this is to decrease the risk of aspiration.

7. Finally, prone and supine abdominal films are taken.

Modification of technique

In patients with malabsorption, especially if an excess of fluid has been shown on the preliminary film, the volume of barium should be increased (240–260 ml). Compression views of bowel loops should be obtained before obtaining double contrast. Flocculation is likely to occur early. It is important to obtain images of the duodenum and the catheter tip should be sited proximal to the ligament of Trietz[1].

Aftercare

1. Nil orally for 5 hours after the procedure.
2. The patient should be warned that diarrhoea may occur as a result of the large volume of fluid given.

Complications

1. Aspiration.
2. Perforation of the bowel owing to manipulation of the guide-wire.

Reference   1. Herlinger, H. (1992) Editorial. Radiology in malabsorption. *Clin. Radiol.* **45**, 73–78.

Further reading   Herlinger, H. (1978) A modified technique for double contrast small bowel enema. *Gastroint. Radiol.* **3**, 201–207.
Herlinger, H. (1983) The small bowel enema and the diagnosis of Crohn's. *Radiol. Clin. N. Am.* **20**, 721–742.
Nolan, D.J. (1979) Rapid duodenal and jejunal intubation. *Clin. Radiol.* **30**, 183–185.
Nolan, D.J. & Cadman, P.J. (1987) The small bowel enema made easy. *Clin. Radiol.* **38**, 295–301.

Barium Enema

Methods
1. *Double contrast* — the method of choice to demonstrate mucosal pattern.
2. *Single contrast* — uses:
   (a) children — since it is usually not necessary to demonstrate mucosal pattern
   (b) reduction of an intussusception (see p. 73).

Indications
1. Change in bowel habit.
2. Pain.
3. Mass.
4. Melaena.
5. Obstruction.

N.B. If a tight stricture is demonstrated, only run a small volume of barium proximally to define the upper margin, for otherwise the barium may impact.

Contraindications

Absolute
1. Toxic megacolon.
2. Pseudomembranous colitis.
3. Rectal biopsy within the previous 3 days (it is preferable to wait for 7 days) if a rectal biopsy has been performed at rigid sigmoidoscopy. Biopsies performed at flexible sigmoidoscopy or colonoscopy are not a contraindication.

Relative
1. Incomplete bowel preparation.
2. Recent barium meal.

Contrast medium
Polibar 125% w/v. 500 ml (or more, as required).

Equipment
Miller disposable enema tube. If the patient is incontinent, it is permissible to use a tube with an inflatable cuff. However, its use should be confined to such cases, owing to the increased risk of perforation (see 'complications' p. 68).

Patient preparation
Many regimens for bowel preparation have been reviewed[1-4]. A suggested regimen is as follows:

For 3 days prior to examination:
Low residue diet.

On the day prior to examination:
1. Fluids only.
2. Picolax – at 8 a.m. and 6 p.m.

On the day of the examination:
A high colonic washout with 2 litres of tepid tap water (outpatients may forgo this if there was no faecal residue present the last time the bowels were opened).

The patient then empties his bowels. At least 1 hour must elapse before starting the barium enema to allow time for the colon to absorb the excess water. In some centres tannic acid has been used in the saline enema to promote evacuation. The concentration must be less than 0.25% in the saline enema, as higher concentrations carry the risk of centrilobular liver necrosis. It must not be used in cases of hepatic failure or inflammatory bowel disease, as it is more easily absorbed[5].

Preliminary film A preliminary plain abdominal film is not necessary unless:
(a) severe constipation renders the effectiveness of bowel preparation doubtful
(b) toxic megacolon is suspected.

Technique
The double contrast method (Figure 3.2)

1. The patient lies on his side on an incontinence sheet, and the catheter is inserted gently into the rectum. It is taped firmly in position. Connections are made to the barium reservoir and the hand pump for injecting air.
2. An i.v. injection of Buscopan (20 mg) or glucagon (1 mg) is given.
3. The infusion of barium is commenced. Intermittent screening is required to check the progress of the barium. The infusion is terminated when the barium reaches the hepatic flexure. The column of barium within the sigmoid colon is run back out by either lowering the infusion bag to the floor or tilting the table erect.
4. Air is gently pumped into the bowel, forcing the column of barium round towards the caecum, and producing the double contrast effect. Some centres

use CO_2 as the negative contrast agent as it has been shown to reduce the incidence of severe post-double contrast enema pain[6].

5. From the prone position, the patient rolls onto his left side and over into an RAO position so that the barium coats the bowel mucosa.

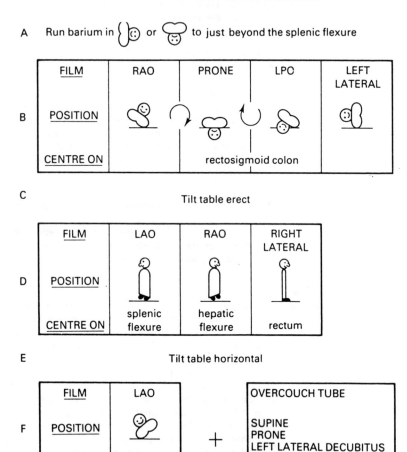

Fig. 3.2 Barium enema sequence.

Films   There is a great variation in views recommended, and the following is only the scheme used in this department. Fewer films may be taken to reduce the radiation dose and cost.

The sequence of positioning enables the barium to flow proximally to reach the caecal pole. Air is pumped in as required to distend the colon.

1. Spot films of the rectum and sigmoid colon (lying):
   (a) RAO
   (b) prone
   (c) LPO
   (d) left lateral of the rectum.
2. Spot films of the hepatic flexure, splenic flexure and rectum (erect):
   (a) LAO to open out the splenic flexure
   (b) RAO to open out the hepatic flexure
   (c) right lateral of the rectum.
3. Spot film of the caecum (lying). Positioning of the patient supine, lying slightly on the right side and with a slight head-down tilt will usually give a double-contrast effect in the caecum. Some compression with a lead-gloved hand may be necessary to persuade a stubborn pool of barium out of the caecal pole.
4. Overcouch films to demonstrate all of the large bowel (lying):
   (a) supine
   (b) prone
   (c) left lateral decubitus
   (d) right lateral decubitus
   (e) prone, with the tube angled 45° caudad and centred 5 cm above the posterior superior iliac spines. This view separates overlying loops of sigmoid colon.

Aftercare
1. The patient should be warned that his bowel motions will be white for a few days after the examination, and to keep his bowels open with laxatives to avoid barium impaction, which can be painful.
2. The patient must not leave the department until any blurring of vision produced by the Buscopan has resolved.

Complications

1. Perforation of the bowel. There is an increased risk of this in:
   (a) infants and the elderly
   (b) obstructing neoplasm
   (c) ulceration of the bowel wall
   (d) inflation of a Foley catheter balloon in a colostomy, or the rectum
   (e) patients on steroid therapy
   (f) hypothyroidism.
2. Venous extravasation. This may result in a barium pulmonary embolus, which carries an 80% mortality.
3. Water intoxication. The symptoms are drowsiness and convulsions. There is an increased risk in megacolon because of the large area of bowel mucosa available for absorption of water.
4. Intramural barium.
5. Cardiac arrhythmias due to rectal distension.
6. Transient bacteraemia.
7. Side-effects of the pharmacological agents used.
8. Severe urticarial reaction to the rubber of the cuff used in self-retaining catheters has been described[7].

References

1. Dodds, W.J., Scanlon, G.T., Shaw, D.K., Stewart, E.T., Youker, J.E. & Metter, J.E. (1977) An evaluation of colon cleansing regimens. *Am. J. Roentg.* **128**, 57–59.
2. Kendrick, R.G.M., MacKenzie, S. & Beckly, D.E. (1981) A comparison of four methods of bowel preparation for barium enema. *Clin. Radiol.* **32**, 95–97.
3. Bartram, C.I., Mootoosamy, I.M. & Lim, K.H. (1984) Washout versus non-washout (Picolax) preparation for double contrast enema. *Clin. Radiol.* **35**, 143–146.
4. Hughes, K., Mann, S., Cooke, M.B.D. & James, W.B. (1983) A new oral bowel evacuant (Picolax) for colon cleansing, *Clin. Radiol.* **34**, 75–77.
5. Kemp Harper, R.A., Pemberton, J. & Tobias, J.S. (1973) Serial liver function studies following barium enemas containing 1% tannic acid. *Clin. Radiol.* **24**, 315–317.
6. Taylor, P.N. & Beckley, D.E. (1991) Use of air in double contrast barium enema — is it still acceptable? *Clin. Radiol.* **44**, 183–184.
7. Sissons, G.R. & Evans, C. (1991) Severe urticarial reaction to rubber: complication of a barium enema. *Clin. Radiol.* **43**(4), 288–289.

Further reading   Margulis, A.R. & Eisenberg, R.L. (1979) The examination of the colon. In: Lodge, T. & Steiner, R.E. (eds) *Recent Advances in Radiology and Medical Imaging 6,* pp. 79–100. Edinburgh: Churchill Livingstone.

Thoeni, R.F. & Margulis, A.R. (1978) The state of radiologic technique in the examination of the colon: a survey. *Radiology* **127**, 317–329.

The 'Instant' Barium Enema

This is performed without bowel preparation because colon involved by inflammatory bowel disease does not contain faecal residue. The technique is better suited to ulcerative colitis, which affects the distal colon and spreads proximally, but the more patchy distribution of Crohn's disease makes it less suitable and small lesions may not be seen. However, it is useful in severe Crohn's disease when bowel preparation is not possible.

Indications To show the extent and severity of mucosal lesions in active ulcerative colitis.

Contraindications
1. Toxic megacolon.
2. Rectal biopsy within the previous 3 days (it is preferable to wait for 7 days).
3. Long-standing ulcerative colitis – should have a formal barium enema to exclude a carcinoma.
4. Crohn's colitis – because assessment is unreliable, but occasionally used if there is severe anal disease which would make bowel preparation intolerable.

Preliminary film Plain abdominal film – to exclude toxic megacolon.

Technique As for normal barium enema.

Films Only three films are required:
1. Prone.
2. Left lateral decubitus.
3. Erect.

N.B. It may be difficult to distinguish mild colitis from normal, because the bowel is poorly coated in the presence of semi-liquid faecal residue. Also the ascending colon is usually poorly visualized because any remaining faecal residue is pushed into this part of the colon during the examination.

Further reading Bartram, C.I. & Kumar, P.J. (1981) *Clinical Radiology in Gastroenterology*. Oxford: Blackwell Scientific.

Balloon Dilatation of Oesophageal Strictures

Indications
1. Peptic strictures.
2. Oesophageal tumours.
3. Anastomotic strictures.
4. Achalasia of the cardia.

Contraindications
Tracheo-oesophageal fistula.

Contrast medium
LOCM 350 should always be used to outline the oesophagus and to define the stricture, as there is a risk of aspiration.

Equipment
1. Fluoroscopy unit, with a facility for spot films.
2. Oesophageal dilatation balloons (15 and 22 mm diameter).
3. Long guide-wire with floppy tip (long enough to allow the wire to traverse the stricture with sufficient outside the mouth to pass and exchange balloons over).
4. Lignocaine local anaesthetic spray.

Patient preparation
An easily accessible intravenous line should be available to allow for the administration of sedative or analgesic agents, as necessary.

Technique
1. The patient is made comfortable on the screening table.
2. A contrast swallow is performed to determine the level and the degree of the stricture. The contrast also outlines the gastrointestinal tract distal to the stricture.
3. The pharynx is anaesthetized using lignocaine spray.
4. The guide-wire is passed, floppy tip first. This manoeuvre may be aided by the use of fluoroscopy and a femorovisceral catheter which allows the wire tip to be directed appropriately.
5. The guide-wire is passed through the stricture, under screening guidance. The wire is passed so that a stable position is attained; placing the tip about 30 cm distal to the stricture is usually possible.

6. The stricture is progressively dilated using the graded balloons. Very tight stenoses may require the use of angioplasty balloons initially. Hand inflation of the balloon using a syringe is performed until the 'waist' in the balloon, caused by the stricture, has been overcome. This inflation is maintained for approx. 60 s. A 22-mm balloon is usually a sufficient maximum diameter.

Aftercare   The patient should remain nil by mouth for at least 4 hours after the procedure, with hourly observations of pulse and blood pressure.

Complications   1. Oesophageal rupture.
2. Mediastinitis secondary to oesophageal injury.

Enema Reduction of an Intussusception

This procedure should only be attempted in full consultation with the surgeon in charge of the case.

Methods
1. Using barium and fluoroscopy.
2. Using air and fluoroscopy.
   Compared with barium this method has the following advantages:
   (a) more rapid reduction, because the low viscosity of air permits rapid filling of the colon
   (b) reduced radiation dose because of the above
   (c) more effective reduction
   (d) in the presence of a perforation, air in the peritoneal cavity is preferable to barium, and gut organisms are not washed into the peritoneal cavity
   (e) there is more accurate control of intraluminal pressure
   (f) less mess, and a dry infant will not lose heat
   (g) cost.
3. Using a water-soluble contrast medium and ultrasound[1].

Contraindications
1. Peritonitis or perforation.
2. Advanced intestinal obstruction. When present, successful reduction is less likely and there is a higher incidence of perforation of gangrenous bowel.
3. The pneumatic method should probably not be used in children over 4 years of age as there is a higher incidence of significant lead points which may be missed[2].

Patient preparation
1. Sedation with papaveretum (Omnopon) 0.2 mg kg^{-1}.
2. Some institutions perform the examination under general anaesthesia. This has the advantages of greater muscle relaxation, which may increase the likelihood of successful reduction, and also

enables the child to go to surgery quickly in the event of a failed radiological reduction.
3. Correction of fluid and electrolyte imbalance. This is especially important when using Gastrografin because of its hyperosmolality effect.

Preliminary film   Plain abdominal film – to assess bowel distension and to exclude perforation. A right-side up decubitus film is often helpful in confirming the diagnosis by showing a failure of caecal filling with bowel gas because of the presence of the soft tissue mass of the intussusception. Normal plain films do not exclude the diagnosis and the clinical findings and/or history should be sufficient indications[3].

Contrast medium   1. Barium sulphate 100 % w/v.
2. Air.
3. Water-soluble contrast, e.g. LOCM 150 or dilute Gastrografin (1 part Gastrografin to 1 part water).

Technique   A 16–22F balloon catheter is inserted into the rectum and the buttocks taped tightly together to provide a seal. It may be necessary to inflate the balloon but if this is done it should be performed under fluoroscopic control so that the rectum is not overdistended.

Barium reduction   1. The child is placed in the prone position so that it is easier to maintain the catheter in the rectum and disturbed as little as possible during the procedure.
2. The bag containing barium is raised 100 cm above the table top and barium run in under gentle hydrostatic pressure. Progress of the column of barium is monitored by inermittent fluoroscopy.
3. If the intussusception does not move after 5 min of sustained pressure, the bag of barium is lowered to table-top height and the child rested for 5 min. If, after three similar attempts, the intussusception is still immovable it is considered irreducible and arrangements are made for surgery.
4. When barium dissects between the two layers of the intussusception, the dissection sign, reduction is less likely[4].
5. The intussusception is only considered to be completely reduced when the terminal ileum is filled

with contrast medium. However, it is not uncommon for there to be a persisting filling defect in the caecum at the end of the procedure, with or without reflux of barium into the terminal ileum. This is often due to an oedematous iliocaecal valve. In the presence of a soft tissue caecal mass, a clinically well and stable child should be returned to the ward to await a further enema after a period of several hours rather than proceed to surgery. A second enema is often successful at complete reduction or showing resolution of the oedematous iliocaecal valve.

Pneumatic reduction
1. Patient positioning is as for the barium method.
2. Air is instilled by a hand-pump and the intussusception is pushed back by a sustained pressure of up to 80 mmHg (approximately equivalent to a bag of 33% w/v barium sulphate at 100 cm)[5]. If this fails the pressure may be increased to 120 mmHg. There should be a pressure release valve in the system to ensure that excessive pressures are not delivered.
3. The points regarding failed or incomplete reduction discussed above also apply to pneumatic reduction.

Ultrasound reduction
1. To facilitate scanning the child must be supine.
2. The intussusception can be identified with ultrasound[6]. The contrast medium is run as far as the obstruction and its passage around the colon and the reducing head of the intussusception monitored by ultrasound.
3. The points regarding failed or incomplete reduction discussed above also apply to this technique

Films
1. Spot films as required.
2. Post-reduction film.

Aftercare Observation in hospital for 24 hours.

Complications
1. Perforation. For the pneumatic method, if a pump is used without a pressure monitoring valve, the presence of a perforation may result in a tension pneumoperitoneum, resulting in respiratory embarrassment.

References

1. Bolia, A.A. (1985) Case report: Diagnosis and hydro-static reduction of an intussusception under ultrasound guidance. *Clin. Radiol.* 36, 655–657.
2. Stringer, D.A. & Ein, S.H. (1990) Pneumatic reduction: advantages, risks and indications. *Pediatr. Radiol.* 20, 475–477.
3. Eklöf, O., Hartelius, H. (1980) Reliability of the abdominal plain film diagnosis in pediatric patients with suspected intussusception. *Pediatr. Radiol.* 9, 199–206.
4. Barr, L.L., Stansberry S.D. & Swischuk, L.E. (1990) Significance of age, duration, obstruction and the dissection sign in intussusception. *Pediatr. Radiol.* 20, 454–456.
5. Sargent, M.A. & Wilson, B.P.M. (1992) Are hydrostatic and pneumatic methods of intussusception reduction comparable? *Pediatr. Radiol.* 22, 346–349.
6. Swischuk, L.E., Hayden, C.K. & Boulden, T. (1985) Intussusception: indications for ultrasonography and an explanation of the doughnut and pseudokidney signs. *Pediatr. Radiol.* 55, 388–391.

Further reading

Katz, M.E. & Kolm, P. (1992) Intussusception reduction 1991: an international survey of pediatric radiologists. *Pediatr. Radiol.* 22, 318–322.

Meyer, J.S. (1992) The current radiological management of intussusception: a survey and review. *Pediatr. Radiol.* 22, 323–325.

Swischuk, L.E. (1992) The current radiological management of intussusception: a survey and review. *Pediatr. Radiol.* 22, 317.

Therapeutic Water-soluble Contrast Enema in Meconium Ileus

Prior to this procedure a diagnostic barium enema is performed to exclude other forms of distal intestinal obstruction, e.g. Hirschsprung's disease.

Contraindications
1. Perforation.
2. Volvulus.

Patient preparation
1. The baby must be well hydrated prior to the procedure, as there may be considerable fluid loss into the bowel, and an i.v. saline drip is mandatory.
2. Antibiotic cover.

Technique
The aim is to run a hypertonic water-soluble contrast medium (usually Gastrografin, but any hypertonic contrast medium is acceptable) through the colon and into the small bowel to surround the meconium. The hypertonic contrast medium then draws water into the bowel and so helps to dislodge the sticky meconium. If successful, meconium should be passed in the next hour. If no result is seen after 1 hour, the procedure is deemed to have failed and surgical intervention will be necessary because prolonged contact of a hyperosmolar solution with the bowel mucosa can cause necrosis. If the passage of meconium is incomplete and the clinical condition remains stable, a second enema may be performed.

Further reading
Noblett, H. (1979) Meconium ileus. In: Ravitch, M.M., Welch, K.J., Benson, C.D., Aberdeen E. & Randolph J.G. (eds) *Paediatric Surgery*, 3rd edn, Vol. 2, pp. 947–949. Chicago: Year Book Medical Publishers.

Sinogram

A water-soluble contrast medium (e.g. Hypaque 45) must be used, unless there is any suspicion of a connection with the pleural cavity, in which case Dionosil aqueous is a safe alternative. A preliminary film is taken to exclude the presence of a radio-opaque foreign body. A fine catheter is then inserted into the orifice of the sinus, next to which a metal marker has been placed. After a gauze pad has been firmly placed over the orifice to discourage reflux, the contrast medium is injected under fluoroscopic control. Spot films are taken as required.

Loopogram

The investigation of the bowel proximal to a colostomy is performed by inserting the tip of a Foley catheter a few centimetres into the appropriate stoma. The balloon may be inflated carefully within the lumen of the bowel proximal to the stoma to provide a seal. The barium is run into the bowel and spot films are taken as required.

The bowel distal to a colostomy may be investigated by barium run in through the rectum in the usual manner, as this is easier and safer.

If there is any suspicion of an anastomotic breakdown, a water-soluble contrast medium must be used.

Ultrasound of the Gastrointestinal Tract

ENDOLUMINAL EXAMINATION OF THE OESOPHAGUS AND STOMACH

Indications
1. Staging of primary malignant disease.
2. Ultrasound-guided biopsy of primary tumours or suspected nodal disease.

Equipment
Echoendoscope with 7.5–10 MHz 360° rotary transducer.

Patient preparation
Slight sedation may be required.

Technique
Monitoring with a pulse oximeter is recommended. If the stomach is to be examined, this is filled with de-aerated water through the working channel before the patient is examined in a left lateral decubitus position. The ultrasound transducer is passed during endoscopy, either combined with direct vision or blind by an experienced endoscopist. A 360° rotary transducer will provide transverse scans with respect to the long axis of the tube.

Aftercare
The patient should be observed by experienced nursing staff until the effects of any sedation have worn off.

Further reading
Botet, J.F. & Lightdale, C. (1991) Endoscopic sonography of the upper gastrointestinal tract. *Am. J. Roentg.* **156**, 63–68.

Botet, J.F. & Lightdale, C. (1992) Endoscopic ultrasonography of the upper gastrointestinal tract. *Radiol. Clin. N. Am.* **30**, 1067–1083.

Shorvon, P.J. (1990) Endoscopic ultrasound in oesophageal cancer: the way forward? *Clin. Radiol.* **42**, 149–151.

TRANSABDOMINAL EXAMINATION OF THE LOWER OESOPHAGUS AND STOMACH

Indications
1. Oesophageal and fundal varices.
2. Gastro-oesophageal reflux.

3. Staging of malignant disease from adjacent organs (endoluminal ultrasound is more accurate).

Equipment 3.5–5 MHz transducer.

Patient preparation None.

Technique
1. A transcutaneous epigastric approach is used, scanning either transversely or longitudinally. The oesophagus can be identified posterior to the liver as it passes through the diaphragmatic hiatus. It can be readily recognized by the presence of high reflectivity air within its lumen.
2. Oesophageal varices are seen as hypo-echoic channels within a thickened oesophageal wall and can be interrogated by colour and duplex Doppler.
3. The normal gastric wall has five recognizable sonographic layers and should not measure more than 6–7 mm.

HYPERTROPHIC PYLORIC STENOSIS

The typical patient is a 6-week-old male infant with non-bilious projectile vomiting.

Equipment 5–7.5 MHz linear or sector transducer.

Technique
1. The right upper quadrant is scanned with the patient supine. If the stomach is very distended, the pylorus will be displaced posteriorly and the stomach should be decompressed with a naso-gastric tube. If the stomach is collapsed, the introduction of some dextrose, by mouth or via a nasogastric tube, will distend the antrum and differentiate it from the pylorus.
2. The pylorus is scanned in its longitudinal and transverse planes and images will resemble an olive and a doughnut, respectively. The poorly echogenic muscle is easily differentiated from the bright mucosa. Antral peristalsis can be seen and the volume of fluid passing through the pylorus with each antral wave can be assessed.
3. A number of measurements can be made. These include muscle thickness, canal length, pyloric

volume and muscle thickness/wall diameter ratio, but there is no universal agreement as to which is the most discriminating parameter.

Further reading
Blumhagen, J.D., Maclin, L., Krauter, D., et al (1988) Sonographic diagnosis of hypertrophic pyloric stenosis. *Am. J. Roentg.* **150**, 1367–1370.
Stunden, R.J., LeQuesne, G.W. & Little, K.E.T. (1986) The improved ultrasound diagnosis of hypertrophic pyloric stenosis. *Pediatr. Radiol.* **16**, 200–205.

SMALL BOWEL

Indications
1. It is infrequent that ultrasound is used as a primary investigation for patients with suspected small-bowel disease, but the small bowel can be included in an examination of the abdomen, especially if the patient has inflammatory bowel disease or suspected small-bowel obstruction.
2. Midgut malrotation[1].

Technique
1. Dilated small-bowel loops and bowel wall thickening may be readily recognized. Doppler examination of the mesenteric vessels may be included to assess activity of inflammatory bowel disease.
2. Malrotation of the small bowel may be diagnosed by alteration of the normal relationship between the superior mesenteric artery and vein.

Reference
1. Gaines, P.A., Saunders, A.J.S. & Drake, D. (1987) Midgut malrotation diagnosed by ultrasound. *Clin. Radiol.* **38**, 51–53.

APPENDIX

Indications Diagnosis of appendicitis and its complications.

Equipment 5–7.5 MHz linear array transducer.

Patient preparation None.

Technique The ultrasound transducer is used to apply graded compression to the right lower quadrant of the abdomen. This displaces bowel loops and compresses the caecum. The normal appendix should be compressible and have a maximum diameter of 6 mm. It should also peristalse.

Further reading

Brown, G.J. (1991) Acute appendicitis – the radiologist's role. *Radiology* **180**, 13–14.

Puylaert, J.B.C.M. (1986) Acute appendicitis – ultrasound evaluation using graded compression. *Radiology* **158**, 355–360.

LARGE BOWEL

Indications

At present, colonoscopy or barium examinations are first line imaging investigations but large-bowel masses can be visualized by ultrasound during a routine abdominal scan. The large bowel can also be examined following installation of normal saline into the large bowel[1].

Reference

1. Limberg, B. (1990) Clinical practice. *Lancet* **335**, 144–146.

RECTUM AND ANUS

Indications

1. Staging of primary rectal carcinoma or suspected local recurrence.
2. Incontinence and suspected anal sphincter defects.
3. Intersphincteric fistula.

Patient preparation

Simple bowel preparation using a small self-administered disposable enema.

Equipment

5–7 MHz radially scanning transducer. A linear transducer can be used but is less satisfactory.

Technique

1. The patient is placed in the left lateral position.
2. A careful digital rectal examination is carried out.
3. The probe is covered with a latex sheath containing contact jelly, and all air bubbles are expelled.
4. More jelly is placed over the latex sheath and the probe is introduced into the rectum.

Aftercare   None.

Further reading   Beynon, J., Feifel, G., Hildebrandt, U. & Mortensen, N.J.Mc.C. (1991) *An Atlas of Rectal Endosonography.* Berlin: Springer-Verlag.

Radionuclide Gastro-oesophageal Reflux Study

Indications
1. Diagnosis and quantification of suspected gastro-oesophageal reflux.
2. Monitoring of the response to treatment for reflux.

Contraindications None.

Radiopharmaceuticals *99mTc-colloid or 99mTc-DTPA* mixed with:
1. *Adults and older children:* 150–300 ml orange juice acidified with an equal volume of 0.1 M hydrochloric acid.
2. *Infants and young children:* normal milk feed.

Typical adult dose is 10–20 MBq, max. 40 MBq.

Equipment
1. Gamma camera.
2. Low-energy general purpose collimator.
3. Imaging computer.
4. Abdominal binder for compression test.

Patient preparation Nil by mouth for 4–6 hours. Infants may be studied at normal feed times.

Technique *Physiological test[1,2] – adults and older children:*
1. The liquid containing the tracer is given and washed down with unlabelled liquid to clear residual activity from the oesophagus.
2. The patient lies semi-recumbent with the camera centred over the stomach and lower oesophagus.
3. Dynamic imaging is commenced with film and computer acquisition of 10–20 s frames for 30–60 min on a 64 × 64 matrix.

Milk scan[1,2] – infants and younger children:
1. The milk feed is divided into two parts and one mixed with the tracer.
2. The radiolabelled milk is given and washed down with the remaining unlabelled milk.
3. After eructation, the child is placed either supine or prone, according to natural behaviour, with the camera anterior over stomach and oesophagus.

4. Imaging as above.
5. If pulmonary aspiration of feed is suspected, later imaging at 4 hours may be performed. The test is specific but not very sensitive for this purpose.

Provocation with abdominal compression[1,3] — *adults and older children:*
1. The abdominal binder is placed around the upper abdomen.
2. The radiolabelled liquid is given as above.
3. The patient lies supine with the camera centred over the stomach and lower oesophagus.
4. A 30-s image is taken.
5. The pressure in the binder is increased in steps of 20 mmHg up to 100 mmHg, being maintained at each step for 30 s while an image is taken.
6. The test is terminated as soon as significant reflux is seen.

Analysis
1. For dynamic studies, regions are drawn round the stomach and lower, middle and upper oesophagus.
2. Time–activity curves of these regions are produced, from which may be calculated the size, extent, frequency and duration of any reflux episodes.

Additional techniques

Oesophageal transit[1]:
The reflux study may be combined with a bolus transport investigation by fast-frame (0.2–0.5 s) dynamic imaging during swallowing and generation of a functional compressed image incorporating information from each frame[4].

Aftercare None.

Complications None.

References
1. (1990) The Oesophagus. In: Harding, L.K. & Robinson, P.J.A. *Clinician's Guide to Nuclear Medicine: Gastroenterology*, pp. 6–21. London: Churchill Livingstone.
2. Guillet, J., Basse-Cathalinat, B., Christophe, E., Ducassou, D., Blanquet, P. & Wynchank, S. (1984) Routine studies of swallowed radionuclide transit in paediatrics: experience with 400 patients. *Eur. J. Nucl. Med.* 9, 86–90.

3. Martins, J.C.R., Isaacs, P.E.T., Sladen, G.E., Maisey, M.N. & Edwards, S. (1984) Gastro-oesophageal reflux scintigraphy compared with pH probe monitoring. *Nucl. Med. Commun.* 5, 201–204.
4. Klein, H.A. & Wald, A. (1984) Computer analysis of radionuclide esophageal transit studies. *J. Nucl. Med.* 25, 957–964.

Further reading Kjellen, G., Brudin, L. & Hakansson, H.O. (1991) Is scintigraphy of value in the diagnosis of gastro-oesophageal reflux disease? *Scand. J. Gastroenterol.* 26, 425–430.

Radionuclide Gastric Emptying Study

Indications

1. Investigation of gastric stasis and dumping syndrome, particularly after peptic ulcer surgery.
2. Diabetic gastropathy.
3. After gastric partitioning for morbid obesity.
4. Investigation of the effects of gastric motility altering drugs.

Contraindications

High probability of vomiting.

Radiopharmaceuticals

Many radiolabelled meals have been designed for gastric emptying studies, but as yet no standard has emerged. Emptying rate measured by radiolabelling is influenced by many variables, for example meal bulk, fat content, calorie content, patient position during imaging and labelling stability in vivo. For this reason, so-called 'normal' emptying times need to be taken in the context of the particular meal and protocol used to generate them. It is important that the meal used is realistic and reproducible. For centres new to the technique, it is better if possible to use a meal for which published data exists than to create yet another formulation with inherently uncertain behaviour.

Both liquid and solid studies may be performed, separately or simultaneously. Liquid emptying times are generally shorter than those for solids. Prolonged solid emptying is highly correlated with prolonged liquid emptying, and there is debate therefore as to whether both studies are necessary[1]. Examples of meals used are:

1. *Liquid meal.* Max. 12 MBq ^{99m}Tc-tin colloid mixed with 200 ml orange juice, or with milk or formula feed for infants.
2. *Solid meal.* Scrambled egg prepared with max. 12 MBq ^{99m}Tc-sulphur colloid[2] or ^{99m}Tc-DTPA[3]. Bulk is made up with other non-labelled foods such as bread and milk. Sulphur colloid is currently unavailable in the UK unless made in-house, but tin colloid should behave similarly.
3. *Dual isotope combined liquid and solid meal*[4].
   (a) *Liquid:* 12 MBq ^{99m}Tc-antimony sulphide colloid mixed with 195 ml orange juice.

Antimony sulphide colloid is currently unavailable in the UK, but tin colloid could be substituted.

(b) *Solid:* 2 MBq [111]indium-labelled resin beads incorporated into a pancake containing 27 g fat, 18 g protein, 625 calories. Bulk is made up with other non-labelled foods. Only 2 MBq of ^{111}In is suggested (ARSAC max. is 12 MBq) in order to minimize the downscatter into the ^{99m}Tc energy window[5].

[113m]In (12 MBq max.) has also been used as a meal label. It is a high-energy γ-emitter (390 keV compared with 171 and 245 keV for ^{111}In) which reduces the attenuation error in anterior imaging (see technique below). It has a shorter $T_{1/2}$ than [111]In (100 min as compared with 2.8 days) and therefore delivers a smaller radiation dose to the colon. [113m]In generators are expensive and currently unavailable.

Equipment
1. Gamma camera.
2. Low-energy general purpose collimator for ^{99m}Tc, medium energy for ^{111}In, high-energy for [113m]In.
3. Imaging computer.

Patient preparation
1. Nil by mouth for 8 hours.
2. No smoking or alcohol from midnight before test.
3. Stop medications such as dopaminergic agonists (e.g. metoclopramide, domperidone), cholinergic agonists (e.g. bethanechol), tricyclic antidepressants and anticholinesterases for 24 hours prior to the study.

Technique
Imaging from a single direction can cause significant errors due to movement of the meal anteriorly as it transfers to the antrum, thereby altering the amount of tissue attenuation of γ-photons. The problem is likely to be exacerbated in obese patients. This can largely be overcome by taking consecutive pairs of opposing views and calculating the geometric mean stomach activity in each pain.
1. The patient eats or drinks the meal as quickly as they comfortably can.
2. The patient is positioned standing in front of the camera.

3. Every 5 min, a pair of 1-min anterior and posterior images are obtained. Care should be taken to accurately reposition the patient for successive images.
4. The patient sits between images.
5. A liquid study should be continued for up to 60 min and a solid study for up to 90 min. If it can be seen that the majority of the meal has emptied inside this time, the study may be terminated.

If this protocol is impractical and an error of up to 20% can be tolerated in the calculated half-emptying time, then a single dynamic study in the anterior position may be performed with the patient sitting or semi-recumbent, or, for an infant, lying prone directly on the surface of a horizontal gamma camera.

Images
1. *Hard copy:* anterior images at 5-min intervals for liquid and 10-min intervals for solid study.
2. *Computer:*
   (a) *anterior only:* dynamic acquisition with 1-min frame time, 64 × 64 matrix size
   (b) *anterior and posterior imaging:* 1-min static images, 128 × 128 matrix size to aid image alignment.

Analysis
1. Stomach region of interest is drawn, aligning frames where necessary.
2. Stomach time-activity curve is produced, using geometric mean if anterior and posterior imaging performed.
3. Half-emptying time is calculated, either from direct observation or by curve-fitting. Liquid emptying normally follows an exponential pattern, whereas solid emptying is normally linear.

Additional techniques
The small bowel transit time can be ascertained by continuing imaging at intervals until the caecum is seen. Since the position of the caecum is often not obvious and may be overlain by small bowel, a 12–24 hour image can be useful to determine the position of the large bowel. This is convenient to perform if a two-stage solid and liquid test is being undertaken on consecutive days. Anatomical mark-

ing of the anterior superior iliac spine may help to locate the caecum.

Aftercare None.

Complications None.

References

1. Siegel, J.A., Krevsky, B., Maurer, A.H., Charkes, N.D., Fisher, R.S. & Malmud, L.S. (1989) Scintigraphic evaluation of gastric emptying: are radiolabeled solids necessary? *Clin. Nucl. Med.* **14**, 40–46.
2. Malmud, L.S., Fisher, R.S., Knight, L.C. & Rock, E. (1982) Scintigraphic evaluation of gastric emptying. *Semin. Nucl. Med.* **12**, 116–125.
3. Jonderko, K. (1987) Radionuclide studies on gastric evacuatory function in health and in the duodenal ulcer disease. I. Types of solid meal distribution within the stomach and their relation to gastric emptying. *Nucl. Med. Commun.* **8**, 671–680.
4. Mather, S.J., Ellison, D., Nightingale, J., Kamm, M. & Britton, K.E. (1991) The design of a two-phase radio-labelled meal for gastric emptying studies. *Nucl. Med. Commun.* **12**, 409–416.
5. Heyman, S. (1988) Gastric emptying, gastroesophageal reflux, and esophageal motility. In: Gelfand, M.J. & Thomas, S.R. (eds) *Effective Use of Computers in Nuclear Medicine*, pp. 412–437. New York: McGraw-Hill.

Further reading

Malmud, L.S. (1990) Gastric emptying. *J. Nucl. Med.* **31**, 1499–1500.

Radionuclide Bile Reflux Study

Indications[1]
1. Persistent symptoms after peptic ulcer surgery or gastrectomy.
2. After gastrectomy.
3. Persistent flatulent dyspepsia after cholecystectomy after other causes have been ruled out.

Contraindications　None.

Radiopharmaceuticals　^{99m}Tc-diethyl iminodiacetic acid (HIDA) or other iminodiacetic acid (IDA) derivative, 75 MBq typical, 150 MBq max.

IDA compounds are rapidly cleared from the circulation by the hepatocytes and secreted into bile in a similar way to bilirubin.

Equipment
1. Gamma camera.
2. Low-energy general purpose collimator.

Patient preparation　Nil by mouth for 6 hours.

Technique　A typical imaging protocol for assessment of bile reflux is described:
1. ^{99m}Tc-HIDA is administered i.v.
2. 20–30 min post-injection, the patient lies supine with the camera anterior. Marker sources may be placed on the iliac crests to monitor patient movement.
3. Imaging is commenced at 2 min per frame for 60–70 min.
4. 30–45 min post-injection when the gallbladder is well visualized, either 70 units of cholecystokinin (CCK) is administered i.v. over 2 min, or a liquid fatty meal is given through a straw to stimulate gallbladder contraction. CCK is more effective at provoking reflux.
5. 80 min post-injection, 200 ml of water is given through a straw to diffuse any activity in the stomach and thereby differentiate it from nearby bowel activity.
6. 4 min before the end of imaging, 100 ml of water containing approx. 5 MBq ^{99m}Tc in non-

absorbable form (e.g. colloid, DTPA, HIDA) is given to outline the stomach.

Additional techniques

1. A standard series of manoeuvres such as Valsalva (forced exhalation against a closed glottis) and coughing may be performed to provoke further reflux into the oesophagus[2].
2. Functional evaluation of the complete oesophagogastroduodenal tract may be performed with a combined ^{99m}Tc-HIDA and radiolabelled swallow study[3].
3. Computer acquisition with region of interest analysis has been used to attempt to quantify reflux[3].

Aftercare   None.

Complications   Possibility of severe colic or hypotension following CCK injection.

References

1. (1990) Hepatobiliary studies: bile reflux, jaundice and acute cholecystitis. In: Harding, L.K. & Robinson, P.J.A. *Clinician's Guide to Nuclear Medicine: Gastroenterology*, pp. 31–48. London: Churchill Livingstone.
2. Bortolotti, M., Abbati, A., Turba, E., Pozzato, R., Bersani, G. & Labò, G. (1985) ^{99m}Tc-HIDA dynamic scintigraphy for the diagnosis of gastroesophageal reflux of bile. *Eur. J. Nucl. Med.* **10**, 549–550.
3. Borsato, N., Bonavina, L., Zanco, P. et al (1991) Proposal of a modified scintigraphic method to evaluate duodenogastroesophageal reflux. *J. Nucl. Med.* **32**, 436–440.

Further reading

Drane, W.E., Karvelis, K., Johnson, D.A. & Silverman, E.D. (1987) Scintigraphic evaluation of duodenogastric reflux: Problems, pitfalls, and technical review. *Clin. Nucl. Med.* **12**, 377–384.

Radionuclide Meckel's Diverticulum Scan

Indications Detection of a Meckel's diverticulum as a cause for gastrointestinal bleeding, obstruction or abdominal pain.

Contraindications Precautions and contraindications to any pre-administered drugs should be observed.

Radiopharmaceuticals ^{99m}Tc-*pertechnetate*, 200 MBq typical, 400 MBq max.

Injected ^{99m}Tc-pertechnetate localizes in ectopic gastric mucosa within a diverticulum.

Equipment
1. Gamma camera.
2. Low-energy general purpose collimator.

Patient preparation
1. Nil by mouth for 6 hours, unless emergency.
2. It may be possible to enhance detection by prior administration of drugs aimed at increasing the uptake of ^{99m}Tc-pertechnetate into gastric mucosa and inhibiting its release into the lumen of the stomach and progression into the bowel. The following regimes have been suggested[1]:
   (a) pentagastrin (subcutaneous 6 μg kg^{-1} 15 min before imaging)
   (b) pentagastrin as above in combination with glucagon (0.25–2 mg i.v.)
   (c) pentagastrin as above with nasogastric suction[2]
   (d) cimetidine (300 mg orally 4 times daily for 48 hr before test, or 300 mg in 100 ml 5% glucose infused i.v. over 20 min, 1 hour before imaging)
   (e) ranitidine (1 mg kg^{-1}, up to a maximum of 50 mg, in sodium chloride 0.9%, infused i.v. over 20 min, 1 hour before imaging).

Technique
1. The bladder is emptied — a full bladder may obscure the diverticulum.
2. The patient lies supine and pertechnetate is administered i.v.
3. Images are obtained with the camera over the

abdomen and pelvis. The stomach must be included in the field of view because diagnosis is dependent on demonstrating excretion of radionuclide in the diverticulum concurrent with excretion by gastric mucosa.

Images Every 5 min up to 50 min:
1. Anterior.
2. Posterior and lateral as required.

The bladder should be emptied before the last image. A final right lateral view may be taken to separate activity in the urinary tract from that in a diverticulum.

Aftercare None.

Complications Pre-administered drug sensitivity and side-effects.

References
1. Datz, F.L., Christian, P.E., Hutson, W.R., Moore, J.G. & Morton, K.A. (1991) Physiological and pharmacological interventions in radionuclide imaging of tubular gastrointestinal tract. *Semin. Nucl. Med.* **21**, 140–152.
2. Feggi, L.M. & Bighi, S.F. (1979) Technical notes for scintigraphy of Meckel's diverticulum. *J. Nucl. Med.* **20**, 888–889.

Further reading Harding, L.K. (1989) Gastrointestinal tract. In: Sharp, P.F., Gemmell, H.G. & Smith, F.W. (eds) *Practical Nuclear Medicine*, pp. 193–209. Oxford: Oxford University Press.

Radionuclide Imaging of Gastrointestinal Bleeding

Indications Gastrointestinal bleeding of unknown origin.

Contraindications
1. No active bleeding at time scheduled for study.
2. Slow bleeding of less than approx. 0.5 ml min^{-1}.
3. Recent barium study (barium causes significant attenuation of γ-photons and may mask a bleeding site).

Radiopharmaceuticals
1. *^{99m}Tc-in-vivo-labelled red blood cells*, 400 MBq max.
   Before radiolabelling with ^{99m}Tc-pertechnetate, the red blood cells are 'primed' with an injection of stannous pyrophosphate. The stannous ions reduce the pertechnetate and allow it to bind to the pyrophosphate which adsorbs on to the red blood cells.
2. *^{99m}Tc-colloid*, 400 MBq max.
   This has been a commonly used alternative to labelled red cells (for a protocol see reference 1), but a number of studies have shown it to be a less sensitive tracer for detecting bleeding sites[2, 3].

Equipment
1. Gamma camera.
2. Low-energy general purpose collimator.
3. Imaging computer.

Patient preparation
1. 'Cold' stannous pyrophosphate (20 μg kg^{-1}) is administered directly into a vein 20–30 min before the ^{99m}Tc-pertechnetate injection. (Injection via a plastic cannula will result in a poor label.)
2. The patient is asked to empty their bladder before each image is taken. Catheterization is ideal if appropriate.

Technique
1. The patient lies supine.
2. The camera is positioned over the anterior abdomen with the symphysis pubis at the bottom of the field of view.
3. ^{99m}Tc-pertechnetate is injected i.v.
4. A 128 × 128 dynamic acquisition on computer is begun immediately with 2-s images for 1 min to

help to localize major blood vessels and kidneys, followed by 1-min images up to 30 mins.

5. Static images are acquired for 1000 kilocounts at 1, 2, 4, 6 and 24 hours or until bleeding site is detected.

6. Oblique and lateral views may help to localize any abnormal collections of activity.

Additional techniques

One problem with ^{99m}Tc-in-vivo-labelled red blood cells is the possibility of false-positive scans caused by accumulation of free ^{99m}Tc-pertechnetate. The best label is produced by an in vitro method, although this is time-consuming. A compromise between these methods can be used where labelling occurs in the syringe as blood is withdrawn from the patient[2,4].

Aftercare None.

Complications None.

References

1. (1990) Hepatobiliary studies: localisation of gastrointestinal bleeding. In: Harding, L.K. & Robinson, P.J.A. *Clinician's Guide to Nuclear Medicine: Gastroenterology*, pp. 116–128. London: Churchill Livingstone.

2. Chaudhuri, T.K. (1991) Radionuclide methods of detecting acute gastrointestinal bleeding. *Nucl. Med. Biol. Int. J. Radiat. Appl. Instrum. Part B* 18, 655–661.

3. Bunker, S.R., Lull, R.J., Tanasescu, D.E. et al (1984) Scintigraphy of gastrointestinal hemorrhage: superiority of ^{99m}Tc red blood cells over ^{99m}Tc sulfur colloid. *Am. J. Roentg.* 143, 543–548.

4. Callahan, R.J., Froelich, J.W., McKusick, K.A., Leppo, J. & Strauss, H.W. (1982) A modified method for the in vivo labeling of red blood cells with Tc-99m: concise communication. *J. Nucl. Med.* 23, 315–318.

Further reading

Bearn, P., Persad, R., Wilson, N., Flanagan, J. & Williams, T. (1992) [99m]Technetium-labelled red blood cell scintigraphy as an alternative to angiography in the investigation of gastrointestinal bleeding: clinical experience in a district general hospital. *Ann. R. Coll. Surg. Engl.* 74, 192–199.

Nicholson, M.L., Neoptolemos, J.P., Sharp, J.F., Watkin, E.M. & Fossard, D.P. (1989) Localization of lower gastrointestinal bleeding using in vivo technetium-99m-labelled red blood cell scintigraphy. *Br. J. Surg.* 76, 358–361.

4 Liver, Biliary Tract and Pancreas

Methods of imaging the hepatobiliary system

1. Plain film.
2. Oral cholecystography.
3. Intravenous cholangiography.
4. Operative cholangiography.
5. Post-operative (T-tube) cholangiography.
6. Endoscopic retrograde cholangiopancreatography (ERCP).
7. Percutaneous transhepatic cholangiography (PTC).
8. Ultrasound.
9. Radionuclide imaging.
   −static, with colloid.
   −dynamic, with iminodiacetic acid derivatives
10. CT.
11. MRI.

Further reading

Bernardino, M.E. (ed.) (1991) Imaging of the liver and biliary tree. *Radiol. Clin. N. Am.* **29**(6).

Burhenne, H.J. (ed.) (1990) Interventional radiology of the biliary tract. *Radiol. Clin. N. Am.* **28**(6).

Ferrucci, J.T. & Stark, D.D. (eds) (1990) *Liver Imaging, Current Trends and New Techniques.* Boston: Andover Medical Publishers Inc.

Kressel, H.Y. (1988) Strategies for magnetic resonance imaging of focal liver disease. *Radiol. Clin. N. Am.* **26**, 607–615.

Wilkins, R.A. & Nunnerley, H.B. (eds) (1990) *Imaging of the Liver, Pancreas and Spleen.* Oxford: Blackwell Scientific Publications.

Methods of imaging the pancreas

1. Chest radiography.
2. Plain abdominal films.
3. Hypotonic duodenography.
4. ERCP.
5. PTC.
6. Arteriography
   − coeliac axis
   − superior mesenteric artery.
7. Venography
   − precutaneous transhepatic method
   − umbilical vein catheterization.
8. Ultrasound
   − transcutaneous
   − intraoperative
   − endoscopic.
9. CT.
10. MRI.

Further reading

Dubbins, P.A. (1990) Pancreatic imaging − general considerations. In: Wilkins, R.A. & Nunnerley, H.B., (eds) *Imaging of the Liver, Pancreas and Spleen*, pp. 367–403. Oxford: Blackwell Scientific Publications.

Freeny, P.C. (ed.) (1989) Radiology of the pancreas. *Radiol. Clin. N. Am.* **27**(1).

Biliary Contrast Media

Like conventional urographic contrast media, biliary contrast media are also tri-iodo benzoic acid derivatives. Iopanoic acid (Telepaque) was introduced in 1951 and the newer compounds are all modifications of it. Differences occur in the prosthetic group (position 1) and the amino group (position 3).

Iopanoic acid
(Telepaque)

Iocetamic acid
(Cholebrin)

The oral agents have a single benzene ring, whilst the i.v. contrast media, e.g. meglumine ioglycamate (Biligram) are dimers which differ only in the length and composition of the polymethylene chain that connects the two rings. The newer i.v. agent, iotroxate (Biliscopin) has a longer linking chain and is less strongly protein bound.

Meglumine ioglycamide (Biligram)

It is the absence of a prosthetic group at position 5 in both the oral and i.v. agents that determines biliary rather than renal excretion.

Metalbolic pathway

1. Absorption of oral contrast media from the gut requires that they have both hydrophilic and lipophilic properties.
2. Passive diffusion occurs across the lipid membrane of the gastrointestinal mucosa. (Intravenous agents, although very water-soluble, are insoluble in lipids and are, therefore, not absorbed when given orally.)
3. After absorption they are bound to albumen and carried in the portal vein to the liver. Intravenous biliary contrast media are also albumen-bound. Toxicity is proportional to albumen binding.
4. In the liver they are taken up by the hepatocyte, possibly via the Y and Z receptors.
5. Intravenous contrast media are not altered in the hepatocyte and are excreted into the bile unchanged. Oral agents are conjugated with glucuronic acid to form more water-soluble conjugates.
6. Excretion into bile is an active transport process which can become saturated and is the rate-limiting step.
7. Oral agents are concentrated in the gallbladder by the absorption of water.
8. Oral agents are finally excreted in the stool. Reabsorption is severely limited because after conjugation they are no longer lipophilic. Intravenous agents, being water-soluble, are excreted by glomerular filtration when the infusion rate is high and biliary excretion is saturated.

Further reading

Gibson, R.N. & Dunn, G.D. (1988) Contrast media in the biliary system and pancreas. In: Carr, D.H. (ed.) *Contrast Media*, pp. 147–159. Edinburgh: Churchill Livingstone.

Loeb, P.M. & Berk, R.N. (1977) Biliary contrast materials. In: Berk, R.N. & Clement, A.R. (eds) *Radiology of the Gallbladder and Bile Ducts*, pp. 71–100. Philadelphia: W.B. Saunders.

Oral Cholecystography

Indications To demonstrate suspected pathology in the gall-bladder.

The cystic duct and common bile duct may also be seen. The examination is unlikely to be successful when the serum bilirubin is greater than 34 μmol litre^{-1}.

Contraindications 1. Severe hepatorenal disease.
2. Acute cholecystitis.
3. Dehydration.
4. An i.v. cholangiogram within the previous week.
5. Previous cholecystectomy.

Contrast medium Any oral cholecystographic agent (see Table 4.1).

Table 4.1 Oral cholecystographic contrast media.

Proprietary name	Chemical name and presentation	Dose	
Telepaque	iopanoic acid, 500 mg tablets	*adult:*	6 tablets
Cholebrin	iocetamic acid, 500 mg tablets	*adult:*	6 tablets
Biloptin	sodium ipodate, 500 mg capsules	*adult:*	6 capsules
		child:	not recommended
Solu-Biloptin	calcium ipodate, 3 g sachets	*adult:*	1 sachet
		child:	under 20 kg − 0.3 g kg^{-1}
			over 20 kg − 0.15 g kg^{-1}

Patient preparation 1. A laxative 2 days prior to the examination.
2. A fat-containing evening meal on the evening prior to the examination. This empties the gall-bladder and allows better subsequent filling. (Fat is also necessary for the absorption of Telepaque.) The cholecystographic agent is taken with water 14 hours prior to the patient's appointment. Food is forbidden until the examination is completed, but water is encouraged.

Preliminary film   Prone 20° LAO, centred 7.5 cm to the right of the spinous processes, 2.5 cm cephalad to the lower costal margin.

This film is taken when the patient makes his appointment. There is controversy regarding the usefulness of this film. Some believe that 5% of calculi will be missed if it is omitted[1], while others believe that virtually all radio-opaque gallstones are seen within the opacified gallbladder[2]. Other pathology, outside the gallbladder, may be found in 5% of patients[3].

Films

1. Prone 20° LAO — contrast medium fills the fundus of the gallbladder.
2. Supine 20° RPO — contrast medium fills the neck and Hartmann's pouch.
3. Erect 20° LAO — may demonstrate floating gallstones.
(4. Overlying bowel shadows may be removed by rotating the patient under fluoroscopic control or by tomography.)
5. Prone 20° LAO, 30 min after a fatty meal (chocolate or a proprietary fat emulsion). The value of this film has been assessed by Harvey et al[4], who found it was:
   (a) essential for the diagnosis of adenomyomatosis[5] and cholesterolosis
   (b) occasionally helpful in diagnosing small stones
   (c) of little value in assessing the biliary ducts or separating the gallbladder from overlying bowel gas
   (d) of no value in the diagnosis of functional biliary tract disorders.

ADDITIONAL FILMS
Tomography after a fatty meal[6]

If the gallbladder is not seen on the first film, the patient is asked the following questions:
1. What time were the tablets taken? (Sufficient time is needed for absorption and concentration in the gallbladder.)
2. How many tablets were taken?

3. Did diarrhoea or vomiting develop after the tablets were taken?

If the tablets have been taken, a 35 × 43 cm supine abdominal film is taken. This may demonstrate:
(a) a gallbladder in an abnormal position, or
(b) unabsorbed contrast medium. This has a flakey appearance and can be distinguished from esterified contrast medium that has passed through the liver and biliary tract, which causes a more uniform, fainter opacification.

If the gallbladder is only poorly seen, the patient is given a further standard dose to be taken that evening and repeat films are taken the following day.

Additional techniques
1. For better visualization of the ducts, manufacturers make the following recommendations:
   (a) Telepaque — 3–6 tablets are taken 4 hours after a fatty lunch on the day preceding the examination, and then a full dose of 6 tablets after a fat-free meal in the evening.
   (b) Biloptin — (i) 12 capsules at the usual time *or* (ii) 6 capsules 10–12 hours before the examination plus another 6 capsules 3 hours before.
   (c) Solu-Biloptin — (i) 2 sachets at the usual time *or* (ii) 1 sachet 10–12 hours before the examination and another 1 sachet 3 hours before.
   (d) Cholebrin — 6 tablets 12–14 hours before the examination plus another 6 tablets 3 hours before.
2. Some radiolucent calculi may only be demonstrated radiographically by prolonged contact with contrast medium — 'the 4-day Telepaque test'. The patient takes 2 Telepaque tablets after each of the three main meals, daily for 4 days. During this time the meals should be relatively fat-free. The examination is performed on the morning of the fifth day, with the patient fasting[7].

Aftercare   None.

Complications

Due to the contrast medium[8]

1. Mild gastrointestinal disturbances — nausea, with or without vomiting, diarrhoea — in 50%. The incidence of diarrhoea is greatest with iopanoic acid.
2. Headache.
3. Skin reactions — urticaria, vasodilatation and pruritus.
4. Uricosuric action.
5. Impaired renal function — more likely if there is coexistent liver impairment, dehydration or repeat, double or multiple doses of contrast medium.
6. Pseudoalbuminuria.
7. Abnormal thyroid function tests.
8. Increased effect of protein-bound drugs because of shared binding with albumen.

References

1. Twomey, B., de Lacey, G. & Gajjar, B. (1983) The plain radiograph in oral cholecystography — should it be abandoned? *Br. J. Radiol.* **56**, 99–100.
2. Anderson, J.F. & Madsen, P.E. (1979) The value of plain radiographs prior to oral cholecystography. *Radiology* **133**, 309–310.
3. Karned, R.K. & LeVeen, R.F. (1978) Preliminary abdominal films in oral cholecystography: are they necessary? *Am. J. Roentg.* **130**, 477–479.
4. Harvey, I.C., Thwe, M. & Low-Beer, T.S. (1976) The value of the fatty meal in oral cholecystography. *Clin. Radiol.* **27**, 117–121.
5. Gajjar, B., Twomey, B. & de Lacey, G. (1976) The fatty meal and acalculous gallbladder disease. *Clin. Radiol.* **35**, 405–408.
6. Pilbrow, W.J. (1980) Tomography of the biliary tract during oral cholecystography: a review of 200 cases. *Clin. Radiol.* **31**, 189–193.
7. Salzman, E. (1976) The 4-day cholecystographic test. In: Felson, B. (ed.) *Roentgenology of the Gall Bladder and Biliary Tract*, pp. 29–31. New York: Grune & Stratton.
8. Ansell, G. (1987) Oral and Intravenous Cholegraphy. In: Ansell, G. & Wilkins, R.A. (eds) *Complications in Diagnostic Imaging*, pp. 205–217. Oxford: Blackwell Scientific Publications.

Intravenous Cholangiography

Indications
1. Further assessment of the non-functioning gall-bladder on oral cholecystography[1].
2. Post-cholecystectomy patients with recurrent symptoms of biliary tract disease.
3. Preoperatively to exclude common bile duct calculi when the gall bladder has been shown by other means to contain calculi.
4. To demonstrate common bile duct abnormalities when the oral cholecystogram is normal.

N.B. The biliary tract is only likely to be visualized when the serum bilirubin is less than $50 \mu\text{mol l}^{-1}$ and, even when there is normal hepatic function, up to 45% of examinations may not provide adequate visualization of the biliary tree and there may be a diagnostic error rate of 40% even in adequate studies[2]. Most of the clinical indications are now better resolved by other imaging methods, particularly ultrasonography, CT, percutaneous transhepatic cholangiography and endoscopic cholangiography[3].

Contraindications
1. Severe hepatorenal disease.
2. Oral cholecystography within the previous week — because the incidence of toxic effects is increased and the ducts are less likely to be visualized[4].

Contrast medium
See Table 4.2.

Equipment
Overcouch tube with tomography facility.

Patient preparation
The patient should be well hydrated.

Preliminary film
Supine 20° RPO of the right side of the abdomen.

Methods
1. A bolus injection of 30 ml Biligram 35% or Biliscopin over at least 5 min.
2. A slow infusion of 100 ml Biligram for infusion over 45–60 min, Endobil for infusion over 15–30 min or Biliscopin for infusion over 15–30 min.

For an adult, infusion of Biligram over 60 min approximates to $3–4 \text{ mg kg}^{-1} \text{ min}^{-1}$, which has been found to give optimum plasma concentration with maximum biliary excretion[5]. It is, therefore, the method of choice. Infusion at slower rates, e.g. $2 \text{ mg kg}^{-1} \text{ min}^{-1}$, increases the number of unsatisfactory i.v. choledochograms with results similar to a bolus injection[6]. A bolus, or infusion of more than $4 \text{ mg kg}^{-1} \text{ min}^{-1}$ does not allow sufficient time for binding to albumen, which is an important step in the metabolic pathway. Renal rather than biliary excretion then occurs.

Table 4.2 Intravenous cholangiographic contrast media.

Proprietary name	Chemical name and dose	Iodine concentration (mg ml^{-1})
Biligram	meglumine ioglycamate 35% w/v *adult:* 30 ml *child:* 2–12 months – 0.8 ml kg^{-1} 1–6 years – 0.6 ml kg^{-1} 6–11 years – 0.45 ml kg^{-1} over 12 years – 0.4 ml kg^{-1}	176
Biligram for infusion	meglumine ioglycamate 17% w/v *adult:* 100 ml *child:* under 12 years – not recommended over 12 years – 1 ml kg^{-1}	85
Endobil infusion	meglumine iodoxamate 9.91% w/v *adult:* 100 ml *child:* not yet recommended	45
Biliscopin	meglumine iotroxate *adult:* 30 ml *child:* dosage not yet established	180
Biliscopin for infusion	meglumine iotroxate *adult:* 100 ml *child:* dosage not yet established	50

The infusion method also results in fewer unpleasant side-effects[6, 7], including hypotension[8]. Hypotension may have serious consequences in the older patient with poor cardiovascular reserve.

Similar comments apply to Endobil infusion.

Biliscopin for infusion exhibits better bile duct visualization and less side-effects than Biligram for infusion[9].

Technique　The patient lies supine for the infusion, which is started at a slow rate and then increased after 5 min.

Films　Taken with the patient 20° RPO or LAO.
1. At the end of the infusion.
2. Every 15 min thereafter until contrast medium reaches the duodenum.
   If the ducts or gallbladder are not seen after 2 hours, further films are taken every 30 min until 4 hours post-infusion. If no opacification has occurred by this time, the examination is terminated.
3. Erect view of the gallbladder.

ADDITIONAL FILM
Tomography at 8–12 cm – often helpful.

Additional technique
Glucagon-enhanced cholangiography　Improved visualization of the common bile duct may be achieved by administering glucagon 1 mg i.v. after the post-infusion film has been taken[10]. Because the effects of glucagon are of short duration the common bile duct is shown best on a 10-min post-infusion film. Glucagon exerts its beneficial effects via the following mechanisms:
1. Contraction of the sphincter of Oddi, followed by relaxation.
2. Increased choleresis.
3. Increased hepatic blood flow.

Aftercare　None.

Complications
Due to the contrast medium　Similar to urographic contrast media but considerably more toxic. In the UK survey[11], the mortality rate of one in 5000 was eight times that of urography. Other complications that may occur are:
1. Impaired liver function – dose-related.
2. Uricosuric action.
3. Precipitation of Bence Jones protein and IgM macroglobulin.
4. Renal impairment – much less common than with oral cholecystographic agents.

References

1. Scholz, F.J., Larsen, C.R. & Wise, R.E. (1976) Intravenous cholangiography: recurring concepts. *Semin. Roentgenol.* 11, 197–202.
2. Goodman, M.W., Ansel, H.J., Vennes, J.A., Lasser, R.B. & Silvis, S.E. (1980) Is intravenous cholangiography still useful? *Gastroenterology* 79, 642–645.
3. Rholl, K.S., Smathers, R.L., McClennan, B.L. & Lee, J.K.T. (1985) Intravenous cholangiography in the CT era. *Gastrointest. Radiol.* 10, 69–74.
4. Finby, N. & Glasberg, G. (1964) A note on the blocking of hepatic excretion during cholangiographic study. *Gastroenterology* 46, 276–277.
5. Bell, G.D., Fayadh, M., Frank, J., McMullin, J. & Kelsey Fry, I. (1978) Ioglycamide (Biligram) studies in man – relation between plasma concentration and biliary excretion. *Br. J. Radiol.* 51, 111–115.
6. Bell, G.D., Frank, J., Fayadh, M., Smith, P.L.C. & Kelsey Fry, I. (1978) Ioglycamide (Biligram) studies in man. Radiological opacification of the bile duct. A comparison of a number of different methods. *Br. J. Radiol.* 51, 191–195.
7. NcNulty, J.G. (1968) Drip infusion cholecystocholangiography. *Radiology* 90, 570–575.
8. Saltzman, G-F. & Sundström, K-A. (1960) The influence of different contrast media for cholegraphy on blood pressure and pulse rate. *Acta Radiol.* 54, 353–364.
9. Doran, J., Clifford K., Martin, P., Knapp, D.R. & Bell, G.D.(1980) Drip infusion cholangiography using iotroxamide. Double blind comparison with ioglycamide. *Br. J. Radiol.* 53, 645–659.
10. Evans, A.F. & Whitehouse, G.H. (1980) Further experience with glucagon enhanced cholangiography. *Clin. Radiol.* 31, 663–665.
11. Ansell, G. (1970) Adverse reactions to contrast agents. *Invest. Radiol.* 5, 374–384.

Peroperative Cholangiography

Indications   During cholecystectomy or bile duct surgery, to avoid surgical exploration of the common bile duct.

Contraindications   None.

Contrast medium   HOCM or LOCM 150 i.e. low iodine content so as not to obscure any calculi. 20 ml.

Equipment   1. Operating table with a film cassette tunnel.
2. Mobile X-ray machine.

Patient preparation   As for surgery.

Technique   The surgeon cannulates the cystic duct with a fine catheter. This is prefilled with contrast medium to exclude air bubbles which might simulate calculi.

Films   1. After 5 ml have been injected.
2. After 20 ml have been injected. Contrast medium should flow freely into the duodenum. Spasm of the sphincter of Oddi is a fairly frequent occurrence and may be due to anaesthetic agents or surgical manipulation. It may be relieved by glucagon, propantheline or amyl nitrite.

The criteria for a normal operative choledochogram are given by Le Quesne[1] as:
  (a) Common bile duct width not greater than 12 mm.
  (b) Free flow of contrast medium into the duodenum.
  (c) The terminal narrow segment of the duct is clearly seen.
  (d) There are no filling defects.
  (e) There is no excess retrograde filling of the hepatic ducts.

Reference   1. Le Quesne, L.P. (1960) Discussion on cholangiography. *Proc. R. Soc. Med.* **53**, 852–855.

Further reading   Chant, A.D.B., Dewbury, K.G., Guyer, P.B. & Goh, H. (1982) Operative cholangiography reassessed. *Clin. Radiol.* **33**, 289–291.

Faris, I., Thomson, J.P.S., Grundy, D.J. & Le Quesne, L.P. (1975) Operative cholangiography: a re-appraisal based on a review of 400 cholangiograms. *Br. J. Surg.* **62,** 966–972.

Millward, S.F. (1982) Post exploratory operative cholangiography: is it a useful technique to check clearance of the common bile duct? *Clin. Radiol.* **33,** 535–538.

Postoperative (T-tube) Cholangiography

Indications To exclude biliary tract calculi where:
(a) operative cholangiography was not performed, or
(b) the results of operative cholangiography are not satisfactory or are suspect.

Contraindications None.

Contrast medium HOCM or LOCM 150. 20–30 ml.

Equipment Fluoroscopy unit with spot film device.

Patient preparation None.

Preliminary film Coned supine PA of the right side of the abdomen.

Technique
1. The examination is performed on or about the tenth postoperative day, prior to pulling out the T-tube.
2. The patient lies supine on the X-ray table. The drainage tube is clamped off near to the patient and cleaned thoroughly with antiseptic.
3. A 23G needle, extension tubing and 20 ml syringe are assembled and filled with contrast medium. After all air bubbles have been expelled the needle is inserted into the tubing between the patient and the clamp. The injection is made under fluoroscopic control, the total volume depending on duct filling.

Films Using a 35 × 35 cm cassette split into three:
1. PA.
2. RAO⎫ positioned under fluoroscopic control
3. LAO⎭ (approx. 45°).

Aftercare None.

Complications

Due to the contrast medium

The biliary ducts do absorb contrast medium and cholangiovenous reflux can occur with high injection pressures. Adverse reactions are, therefore, possible but the incidence is small.

Due to the technique

Injection of contrast medium under high pressure into an obstructed biliary tract can produce septicaemia.

Percutaneous Extraction of Retained Biliary Calculi (Burhenne Technique)

Indications   Retained biliary calculi seen on the T-tube cholangiogram (incidence 3%).

Contraindications
1. Small T-tube (< 12F).
2. Tortuous T-tube course in soft tissues.
3. Acute pancreatitis.
4. Drain in situ (cross connections exist between the drain tract and the T-tube tract).

Contrast medium   HOCM or LOCM 150. (Low-density contrast medium is used to avoid obscuring the calculus.)

Equipment
1. Fluoroscopy unit with spot film device.
2. Medi-Tech steerable catheter system with wire baskets.

Patient preparation
1. T-tube should be greater than 12F.
2. T-tube should be brought out obliquely towards the right flank (to avoid irradiation of the radiologist's fingers).
3. Following discovery of the retained stone on the tenth day T-tube cholangiogram, the patient should be discharged with the T-tube clamped for at least 4 weeks to allow the formation of a solid fistulous tract.
4. Admission to hospital on the day prior to the procedure.
5. Prophylactic antibiotics and pre-medication 1 hour prior to the procedure.
6. Analgesia during the procedure.

Technique
1. The patient lies supine on the X-ray table. A T-tube cholangiogram is performed to accurately localize the retained calculus.
2. The T-tube is slowly withdrawn from the patient.
3. The steerable catheter is advanced down the T-tube track and its tip is positioned just beyond the calculus. A basket is then inserted through the catheter and opened beyond the stone. The opened basket and catheter are then slowly withdrawn and the stone engaged. The basket should

not be closed as the stone may be disengaged or fragmented. The catheter system with the engaged stone in the basket should be slowly withdrawn to the skin surface in one movement.

4. The duct system is opacified by intermittent injections of contrast through the steerable catheter.

5. At the end of the procedure a suction catheter or similar is manipulated into the duct system and sutured to the skin.

6. Stones up to 10 mm in diameter may be extracted through a 14F tract. Stones greater than 10 mm will require fragmentation (if soft) or endoscopic sphincterotomy/surgery. Multiple stones may require repeated procedures.

7. A completion cholangiogram should be performed via the suction catheter on the day following the procedure, when the gas bubbles have cleared.

Aftercare
1. Pulse and blood pressure half-hourly for 6 hours.
2. Bed rest for 12 hours.

Complications Morbidity 4%.

Due to the contrast medium
1. 'Allergic' reactions – rare.
2. Pancreatitis.

Due to the technique
1. Fever.
2. Perforation of the T-tube tract.

Further reading
Burhenne, H.J. (1980) Percutaneous extraction of retained biliary stones: 661 patients. *Am. J. Roentg.* **134**, 888–898.

Mason, R. (1980) Percutaneous extraction of retained gallstones via the T-tube track – British experience of 131 cases. *Clin. Radiol.* **31**, 497–499.

Endoscopic Retrograde Cholangiopancreatography

Compared with percutaneous transhepatic cholangiography ERCP has three advantages[1]:
1. The ability to visualize and biopsy ampullary lesions.
2. The demonstration of biliary tree and pancreatic duct.
3. Better therapeutic potential.

Indications
1. Investigation of extrahepatic biliary obstruction.
2. Post-cholecystectomy syndrome.
3. Investigation of diffuse biliary disease, e.g. sclerosing cholangitis.
4. Pancreatic disease.

Contraindications
1. Australia antigen positive; AIDS-positive.
2. Oesophageal obstruction; varices; pyloric stenosis.
3. Previous gastric surgery.
4. Acute pancreatitis.
5. Pancreatic pseudocyst.
6. When glucagon or Buscopan are contraindicated.
7. Severe cardio/respiratory disease.

Contrast medium
Pancreas   LOCM 240.

Bile ducts   LOCM 150; dilute contrast medium ensures that calculi will not be obscured.

Equipment
1. Side-viewing endoscope.
2. Polythene catheters.
3. Fluoroscopic unit with spot film facilities.

Patient preparation
1. Nil orally for 4 hours prior to procedure.
2. Premedication: see Chapter 1.
3. Antibiotic cover.

Preliminary film   Prone AP and LAO of the upper abdomen, to check for opaque gallstones and pancreatic calcification/calculi.

Technique The pharynx is anaesthetized with 4% Xylocaine spray and the patient is given diazepam 5 mg min^{-1} i.v. until sedated. He then lies on his left side and the endoscope is introduced. The ampulla of Vater is located and the patient is turned prone. A polythene catheter prefilled with contrast medium is inserted into the ampulla, having ensured that all air bubbles are excluded. A small test injection of contrast under fluoroscopic control is made to determine the position of the cannula. It is important to avoid overfilling of the pancreas. If it is desirable to opacify both the biliary tree and pancreatic duct, then the latter should be cannulated first. A sample of bile should be sent for culture and sensitivity if there is evidence of biliary obstruction.

Films

Pancreas (using fine focal spot)

1. Prone, both posterior obliques.

Bile ducts

1. Early filling films to show calculi
    (a) Prone — straight and posterior obliques
    (b) Supine — straight, both obliques; Trendelenburg to fill intrahepatic ducts; semi-erect to fill lower end of common bile duct and gallbladder.
2. Films following removal of the endoscope, which may obscure the duct.
3. Delayed films to assess the gallbladder and emptying of the common bile duct.

Aftercare

1. Nil orally until sensation has returned to the pharynx (½–3 hours).
2. Pulse, temperature and blood pressure half-hourly for 6 hours.
3. Maintain antibiotics if there is biliary or pancreatic obstruction.
4. Serum/urinary amylase if pancreatitis is suspected.

Complications

Due to the contrast medium

1. 'Allergic reactions' — rare.
2. Acute pancreatitis — more likely with large volumes, high-pressure injections.

Due to the technique

LOCAL
Damage by the endoscope, e.g. rupture of the oesophagus, damage to the ampulla, proximal pancreatic duct and distal common duct.

DISTANT
Bacteraemia, septicaemia, aspiration pneumonitis, hyperamylasaemia (approx. 70%). Acute pancreatitis (0.7–7.4%).

Reference

1. Summerfield, J.A. (1988) Biliary obstruction is best managed by endoscopists. *Gut* **29**, 741–745.

Further reading

Freeman, A. & Martin, D. Editorial (1991) New trends with endoscopic retrograde cholangiopancreatography. *Clin. Radiol.* **43**, 223–226.

Lawrie, B.W.E. (1987) Endoscopy and endoscopic retrograde cholangiopancreatography. In: Ansell, G. & Wilkins, R.A. (eds) *Complications in Diagnostic Imaging*, pp. 186–204. Oxford: Blackwell Scientific Publications.

Percutaneous Transhepatic Cholangiography

Indications
1. Cholestatic jaundice, to confirm or exclude extrahepatic bile duct obstruction.
2. Prior to therapeutic intervention, e.g. biliary drainage procedure.

Contraindications
1. Bleeding tendency:
   (a) platelets less than 100 000
   (b) prothrombin time 2 s greater than control.
2. Biliary tract sepsis.
3. Non-availability of prompt surgical facilities should they be necessary, or a patient who is unfit for surgery.
4. Hydatid disease.

Contrast medium
LOCM or HOCM 150; 20–60 ml.

Equipment
1. Fluoroscopy unit with spot film device and tilting table.
2. Chiba needle (a fine, flexible 22G needle, 18 cm long).

Patient preparation
1 Haemoglobin, prothrombin time and platelets are checked, and corrected if necessary.
2. Prophylactic antibiotics — ampicillin 500 mg q.d.s. — to commence 24 hours before and continue for 3 days after the examination.
3. Nil by mouth for 5 hours prior to the procedure.
4. Premedication — see Chapter 1.

Preliminary film
Supine PA of the right side of the abdomen.

Technique
1. The patient lies supine. Under fluoroscopic control a metal marker is placed on the skin in the right mid-axillary line such that its position overlies the liver during full inspiration and expiration. A second metal marker is placed on the xiphisternum.
2. Using aseptic technique the skin, deeper tissues and liver capsule are anaesthetized at the site of the first metal marker.
3. During suspended respiration the Chiba needle is

inserted into the liver, but once it is within the liver parenchyma the patient is allowed shallow respirations. It is advanced parallel to the table top in the direction of the xiphisternum until just short of the right lateral margin of the spine.

4. The stilette is withdrawn and the needle connected to a syringe and extension tubing prefilled with contrast medium. Contrast medium is injected under fluoroscopic control while the needle is slowly withdrawn. If a duct is not entered at the first attempt, the needle tip is withdrawn to approximately 2–3 cm from the liver capsule and further passes are made, directing the needle tip more cranially, caudally, anteriorly or posteriorly until a duct is entered. If a duct has not been entered after ten attempts, the procedure is terminated and the assumption is made that the ducts are not dilated. The number of passes is not related to the incidence of complications and the likelihood of success is directly related to the degree of duct dilatation and the number of passes made.

5. Excessive parenchymal injection should be avoided and when it does occur it results in opacification of intrahepatic lymphatics. Injection of contrast medium into a vein or artery is followed by rapid dispersion.

6. If the intrahepatic ducts are seen to be dilated, bile should be aspirated and sent for microbiological examination. (The incidence of infected bile is high in such cases.)

7. Contrast medium is injected to fill the duct system and define the lower end of an obstruction (if present). The needle is withdrawn. Care should be taken not to overfill an obstructed duct system because septic shock may be precipitated.

Films   Contrast medium is heavier than bile and the sequence of duct opacification is, therefore, gravity-dependent and determined by the site of injection and the position of the patient.

Using the undercouch tube with the patient *horizontal*:
1. PA.
2. 45° RPO.
3. Right lateral.

4. Trendelenburg.
5. Spot views of the gallbladder, if this has been opacified.

Using the undercouch tube with the patient *erect*:
1. PA.
2. 45° RPO.
3. Right lateral.
4. Spot views of the gallbladder.
5. When the above films have shown an obstruction at the level of the porta hepatis, a further film after the patient has been in the erect position for 30 min may show the level of obstruction to be lower than originally thought.

ADDITIONAL FILMS
Hypotonic duodenography — this may be performed to give additional information regarding the site of an obstruction and its position relative to the duodenum. (For method and films see p. 53.)

Delayed films — films taken after several hours, or the next day, may show contrast medium in the gallbladder if this was not achieved during the initial part of the investigation.

Aftercare Pulse and blood pressure half-hourly for 6 hours.

Complications Morbidity approximately 5%; mortality less than 0.1%.

Due to the contrast medium Allergic/idiosyncratic reactions — very uncommon.

Due to the technique LOCAL
1. Puncture of extrahepatic structures — usually no serious sequelae.
2. Intrathoracic injection.
3. Cholangitis.
4. Bile leakage — may lead to biliary peritonitis. Incidence 2%; mortality 1%. More likely if the ducts are under pressure and if there are multiple puncture attempts. Less likely if a drainage catheter is left in situ prior to surgery. (See 'Biliary drainage', p. 123.)
5. Subphrenic abscess.

6. Haemorrhage.
7. Shock — owing to injection into the region of the coeliac plexus.

GENERALIZED
Bacteraemia, septicaemia and endotoxic shock.

Further reading
Fraser, G.M., Cruickshank, J.G., Sumerling, M.D. & Buist, T.A.S. (1978) Percutaneous transhepatic cholangiography with the Chiba needle. *Clin. Radiol.* **29**, 101–112.

Harbin, W.P., Mueller, M.D. & Ferrucci Jr., J.T. (1980) Transhepatic cholangiography: complications and use patterns of the fine needle technique. *Radiology* **135**, 15–22.

Jacques, P.F. & Bream, C.A. (1978) Barium duodenography as an adjunct to percutaneous transhepatic cholangiography. *Am. J. Roentg.* **130**, 693–696.

Jacques, P.F., Mauro, M.A. & Scatliff, J.H. (1980) The failed transhepatic cholangiogram. *Radiology* **134**, 33–35.

Jain, S., Long, R.G., Scott, J., Dick, R. & Sherlock, S. (1977) Percutaneous transhepatic cholangiography using the Chiba needle. *Br. J. Radiol.* **50**, 175–180.

Lintott D.J. (1992) Direct cholangiography. In: Wilkins, R.A. & Nunnerley, H.B. (eds) *Imaging of the Liver, Pancreas and Spleen*, pp. 278–308. Oxford: Blackwell Scientific Publications.

Biliary Drainage

External drainage   This is achieved following transhepatic cannulation of the biliary tree. It has been used to reduce operative morbidity in jaundiced patients but this has not gained widespread acceptance.

Internal drainage   This is achieved following transhepatic or endoscopic cannulation of the biliary tree. An endoprosthesis with proximal and distal side-holes or a transhepatic catheter is sited across a stricture. The endoprosthesis method is preferable because of the complications of long-term transhepatic catheterization.

Indications
1. Proven malignant biliary stricture, not amenable to surgery.
2. Benign stricture following balloon dilatation.

Contraindications   As for percutaneous transhepatic cholangiography.

Contrast media   LOCM or HOCM 200 20–60 ml.

Equipment
1. Wide-channelled endoscope for introduction of endoprosthesis.
2. A biplane fluoroscope facility is useful but not essential for transhepatic puncture.
3. Set including guide-wires, dilators and endoprosthesis.

Patient preparation
1. Nil orally for 4 hours before procedure.
2. Premedication including analgesia, e.g. pethidine 75 mg i.v., and pethidine 25 mg i.v. during the procedure, if necessary. An antiemetic, e.g. Stemetil 12.5 mg, may be added.
3. Antibiotic before and for at least 3 days following, e.g. Cefuroxine 750 mg i.v. 6-hourly.
4. Intravenous line for fluids to avoid dehydration and as a route for i.v. drugs during the procedure.

Technique
Transhepatic
1. A percutaneous transhepatic cholangiogram is performed.
2. A duct in the right lobe of the liver is chosen that has a horizontal or caudal course to the porta

hepatis. This duct is studied on AP and lateral fluoroscopy (if possible) to judge its depth and then an 18G 25 cm sheathed needle is introduced following percutaneous puncture through an intercostal space in the mid-axillary line. The chosen duct is punctured on fluoroscopy, care being taken not to push the needle tip through the medial wall of the duct. If the duct is not successfully punctured, the needle is reinserted into the sheath and a further pass is made without removing the sheath from the liver, thus minimizing the number of punctures of the capsule.

3. Upon successful puncture a J guide-wire is inserted through the sheath and manoeuvred towards or through the obstruction, if possible. The sheath is then advanced over the guide-wire as far as possible. The wire is exchanged for a more rigid Lunderquist guide-wire and over this dilators are passed to facilitate passage of the catheter/endoprosthesis. If passage through the stricture with the internal guide is not possible other wires that can be shaped may be successful. Failing this, external drainage is instituted and further attempts are made to pass the stricture a few days later.

4. An endoprosthesis is pushed through the stricture and sited with its side-holes above and below the stricture so that internal drainage is instituted. An internal/external catheter may be placed across the stricture and secured to the skin with sutures or a locking disc device.

Endoscopic 1. Cholangiography following cannulation of the biliary tree.

2. Endoscopic sphincterotomy.

3. A guide-wire is placed via the channel of the endoscope through the sphincter and pushed past the stricture using fluoroscopy to monitor progress.

4. Following dilatation of the stricture the endoprosthesis is pushed over the guide-wire and sited with its side-holes above and below the stricture.

Aftercare 1. As for percutaneous transhepatic cholangiography.

2. Antibiotics for at least 3 days.
3. An externally draining catheter should be regularly flushed through with normal saline and exchanged at 3-monthly intervals.

Complications
1. As for percutaneous transhepatic cholangiography, endoscopic retrograde cholangiopancreatography and sphincterotomy.
2. Sepsis — particularly common with externally draining catheters.
3. Dislodgement of catheters, endoprostheses.
4. Blockage of catheters/endoprostheses.
5. Perforation of bile duct above the stricture on passage of guide-wires.

Further reading
Braasch, J.W. & Gray, B.N. (1977) Considerations that lower pancreatoduodenectomy mortality. *Am. J. Surg.* **129**, 480–483.

Dooley, J.S. Dick, R. Irving, D., Olney, J. & Sherlock, S. (1981) Relief of bile duct obstruction by the percutaneous transhepatic insertion of an endoprosthesis. *Clin. Radiol.* **32**, 163–172.

Ferrucci, J.T., Mueller, P.R. & Harbin, W.P. (1980) Percutaneous transhepatic biliary drainage. Technique, results and applications. *Radiology* **135**, 1–13.

Molnar, W. & Stockum, A.E. (1974) Relief of obstructive jaundice through percutaneous transhepatic catheter — a new therapeutic method. *Am. J. Roentg.* **122**, 356–367.

Ring, E.J., Oleaga, J.A., Freiman, D.B., Husted, J.W. & Lunderquist, A. (1978) Therapeutic applications of catheter cholangiography. *Radiology* **128**, 333–338.

Ring, E.J., Husted, J.W., Oleaga, J.A. & Freiman, D.B. (1979) A multihole catheter for maintaining longterm percutaneous antegrade biliary drainage. *Radiology* **132**, 752–754.

Ultrasound of the Liver

Indications
1. Suspected focal or diffuse liver lesion.
2. Staging known extrahepatic malignancy.
3. Right upper quadrant pain or mass.
4. Hepatomegaly.
5. Jaundice.
6. Abnormal liver function tests.
7. Pyrexia of unknown origin.
9. To facilitate the placement of needles for biopsy, etc.

Contraindications None.

Patient preparation Not imperative but fasting is required if the gall-bladder is also to be studied.

Equipment 3–5 MHz transducer. Small scan head is necessary for an intercostal approach, eg phased or annular array.

Technique
1. Patient supine.
2. Time-gain compensation set to give uniform reflectivity throughout the right lobe of the liver.
3. Suspended inspiration.
4. Longitudinal scans from epigastrium or left subcostal region across to right subcostal region. The transducer should be angled up to include the whole of the left and right lobes.
5. Transverse scans, subcostally, to visualize the whole liver.
6. If visualization is incomplete, due to a small or high liver, then right intercostal, longitudinal, transverse and oblique scans may be useful. Suspended respiration without deep inspiration may suffice for intercostal scanning. In patients who are unable to hold their breath, real time scanning during quiet respiration is often adequate. Upright or left lateral decubitus positions are alternatives if visualization is still incomplete.

Additional views
Hepatic veins Best seen using a transverse intercostal or epigastric approach. During inspiration, in real time, these can be seen traversing the liver to enter the inferior

vena cava (IVC). Hepatic vein walls do not have increased reflectivity in comparison to normal liver parenchyma.

Portal vein Longitudinal view of the portal vein is shown by an oblique subcostal or intercostal approach. Portal vein walls are of increased reflectivity in comparison to parenchyma.

Hepatic artery May be traced from the coeliac axis, which is recognized by the 'seagull' appearance of the origins of the common hepatic artery and splenic artery.

Common bile duct See 'Ultrasound of the Gallbladder and Biliary System'.

The spleen size should be measured in all cases of suspected liver disease or portal hypertension. 95% of normal adult spleens measure 12 cm or less in length, and less than 7 cm × 5 cm in thickness. The spleen size is commonly assessed by 'eyeballing' and measurement of the longest diameter[1].

Reference 1. Rumack, C.M., Wilson, S.R. & Charboneau, J.W. (1991) *Diagnostic Ultrasound*, Vol. 1, p. 92. St Louis: Mosby Year Book.

Ultrasound of the Gallbladder and Biliary System

Indications
1. Suspected gallstones.
2. Right upper quadrant pain.
3. Jaundice.
4. Fever of unknown origin.
5. Acute pancreatitis.
6. To assess gallbladder function.
7. Guided percutaneous procedures.

Contraindication   None.

Patient preparation   Fasting for at least 6 hours, preferably overnight. Water may be permitted.

Equipment   3–5 MHz transducer. A stand-off may be used for a very anterior gallbladder. Small scan head may be optimal.

Technique
1. Patient supine.
2. The gallbladder can be located by following the reflective main lobar fissure from the right portal vein to the gallbladder fossa.
3. Developmental anomalies are rare but the gall-bladder may be intrahepatic or on a long mesentery.
4. The gallbladder is scanned slowly along its long axis and transversely from the fundus to the neck leading to the cystic duct.
5. It must be re-scanned in the left lateral decubitus or erect positions because stones may be missed if only supine scans are used.
6. Visualization of the neck and cystic ducts may be improved by head down tilt.

The normal gallbladder wall is never more than 3 mm thick.

Additional views
Assessment of gallbladder function
1. Fasting gallbladder volume may be assessed by measuring longitudinal, transverse and AP diameters.

2. Normal gallbladder contraction reduces the volume by more than 25%, 30 min after a standard fatty meal. Somatostatin, calcitonin, indomethacin and nifedipine antagonize this contraction.

Intrahepatic bile ducts

1. Left lobe: transverse epigastric scan.
2. Right lobe: subcostal or intercostal longitudinal oblique.

Normal intrahepatic ducts may be visualized with modern scanners. Intrahepatic ducts are dilated if their diameter is more than 40% of the accompanying portal vein branch. There is normally acoustic enhancement posterior to dilated ducts but not portal veins. Dilated ducts have a beaded branching appearance.

Extrahepatic bile ducts

1. Patient supine or in the right anterior oblique position.
2. The upper common duct is demonstrated on a longitudinal oblique, subcostal or intercostal scan running anterior to the portal vein. The right hepatic artery is often seen crossing transversely between the two.
3. The common duct may be followed downwards along its length through the head of the pancreas to the ampulla and, when visualized, transverse scans should also be performed to improve detection of intraduct stones.

The internal diameter of the common hepatic duct is 4 mm or less in a normal adult; 5 mm is borderline and 6 mm considered dilated. The lower common duct (common bile duct) is normally 6 mm or less. Distinction of the common hepatic duct from the common bile duct depends on identification of the junction with the cystic duct. This is usually not possible with ultrasound. Colour flow Doppler enables quick distinction of bile duct from ectatic hepatic artery. In 17% of patients the artery lies anterior to the bile duct[1].

Post-cholecystectomy

There is disagreement as to whether the normal common duct dilates after cholecystectomy. Symptomatic patients and those with abnormal liver function tests should have further investigation if the common duct measures more than 6 mm.

References   1. Berland, L.L., Lawson, T.L. & Foley, W.D. (1982) Porta hepatis: sonographic discrimination of bile ducts from arteries with pulsed doppler with new anatomic criteria. *Am. J. Roentg.* **138**, 833–840.

Further reading   Laing, F.C. (1987) Ultrasonography of the gallbladder and biliary tree. In: Sarti, D.A. (ed.) *Diagnostic Ultrasound Text and Cases*, 2nd edn, pp. 142–146. St Louis: Year Book Medical Publishers.

Mittelstaedt, C.A. (1987) The biliary system. In: *Abdominal Ultrasound*, pp. 81–89. Edinburgh: Churchill Livingstone.

Ultrasound of the Pancreas

Indications
1. Suspected pancreatic tumour.
2. Pancreatitis or its complications.
3. Epigastric mass.
4. Epigastric pain.
5. Jaundice.
6. To facilitate guided biopsy.

Contraindications   None.

Patient preparation   Nil by mouth, preferably overnight.

Equipment   3–5 MHz transducer. A stand-off may be required in thin patients.

Technique
1. Patient supine.
2. The body of the pancreas is located anterior to the splenic vein in a transverse epigastric scan.
3. The transducer is angled transversely and obliquely to visualise the head and tail.
4. The tail may be demonstrated from a left intercostal view using the spleen as an acoustic window.
5. Longitudinal epigastric scans may be useful.
6. The pancreatic parenchyma increases in reflectivity with age, being equal to liver reflectivity in young adults.
7. Gastric or colonic gas may prevent complete visualization. This may be overcome by left and right oblique decubitus scans or by scanning with the patient erect. Water may be drunk to improve the window through the stomach and the scans repeated in all positions. One cup is usually sufficient. Degassed water preferable.

The pancreatic duct should not measure more than 3 mm in the head or 2 mm in the body.

Radiolabelled Colloid Liver Scan

Indications
1. Hepatic space occupying lesions – primary and secondary tumours, abscesses and cysts.
2. Diffuse liver disease.

Contraindications   None.

Radiopharmaceuticals   ^{99m}Tc-colloid, 80 MBq max. Cleared by phagocytosis into the reticuloendothelial cells, where it is retained. Spleen is demonstrated as well as liver.

Equipment
1. Gamma camera.
2. Low-energy general purpose collimator (high sensitivity collimator for flow studies).
3. Imaging computer for flow studies.

Patient Preparation   Nil by mouth for 4–6 hours for flow study.

Technique
1. ^{99m}Tc-colloid is administered i.v.
2. With the patient supine, images are obtained after 15 min, or longer in patients with very poor clearance.

Images   500 kilocounts for first view, others for same length of time:
1. Anterior, with costal margin markers.
2. Posterior.
3. Left lateral.
4. Right lateral.

Additional techniques
1. A first-pass dynamic flow study may be performed to improve differential diagnosis of liver masses:
   (a) The fasted patient is positioned supine with the camera anterior or posterior depending upon analysis method to be employed[1].
   (b) A fast bolus injection of ^{99m}Tc-colloid is given using the Oldendorf technique (see p. 14) if the patient has good veins.
   (c) 1-s images are collected on computer for 60 s.
   (d) Analysis of regional time-activity curves may be performed to provide an index of liver arterial and portal perfusion[1].

(e) Static images are acquired as above.

2. Tomography may be used for assessment of diffuse liver disease[2] and to improve detection of small and deep-seated lesions. The injected activity may be increased up to 200 MBq max. for tomography.

Aftercare None.

Complications None.

References 1. Britten, A.J., Fleming, J.S., Flowerdew, A.D.S. et al (1990) A comparison of three indices of relative hepatic perfusion derived from dynamic liver scintigraphy. *Clin. Phys. Physiol. Meas.* 11, 45–51.

2. Delcourt, E., Vanhaeverbeek, M., Binon, J.P. et al (1992) Emission tomography for assessment of diffuse alcoholic liver disease. *J. Nucl. Med.* 33, 1337–1345.

Further reading Wraight, E.P. (1989) The hepato-biliary system, In: Sharp, P.F., Gemmell, H.G. & Smith, F.W. (eds) *Practical Nuclear Medicine*, pp. 179–192. Oxford: Oxford University Press.

(1990) Liver disease. In: Harding, L.K. & Robinson, P.J.A. *Clinician's Guide to Nuclear Medicine: Gastroenterology*, pp. 49–79. London: Churchill Livingstone.

Dynamic Radionuclide Hepatobiliary Imaging (Cholescintigraphy)

Indications
1. Suspected acute cholecystitis[1].
2. Diagnosis and location of biliary obstruction after negative ultrasound investigation[2].
3. Assessment of neonatal jaundice where biliary atresia is considered[3].
4. Suspected bile leaks after trauma or surgery[4].

Contraindications   None.

Radio-pharmaceuticals
1. ^{99m}Tc-diethyliodo-iminodiacetic acid (IODIDA).
2. ^{99m}Tc-trimethylbromo-iminodiacetic acid (TBIDA).
3. ^{99m}Tc-diisopropyl-iminodiacetic acid (DISIDA).
4. ^{99m}Tc-diethyl-iminodiacetic acid (HIDA).

75 MBq typical, 150 MBq max.

These ^{99m}Tc-labelled derivatives of iminodiacetic acid (IDA) are rapidly cleared from the circulation by hepatocytes and secreted into bile in a similar way to bilirubin[5]. IODIDA, TBIDA and DISIDA show more rapid hepatic uptake and less urinary excretion than HIDA. With some of the lowest urinary excretion rates of all the IDA derivatives, IODIDA and TBIDA have significant advantages at high bilirubin levels ($>80–100\ \mu$mol l^{-1}) because of non-visualization of the urinary tract and better biliary contrast[6]. A number of other IDA derivatives have been developed with similar kinetics to those mentioned.

Equipment
1. Gamma camera.
2. Low-energy general purpose collimator.

Patient preparation
1. Nil by mouth for 4–6 hours.
2. For the investigation of biliary atresia, infants are given phenobarbitone orally 5 mg kg^{-1} day^{-1} in 2 divided doses for 3–5 days prior to the study to enhance hepatic excretion of radiopharmaceutical[7].

Technique
:   The imaging protocol depends upon the clinical quesion being asked. A dynamic study should be performed where it is important to visualize the progress of the bile in detail, e.g. post-surgery:
    1. The patient lies supine with the camera anterior and the liver at the top of the field of view.
    2. The radiopharmaceutical is injected i.v.
    3. 2-min dynamic images are acquired for 30–40 min, followed by static images as below.

Images
:   1. 3-min anterior views every 15 min for 1 hour starting 2 min after injection.
    2. If the gallbladder and duodenum are not seen, images are obtained at hourly intervals up to 4–6 hours.
    3. A right lateral or right lateral oblique view may be useful in doubtful cases to distinguish the gallbladder from duodenal activity.
    4. If no bowel activity is seen by 4–6 hours and it is important to detect any flow of bile at all, e.g. in suspected biliary atresia, a 24-hour image should be taken.

Additional techniques
:   *Quantitative analysis*
    1. It has been proposed that a liver-to-heart activity ratio, from 2.5 to 10 min after injection, of greater than 5 excludes biliary atresia[8], although others have failed to confirm this[9].
    2. Some investigators have calculated liver function parameters from dynamic studies, e.g. to attempt to differentiate between transplant rejection and hepatocyte dysfunction[10].

Aftercare
:   None.

Complications
:   None.

References
:   1. Dykes, E.H., Wilson, N., Gray, H.W. & McArdle, C.S. (1986) The role of ^{99m}Tc HIDA cholescintigraphy in the diagnosis of acute gallbladder disease: Comparison with oral cholecystography and ultrasonography. *Scott. Med. J.* **31**, 170–173.
    2. Wraight, E.P. (1989) The hepato-biliary system. In: Sharp, P.F., Gemmell, H.G. & Smith, F.W. (eds) *Practical Nuclear Medicine*, pp. 179–192. Oxford: Oxford University Press.

3. Johnston, G.S., Rosenbaum, R.C., Hill, J.L. & Diaconis, J.N. (1985) Differentiation of jaundice in infancy: an application of radionuclide biliary studies. *J. Surg. Oncol.* **30**, 206–208.

4. Rayter, Z., Tonge, C., Bennett, C., Thomas, M. & Robinson, P. (1991) Ultrasound and HIDA: Scanning in evaluating bile leaks after cholecystectomy. *Nucl. Med. Commun.* **12**, 197–202.

5. Krishnamurthy, G.T. & Turner F.E. (1990) Pharmacokinetics and clinical application of technetium 99m-labelled hepatobiliary agents. *Semin. Nucl. Med.* **20**, 130–149.

6. Schwarzrock, R., Kotzerke, J., Hundeshagen, H. et al (1986) ^{99m}Tc-diethyl-iodo-HIDA (JODIDA): a new hepatobiliary agent in clinical comparison with ^{99m}Tc-diisopropyl-HIDA (DISIDA) in jaundiced patients. *Eur. J. Nucl. Med.* **12**, 346–350.

7. Hepatobiliary studies: Bile reflux, jaundice and acute cholecystitis. In: Harding, L.K. & Robinson, P.J.A. *Clinician's Guide to Nuclear Medicine: Gastroenterology*, pp. 31–48. London: Churchill Livingstone.

8. El Tumi, M.A., Clarke, M.B., Barrett, J.J. & Mowat, A.P. (1987) Ten minute radiopharmaceutical test in biliary atresia. *Arch. Dis. Child.* **62**, 180–184.

9. Charlton, C.P.J., Tarlow, M.J., Tulley, N.J. & Harding, L.K. (1988) Biliary atresia: is a 10 minute test useful? *Nucl. Med. Commun.* **9**, 159.

10. Merion, R.M., Campbell, D.A. Jr, Dafoe, D.C., Rosenberg, L., Turcotte, J.G. & Juni, J.E. (1988) Observations on quantitative scintigraphy with deconvolutional analysis in liver transplantation. *Transplant Proc.* **20**(Suppl. 1) 695–697.

Further reading   Jamieson, N.V., Friend, P.J. & Wraight, E.P. (1986) A two year experience with ^{99m}Tc HIDA cholescintigraphy in teaching hospital practice. *Surg. Gynecol. Obstet.* **163**, 29–32.

The Investigation of Jaundice

The aim is to separate haemolytic causes of jaundice from obstructive jaundice or hepatocellular jaundice. Clinical history and examination are followed by biochemical tests of blood and urine and haematological tests.

Imaging investigations

1. OBSTRUCTIVE JAUNDICE
Ultrasound is the primary imaging modality and achieves accuracy figures of 95% for the level of obstruction and 88% for the cause[1]. Dilated ducts suggest obstructive jaundice. The bile ducts, gallbladder and pancreas should be examined to determine the level and cause of obstruction. ERCP or, if that is not possible, PTC are often required to confirm the cause of the obstruction. They may also offer the opportunity for therapy. If the suspected cause is tumour, a CT scan to assess the pancreas and related lymph nodes is often required. In some cases, angiography is used to exclude involvement of the mesenteric and portal veins prior to surgery.

In some cases due to high bile-duct tumours PTC may be required as well as ERCP to fully evaluate the bile ducts.

2. NON-OBSTRUCTIVE JAUNDICE
When ultrasound shows no dilated ducts and hepatocellular jaundice is suspected, liver biopsy is considered. There may be other ultrasound evidence of parenchymal liver disease or signs of portal hypertension.

If obstructive jaundice is still suspected despite the ultrasound result, then ERCP or PTC is required. Extrahepatic obstruction may be present in the absence of duct dilatation[2], and patients with primary sclerosing cholangitis or widespread intrahepatic metastases may have obstruction without duct dilatation.

References

1. Gibson R.N., Yeung, E., Thompson, J.N. et al (1986) Bile duct obstruction: radiologic evaluation of level, cause and tumour resectability. *Radiology* **160**, 43–47.

2. Muhletaler, C.A., Gerlock, A.J., Fleischer, A.C. & James, A.E. (1980) Diagnosis of obstructive jaundice with non-dilated bile ducts. *Am. J. Roentg.* **134,** 1149–1152.

The Investigation of Liver Tumours

Introduction

Investigation falls into three stages:
1. Detection
2. Characterization of the tumour
3. Assessment for surgical resection or staging for chemotherapy.

The clinical context and proposed management course usually determine the extent of investigation. Liver metastases are much commoner than primary liver cancers. Benign haemangiomas are also common, being present in 5–10% of the population. Other benign liver tumours are uncommon.

The clinical data correlated with the radiological investigations usually enable the character of a liver tumour to be determined with a high degree of probability. This can be confirmed with image-guided or surgical biopsy when appropriate. Some surgeons are averse to preoperative biopsy because of the small risk of disseminating malignant cells and the possibility of misleading sampling error[1]. If biopsy is performed, it is often important to sample the 'normal' liver as well as the lesion. The presence of, for example, cirrhosis may have a major impact on management.

Hepatic resection is an established procedure for the management of hepatic metastases and primary liver tumours. Various imaging methods are used to assess the number and location of tumours. Variation in imaging equipment makes comparison of sensitivities of techniques difficult. A recent study[2] gave the following results:

	Sensitivity
Contrast-enhanced CT	68%
MRI	63%
Ultrasound	53%

However, at present, CT arterial portography (CTAP) and intraoperative ultrasound are the most sensitive techniques for detecting liver tumours, with sensitivities of 91 and 96%, respectively[3, 4].

Ultrasound Widely used for general screening for metastases and often the first modality to detect an unsuspected focal liver lesion.

CT There are various techniques. Used for general screening and staging. The remainder of the abdomen and chest may also be imaged for full staging.

The pattern of contrast enhancement may confirm haemangioma and help characterize other liver tumours.

Angiography May provide diagnostic characterization of various tumours, including haemangioma, hepatoma and focal nodular hyperplasia. It is also used to provide a 'road map' to plan surgery.

Arteriography is a pre-requisite for *Lipiodol-enhanced CT*. Follow-up CT scans are obtained 7–10 days after the injection of 7–10 ml of Lipiodol through the hepatic arterial catheter. This may show small hepatoma nodules not visualized by standard CT or ultrasound.

Arteriography is also a pre-requisite for CT arterial portography, a technique usually limited to potential candidates for surgical resection of tumour. A 5F catheter is left with its tip positioned in the superior mesenteric artery and the patient is transferred immediately to the CT scanner. A pump injector is used to deliver 100–150 ml of LOCM 300 at 1–2 ml s^{-1}. An intra-arterial injection of 40 mg papaverine hydrochloride may be given prior to the pump injection to increase portal vein flow. Scanning is commenced 10–20 s after initiation of the pump injection and contiguous 10-mm slices are taken through the liver using a fast scan mode. Normal hepatic tissue is perfused by the portal vein, whereas tumours obtain their blood supply predominantly from the hepatic artery. Consequently, they appear as low density on CTAP. This is the most sensitive method of preoperative liver metastasis detection with spatial display of their segmental distribution. If the hepatic artery arises from the superior mesenteric artery (SMA), there may be confusing hepatic arterial enhancement.

MRI   With modern equipment liver lesions are readily detected, at least as well as with CT, but its true role has yet to be clarified. The characteristics of some tumours may be determined.

Radionuclide scans   Standard colloid scans are of little value because defects are non-specific. Uptake of isotope in focal nodular hyperplasia may distinguish this condition from other liver tumours. Labelled red cell scans may confirm haemangioma with a high degree of specificity. Radionuclide bone scans may be required for staging possible bony spread of hepatocellular carcinoma.

Image-guided biopsy   When clinically justified, ultrasound or CT-guided biopsy is possible for virtually any liver lesion that can be imaged. Vascular lesions such as haemangioma are best approached through normal liver to reduce the risk of bleeding.

Intraoperative techniques   Laparoscopy is now widely used in surgical practice. Intraoperative ultrasound may detect intrahepatic lesions not palpable at laparotomy. Laparoscopic ultrasound is not widely available but may ultimately prove the favoured surgical staging technique.

References

1. Pain, J.A., Karani, J. & Howard, E.R. (1991) Preoperative radiological and clinical assessment of hepatic tumours — is biopsy necessary? *Clin. Radiol.* **44**, 181–182.
2. Wernecke, K., Rummeny, E., Bongartz, G. et al (1991) Detection of hepatic masses in patients with carcinoma: comparative sensitivities of sonography, CT and MR imaging. *Am. J. Roentg.* **157**, 731–739.
3. Soyer, P. Levesque, M., Elias, D., Zeitoun, G. & Roche, A. (1992) Detection of liver metastases from colo-rectal cancer: comparison intraoperative ultrasound during arterial portography. *Radiology* **183**, 541–544.
4. McGrath, F.P., Malone, D.E., Dobranowski, J. & Stevenson, G.W. (1993) Editorial. CT Portography and delayed high dose iodine CT. *Clin. Radiol.* **47**, 1–6.

Pancreatitis

Ultrasound is the first-line investigation but in acute pancreatitis the presence of a sentinel loop will often obscure the pancreas and prevent good visualization. Even if the pancreas is seen, it can appear normal in acute pancreatitis. The gallbladder and biliary tree should always be examined in the fasted patient to exclude the presence of gallstones which may be causing the pancreatitis.

CT is the next investigation. It should be performed initially without oral or i.v. contrast enhancement to look for the presence of calcification within the pancreas itself and to look for small gallstones which can be obscured by the presence of oral contrast medium. Scans of the pancreas should then be obtained during dynamic incremental scanning following rapid infusion of intravenous contrast medium (100 ml of LOCM 300–350). This will enable identification of non-perfused areas of pancreas, and the presence of pseudocysts, abscesses and phlegmons should be sought.

PANCREATIC PSEUDOCYSTS
Initial investigation should be with ultrasound. It should be remembered that pseudocysts can occur anywhere in the abdomen or pelvis and can even be found in the thorax. The spleen and left kidney provide acoustic windows to visualize the region of the tail of the pancreas.

CT scanning may also be performed if bowel loops prevent adequate visualization. It should always be performed prior to radiologically guided intervention to prevent drainage of a pseudoaneurysm. (During ultrasonography supposed fluid collections can be interrogated with colour or duplex Doppler).

Further reading   Freeny, P.C. (ed.) (1989) Radiology of the pancreas. *Radiol. Clin. N. Am.* **27**(1).
Jones, S.N. (1991) Editorial. The drainage of pancreatic fluid collections. *Clin. Radiol.* **43**, 153–155.

Pancreatic Carcinoma

First-line investigation is usually ultrasound. Having diagnosed a pancreatic mass, local extension should be determined with special reference to the portal vein; patency should be verified with duplex or colour flow Doppler. Other features to be ascertained are encasement of vessels, relationship of tumour to inferior vena cava, spread to adjacent bowel, regional lymphadenopathy and any distant metastases. If the mass is easily visible on ultrasound it can be used to guide biopsy.

If ultrasound fails to diagnose a lesion or suggests that surgery is possible, CT should be performed either to identify a focal pancreatic lesion or to confirm surgical resectability. When the patient presents with jaundice, ultrasound is usually followed by ERCP. If surgery is not planned, endoscopic stenting may be performed to relieve the jaundice.

Angiography is performed in some cases prior to surgery to exclude encasement of the portal and superior mesenteric veins in particular.

Further reading

Freeny, P.C. (1989) Radiologic diagnosis and staging of pancreatic ductal adenocarcinoma. *Radiol. Clin. N. Am.* **27**, 121–128.

Thompson, J.N. (1990) Diagnosing cancer of the pancreas. *BMJ* **301**, 775–776.

Zollinger–Ellison Syndrome

Caused by a gastrin-secreting tumour, usually within the pancreas or adjacent duodenum. 60% are malignant and may metastasize. Gastrinoma may be associated with parathyroid adenoma or pituitary adenoma in multiple endocrine neoplasia syndrome. Gastrinoma may present with recurrent severe peptic ulceration and is diagnosed by elevated gastrin levels in association with an elevated basal acid output.

Barium studies (or endoscopy) may show thickened gastric and duodenal folds and ulceration continuing beyond the first part of the duodenum. Having confirmed the tumour by elevated gastrin levels, investigations are directed at localization of the tumour before surgery. Ultrasound and CT may show a larger tumour in the pancreas or duodenum and indicate liver or nodal metastases if present. Selective pancreatic angiography and transhepatic pancreatic venous sampling have been more likely to localize a small primary tumour. Intraoperative ultrasound shows great promise in demonstrating the tumour and endoscopic ultrasound is also likely to be effective.

Further reading
Rossi, P., Allison, D.J., Bezzi, M. et al (1989) Endocrine tumours of the pancreas. *Radiol. Clin. N. Am.* **27**, 129–161.

5 Urinary Tract

Methods of imaging the urinary tract

1. Plain films, including tomography.
2. Excretion urography.
3. Micturating cystourethrography.
4. Ascending urethrography.
5. Retrograde pyeloureterography.
6. Percutaneous renal puncture.
7. Arteriography.
8. Venography – including renal vein sampling.
9. Ultrasound.
10. Radionuclide imaging
    – static
    – dynamic
    – radionuclide cystography – direct and indirect.
11. CT.
12. MRI.

Further reading

Amis, E.S. Jr (ed.) (1991) Contemporary Uroradiology. *Radiol. Clin. N. Am.* **29**(3).

Clements, R., Griffiths, G.J. & Peeling, W.B. (1991) Review article. 'State of the art' transrectal ultrasound imaging in the assessment of prostatic disease. *Br. J. Radiol.* **64**, 193–200.

Clements, R., Griffiths, G.J. & Peeling, W.B. (1992) Review. Staging prostatic cancer. *Clin. Radiol.* **46**, 225–231.

Evans, C. (1987) Annotation: renal failure radiology – 1987. *Clin. Radiol.* **38**, 457–462.

Friedland, G.W. (1990) Editorial. The urethra – imaging and intervention in the 1990s. *Clin. Radiol.* **42**, 157–160.

Husband, J.E. (1992) Review. Staging bladder cancer. *Clin. Radiol.* **46**, 153–159.

Lang, E.K. (ed.) (1986) Interventional Radiology. *Radiol. Clin. N. Am.* **24**(4).

Rees, J.I.S. & Evans, C. (1991) Editorial. Imaging after renal transplantation. *Clin. Radiol.* **43**, 4–7.

Excretion Urography

Indications   Suspected urinary tract pathology.

Contraindications   See p. 4 — general contraindications to water-soluble contrast media.

Dehydration is contraindicated in the following situations:
1. Renal failure.
2. Myeloma.
3. Infancy.

Contrast medium   HOCM or LOCM 370 are acceptable but the following 'high-risk' groups should receive LOCM:
1. Infants and small children and the elderly.
2. Those with renal and/or cardiac failure.
3. Poorly hydrated patients.
4. Patients with diabetes, myelomatosis or sickle-cell anaemia.
5. Patients who have had a previous severe contrast medium reaction with LOCM or those with a strong allergic history.

Adult dose   50 ml.

Paediatric dose[1]   1 ml kg^{-1}.

Patient preparation
1. No food for 5 hours prior to the examination. Dehydration is not necessary and does not improve image quality[2].
2. Patients should, preferably, be ambulant for 2 hours prior to the examination to reduce bowel gas.
3. The routine administration of bowel preparation fails to improve the diagnostic quality of the examination and its use makes the examination more unpleasant for the patient[3].
4. If the examination is to be performed on a patient who has previously had a severe contrast medium reaction, consideration should be given to administering methyl prednisolone 32 mg orally 12 and 2 hours prior to injection of contrast medium in addition to ensuring that a LOCM is used.

Preliminary films
1. Supine, full-length AP of the abdomen, in inspiration. The lower border of the cassette is at the level of the symphysis pubis and the X-ray beam is centred in the mid-line at the level of the iliac crests.
2. Supine AP of the renal areas, in expiration. The X-ray beam is centred in the mid-line at the level of the lower costal margin.

The position of overlying opacities may be further determined by:

3. 35% posterior oblique views, or
4. Tomography of the kidneys[4, 5] at the level of a third of the AP diameter of the patient (approx. 8–11 cm) The optimal angle of swing is 25–40°.

The examination should not proceed further until these films have been reviewed by the radiologist and deemed satisfactory.

Technique
The median antecubital vein is the preferred injection site because flow is retarded in the cephalic vein as it pierces the clavipectoral fascia. A 19G needle is advanced up the vein to reduce the risk of a perivenous injection and the injection is given rapidly as a bolus to maximize the density of the nephrogram.

Upper arm or shoulder pain may be due to stasis of contrast medium in the vein. This is relieved by abduction of the arm.

Films
1. *Immediate film*. AP of the renal areas. This film is exposed 10–14 s after the injection (arm-to-kidney time). It aims to show the nephrogram, i.e. the renal parenchyma opacified by contrast medium in the renal tubules.
2. *5-min film*. AP of the renal areas. This film is taken to determine if excretion is symmetrical and is invaluable for assessing the need to modify technique, e.g. a further injection of contrast medium if there has been poor initial opacification.

A compression band is now applied around the patient's abdomen and the balloon positioned midway between the anterior superior iliac spines,

i.e. precisely over the ureters as they cross the pelvic brim. The aim is to produce better pelvicalyceal distension. Compression is contraindicated:
(a) after recent abdominal surgery
(b) after renal trauma
(c) if there is a large abdominal mass
(d) when the 5-minute film shows already distended calyces.

3. *15-min film.* AP of the renal areas. There is usually adequate distension of the pelvicalyceal systems with opaque urine by this time. Compression is released when satisfactory demonstration of the pelvicalyceal system has been achieved.

4. *Release film.* Supine AP abdomen. This film is taken to show the whole urinary tract. If this film is satisfactory, the patient is asked to empty his bladder.

5. *After micturition film.* Based on the clinical findings and the radiological findings on the earlier films, this will be either a full-length abdominal film or a coned view of the bladder with the tube angled 15° caudad and centred 5 cm above the symphysis pubis. The principal value of this film is to assess bladder emptying, to demonstrate a return to normal of dilated upper tracts with relief of bladder pressure, to aid the diagnosis of bladder tumours, to confirm ureterovesical junction calculi and, uncommonly, to demonstrate a urethral diverticulum in females[6, 7].

ADDITIONAL FILMS
1. 35° posterior obliques of the kidneys, ureters or bladder.
2. Tomography — when there are confusing overlying shadows.
3. 30° caudad angulation of the tube for the renal area. This may throw a faecal laden transverse colon clear of the kidneys.
4. Prone abdomen — may provide better visualization of the ureters by making them more dependent.
5. Delayed films — may be necessary for up to 24 hours after injection in cases of obstructive uropathy.

The infant   1. As in all paediatric work the technique should be flexible to suit the problem. The radiologist should inspect each film and decide on any modification of technique before the next film. A typical basic film sequence is:
(a) a 2-min film of the renal areas
(b) a 5-min film of the renal areas
(c) a 15-min full-length abdominal film.

We do not use abdominal compression on the young infant.

Excretion of contrast medium during the first month of life is delayed and prolonged. Optimum visualization of the upper urinary tract may not occur until 1–3 hours. Therefore, if the initial 2- and 5-min films show little opacification, further films at 1, 2 and 3 hours may provide more information than multiple films in the first hour[8].

For the older child the adult film sequence is used.

2. Excessive bowel gas may interfere with satisfactory visualization of the kidneys. A fizzy drink will produce a gas-filled stomach, which acts as a window through which the kidneys can be seen[9]. If the gas-filled stomach is not large enough to reveal the right kidney, the patient can be turned into the RPO position.

If this technique is unsuccessful, tomography may be employed. The radiation dose can be limited by the use of a multi-layer cassette.

A lateral abdominal film may also be useful by enabling the kidney to be viewed behind the bowel gas shadows.

Excretory
micturating
cystourethrography

This technique is used when further information is required regarding the urethra or the act of micturition. However, opacification is not as great as when contrast medium is instilled retrogradely. Excretion urography is performed in the usual manner and when the bladder is full spot films are taken of the bladder and urethra during micturition. (See p. 163 for details of positioning, etc.)

Complingications

Due to the contrast medium   See pp. 9 and 24.

Due to the technique   Malplaced abdominal compression may produce intolerable discomfort or hypotension.

References   1. Cohen, M.D. (1979) Intravenous urography in neonates and infants. What dose of contrast should be used? *Br. J. Radiol.* **52**, 942–944.
2. Bell, K.E. & McIlrath, E.M. (1985) Dehydration in urography: is it really necessary? *Clin. Radiol.* **36**, 311–312.
3. Bailey, S.R., Tyrrell, P.N.M. & Hale, M. (1991) A trial to assess the effectiveness of bowel preparation prior to intravenous urography. *Clin. Radiol.* **44**, 335–337.
4. Dure-Smith, P. & McArdle, G.H. (1972) Tomography during excretory urography: technical aspects. *Br. J. Radiol.* **45**, 896–901.
5. Hattery, R.R., Williamson, B. Jr. & Hartman, G.W. (1976) Urinary tract tomography. *Radiol. Clin. N. Am.* **14**, 23–49.
6. Gerber, W.L. & Brown, R.C. (1985) The value of post-void radiographs in excretion urography. *Clin. Radiol.* **36**, 525–527.
7. Morewood, D.J.W. & Scally, J.K. (1986) An evaluation of the post-micturition radiograph following intravenous urography. *Clin. Radiol.* **37**, 499–500.
8. Nogrady, M.B. & Scott Dunbar, J. (1968) Delayed concentration and prolonged excretion of urographic contrast medium in the first month of life. *Am. J. Roentg.* **104**, 189–195.
9. Hope, J.W. & Campoy, F. (1955) The use of carbonated beverages in paediatric excretory urography. *Radiology*, **64**, 66–71.

Percutaneous Renal Puncture

Indications

1. Renal cyst puncture. At autopsy 50% of those over 50 years have grossly detectable renal cysts. 4.5% of all patients undergoing excretion urography have asymptomatic renal lesions but only 2.5% of these will be primary malignant tumours[1]. Using strict diagnostic criteria ultrasound or CT are very accurate in diagnosing the uncomplicated renal cyst which does not need further evaluation[2, 3]. Nevertheless, approximately 5% of all renal lesions will be of indeterminate aetiology on initial ultrasound or CT examination. Indications for cyst puncture, therefore, include:
   (a) indeterminate mass
   (b) ultrasound and CT results inconclusive or conflicting
   (c) calcification within a cyst wall.
   Clinical signs or symptoms may not correlate with the diagnosis of a simple cyst and the following are also indications for cyst puncture:
   (d) unexplained haematuria with an apparent cyst
   (e) unexplained fever with an apparent cyst.
   Therapeutic indications for cyst puncture are:
   (f) to relieve local symptoms attributable to a cyst.

2. Antegrade pyelography:
   (a) when other less invasive imaging modalities fail to delineate the cause and/or level of an obstruction
   (b) when retrograde pyelography is unsuccessful or not possible, e.g. internal ureteral diversion
   (c) to facilitate renal pressure/flow studies. This is performed when other modalities, particularly diuretic renography, have failed to demonstrate whether the dilated upper urinary tract is truly obstructed.

3. Prior to, or as part of, percutaneous nephrostomy (see p. 156).

Contraindications
1. As for water-soluble contrast medium in the radiographic method (see p. 4).
2. Bleeding diathesis.
3. The possibility of renal hydatid disease.

Contrast medium
1. For preliminary visualization of the kidneys — as for excretion urography.
2. To outline the pelvicalyceal system or renal cyst — any HOCM or LOCM 200. Volume is dependent on the size of the cyst or collecting system.

Equipment
1. Fluoroscopy unit, ultrasound machine or CT scanner
2. Overcouch tube.
3. 22G needle, e.g. Chiba or Greenburg.

Patient preparation
1. As for excretion urography if this method is used to outline the kidney.
2. Confirm normal blood coagulation.
3. Nervous patients may need sedation; children will need general anaesthesia.

Preliminary film
Supine AP of the renal area for the radiographic method.

Technique
Insertion of the needle can be controlled by three imaging methods:
1. Fluoroscopy.
2. Ultrasonography
3. CT

RENAL CYST PUNCTURE

1. The patient is placed in the prone position. A radiolucent pad is placed under the abdomen to limit anterior movement of the kidney.
2. The cyst is located indirectly after opacification of the kidneys with i.v. contrast medium or directly with ultrasound. The optimum site for puncture is marked on the skin.
3. The skin and subcutaneous tissues are infiltrated with 1% lignocaine.
4. The needle is passed directly into the lesion during suspended respiration. Intermittent fluoroscopy, ultrasound or CT is used to monitor the path of the needle. The combined use of ultrasound and

fluoroscopy is often very helpful[4]. The needle may be deflected around the cyst and, if this happens, it will be necessary to advance it into the cyst with a quick thrust.

5. The stillette is removed and the cyst contents aspirated and examined
   - (a) biochemically – fat, protein ⎫ as
   - (b) bacteriologically ⎬ clinically
   - (c) cytologically ⎭ indicated.

   Simple cyst fluid is clear and straw-coloured. Some authors have suggested that if such fluid is aspirated then no further investigation is necessary[5, 6]. If no fluid can be aspirated, the position of the needle can be confirmed with ultrasound or CT, and adjustment of position made. If the procedure is performed with fluoroscopy only, the needle is withdrawn until fluid is obtained. If that is unsuccessful, a further attempt at puncture is made.

6. When approximately 75% of the cyst contents have been aspirated, 25% of the aspirated volume is replaced with contrast medium and 50% with air. This enables dual contrast pictures to be obtained. The needle is removed.

FILMS

The choice of films is designed to outline all the walls of the cyst with both air and contrast medium. Using the overcouch tube with the beam centred on and collimated to the affected kidney:

1. Prone lateral.
2. Supine lateral.
3. Right and left lateral decubitus.
4. Supine AP
5. Erect AP.

Modification of technique

1. If after correct needle placement, either no fluid or only grossly haemorrhagic aspirate is obtained then it can be presumed that the mass is solid in nature. Cytological examination of the aspirate is most important as there is a 25% chance of carcinoma being present[7]. A small amount of contrast medium is injected into the lesion and AP and lateral radiographs exposed. These will demonstrate contrast material within the interstices of the lesion.

ANTEGRADE PYELOGRAPHY

1. The needle is introduced as for cyst puncture but directed through the renal parenchyma into a minor calyx. This reduces the risk of laceration of the pelvis and extravasation of urine.
2. Contrast medium is introduced until the level of obstruction is outlined.

FILMS
(a) AP
(b) both 35° posterior obliques.

Contrast medium should be removed from an obstructed pelvis to prevent the development of chemical pyelitis.

RENAL PRESSURE/FLOW STUDY

1. Vesicoureteric reflux should already have been excluded.
2. Catheters in the bladder and rectum are used to measure true intravesical pressure. Following antegrade puncture of the renal pelvis, the needle is connected to equipment that will infuse saline and measure intrapelvic pressure. *Absolute* intrapelvic pressure and *relative* pressure (bladder pressure subtracted from renal pressure) can be recorded during the infusion.
3. In the normal urinary tract, infusion at a rate of 10 ml min^{-1} produces a relative pressure in the renal pelvis less than 13 cmH_2O. Pressures greater than 20 cmH_2O indicate obstruction while those in the range 14–20 cmH_2O are equivocal[8].

Aftercare Chest radiograph to exclude a pneumothorax or haemopneumothorax[9].

Complications Major (1%), minor (10%)[10].

Due to the contrast medium
1. Contrast medium can be absorbed from the intact renal pelvis and give rise to adverse reactions.
2. Chemical pyelitis from prolonged contact of contrast medium with the obstructed pelvis.

Due to the technique
1. Perirenal and intrarenal haemorrhage.
2. Haematuria.

3. Pneumothorax.
4. Infection – new or an exacerbation by puncture of a pyonephrosis.
5. Pain.
6. Urinoma.
7. Arteriovenous fistula.
8. Puncture of adjacent organs.

References

1. Lang, E.K. (1980) Roentgenologic approach to the diagnosis and management of cystic lesions of the kidney: Is cyst exploration mandatory? *Urol. Clin. N. Am.* **7**, 677–688.
2. Pollack, H.M., Banner, M.P., Arger, P.H. et al (1982) The accuracy of gray-scale renal ultrasound in differentiating cystic neoplasms from benign cysts. *Radiology* **143**, 741–745.
3. McClennan, B.L., Stanley, R.J., Melson, G.L. et al (1979) CT of the renal cyst: Is cyst aspiration necessary? *Am. J. Roentg.* **133**, 671–675.
4. Raskin, M.M., Roen, S.A. & Serafini, A.N. (1974) Renal cyst puncture: combined fluoroscopic and ultrasonic technique. *Radiology* **113**, 425–427.
5. Stewart, B.H. & Pasalis, J.K. (1976) Aspiration and cytology in the evaluation of renal mass lesions. *Cleve. Clin. Q.* **43**, 1–6.
6. Levine, S.R., Emmet, J.L. & Woolner, L.B. (1964) Cyst and tumour occuring in the same kidney. *J. Urol.* **91**, 8–9.
7. Ainsworth, W.L. & Vest, S.A. (1951) The differential diagnosis between renal tumours and cysts. *J. Urol.* **64**, 740–749.
8. Whitaker, R.H. (1979) An evaluation of 170 diagnostic pressure flow studies in the upper urinary tract. *J. Urol.* **121**, 602–604.
9. Jeans, W.D., Penry, J.N. & Roylance, J. (1972) Renal puncture. *Clin. Radiol.* **23**, 298–311.
10. Lang, E.K. (1977) Renal cyst puncture and aspiration: a survey of complications. *Am. J. Roentg.* **128**, 723–727.

Further reading

Pfister, R. & Newhouse, J. (1979) Interventional percutaneous pyeloureteral techniques. I Antegrade pyelography and ureteral perfusion. II Percutaneous nephrostomy and other procedures. *Radiol. Clin. N. Am.* **17**, 341–363.

Sandler, C.M., Houston, G.K., Hall, J.T. & Morettin, L.B. (1986) Guided cyst puncture and aspiration. *Radiol. Clin. N. Am.* **24**, 527–537

Percutaneous Nephrostomy

The introduction of a drainage catheter into the collecting system of the kidney.

Indications
1. Obstructive uropathy.
2. Prior to percutaneous nephrolithotomy.
3. Ureteric fistulae; external drainage may allow closure.

Contraindications   Uncontrolled bleeding diathesis.

Contrast medium   As for percutaneous renal puncture.

Equipment
1. Puncturing needle (18G); Longdwell, or equivalent.
2. Drainage catheter: at least 7F pigtail with multiple side holes.
3. Guide-wires: conventional angiographic and Lunderquist.
4. Fluoroscopy and real-time ultrasound, if possible.

Patient preparation
1. Fasting for 4 hours.
2. Premedication.
3. Prophylactic antibiotic.
4. Surgical backup in view of clinical workup, possible complications and further management.
5. The patient should empty the bladder just prior to the procedure.

Technique
Patient position   With the patient lying in the prone position on the fluoroscopic table, a foam pad or non-opaque pillow is placed under the abdomen so that the kidney lies in a fixed posterior position. An oblique position with the kidney to be punctured raised is sometimes used.

Identifying the collecting system
1. Excretion urography, if adequate residual function.
2. Antegrade pyelography.
3. Real-time ultrasound may be used to identify the renal pelvis for antegrade pyelography and to determine the plane of definitive puncture of the collecting system. With a biopsy needle attachment, a real-time ultrasound probe may be used to

guide the puncturing needle into the collecting system.

Site/plane of puncture

A point on the posterior axillary line is chosen below the twelfth rib. Having identified the mid/lower pole calyces with contrast/ultrasound, the plane of puncture is determined. This will be via the soft tissues and renal parenchyma, in which plane vessels around the renal pelvis will be avoided and the drainage catheter will gain some purchase on the renal parenchyma. The drainage catheter is also more comfortable for the patient in this plane, and is less likely to be kinked when he/she lies supine.

Techniques of puncture, catheterization

The skin and soft tissues are infiltrated with local anaesthetic using a spinal needle. Puncture may then be made using one of the following systems (depending on preference):

1. An 18G sheathed needle, a cyst puncture or a Longdwell needle, in conjunction with the Seldinger technique for catheterization. Upon successful puncture a J guide-wire is inserted and coiled within the collecting system; the sheath is then pushed over the wire, which is exchanged for a more rigid Lunderquist wire. If possible the guide-wire is manipulated into the ureter. Dilatation is then performed to 1F greater than the size of the drainage catheter, which is then inserted. During all manipulation, care must be taken not to kink the guide-wire within the soft tissues. A substantial amount of guide-wire should be maintained within the collecting system so that position is not lost and if kinking does occur, then the kinked portion of the wire can be withdrawn outside the skin.
2. *The Cope needle system*, using a 21G puncturing needle that takes a special guide-wire. This affords a single puncture with a fine needle, leading on to eventual catheterization.
3. *The trocar-cannula system*, in which direct puncture of the collecting system is made with the drainage catheter already assembled over a trocar. On removal of the trocar the drainage catheter is pushed further into the collecting system.

Having successfully introduced a catheter, the latter is securely fixed to the skin and drainage commenced.

Aftercare
1. Bed rest for 12 hours.
2. Both blood pressure and temperature half-hourly for 6 hours.
3. Urine cultures and sensitivity.

Complications
1. Unsuccessful drainage.
2. Haemorrhage.
3. Perforation of the collecting system.
4. Septicaemia.

Percutaneous Nephrolithotomy

The removal of renal calculi through a nephrostomy tract.

Indications
1. Removal of renal calculi.
2. Disintegration of large renal calculi.

Contraindications
Uncontrolled bleeding diathesis.

Contrast medium
As for percutaneous renal puncture.

Equipment
1. Puncturing needle (18G): Longdwell or equivalent.
2. Guide-wires, including J-angiographic and Lunderquist.
3. Tract dilating equipment; Teflon dilators (from 7F to 30F), metal coaxial dilators or a special angioplasty balloon catheter.
4. Fluoroscopy facilities with rotating C arm if possible.

Patient preparation
1. Full discussion between radiologist/urologist concerning indications, etc.
2. Admission on the day prior to the procedure. A general anaesthetic is usually required.
3. Coagulation screen.
4. Two units of blood cross matched.
5. Antibiotic cover.
6. Premedication.
7. Bladder catheterization.

Technique
Patient position
As for a percutaneous nephrostomy (see p. 156).

Methods of opacification of the collecting system
1. Excretion urography.
2. Retrograde ureteric catheterization; distension of the collecting system may be achieved.
3. Antegrade pyelography; this also enables distension of the collecting system.

Puncture of the collecting system
A lower pole posterior calyx is chosen if the calculus is situated in the renal pelvis. Otherwise the calyx in which the calculus is situated must be punctured. Special care must be taken if puncturing above the

twelfth rib because of the risk of perforating the diaphragm and pleura. Puncture is in an oblique plane from the posterior axillary line through the renal parenchyma. Puncture of the selected calyx is made using either a rotating C-arm fluoroscopic facility or rocking the patient to determine the depth of the calyx in relation to the needle tip. On successful puncture a J guide-wire is inserted through the sheath and as much wire as possible is guided into the collecting system. The sheath is then pushed over the wire, which is exchanged for a more rigid Lunderquist wire. If possible, the wire is manipulated into the ureter. At this stage full dilation may be performed (single stage) or a nephrostomy tube left in situ with dilatation later (two-stage procedure).

Dilatation   This is carried out under general anaesthesia. It is performed using Teflon dilators from 7F to 30F which are introduced over the guide-wire. Alternatively, metal coaxial dilators or a special angioplasty balloon (10 cm long) are used. A sheath is inserted over the largest dilator or balloon and through the sheath lumen removal of the calculus or disintegration is performed.

Removal/
disintegration   Removal of calculi of less than 1 cm is possible using a nephroscope and forceps. Larger calculi must be disintegrated using an ultrasonic or electrohydraulic disintegrator.

Aftercare   1. Usually determined by the anaesthetist/urologist.
2. Plain radiograph of renal area to ensure that all calculi/fragments have been removed.

Complications   IMMEDIATE
1. Failure of access, dilatation or removal.
2. Perforation of the renal pelvis on dilatation.
3. Haemorrhage.
4. Damage to surrounding structures, i.e. diaphragm, colon, spleen and liver.
5. Problems related to the irrigating fluid, i.e. haemolysis.

DELAYED
Aneurysm of an intrarenal artery.

Retrograde Pyeloureterography

Indications	1. Demonstration of the site, length, lower limit and, if possible, the nature of an obstructive lesion. 2. Demonstration of the pelvicalyceal system after an unsatisfactory excretion urogram. Seldom necessary with modern imaging methods.
Contraindications	Acute urinary tract infection.
Contrast medium	HOCM or LOCM 150–200, i.e. not too dense to obscure small lesions. 10 ml.
Equipment	Fluoroscopy unit.
Patient preparation	As for surgery.
Preliminary film	Full-length supine AP abdomen when the examination is performed in the X-ray department.

Technique

In the operating theatre

The surgeon catheterizes the ureter via a cystoscope and advances the ureteric catheter to the desired level. Contrast medium is injected under fluoroscopic control and spot films exposed.

In the X-ray department

1. With ureteric catheter(s) in situ, the patient is transferred from the operating theatre to the X-ray department.
2. Urine is aspirated and under fluoroscopic control contrast medium is slowly injected. About 3–5 ml are usually enough to fill the pelvis but the injection should be terminated before this if the patient complains of pain or fullness in the loin.

FILMS
Using the undercouch tube:
(a) supine PA of the kidney
(b) both 35° anterior obliques of the kidney.

3. If there is pelviureteric junction obstruction, the contrast medium in the pelvis is aspirated. The films are examined and if satisfactory, the catheter is withdrawn, first to 10 cm below the renal pelvis, and then to lie just above the ureteric orifice.

About 2 ml of contrast medium are injected at each of these levels and films taken.

FILMS
Using the undercouch tube:
(a)　supine PA of the ureter
(b)　both 35° anterior obliques of the ureter.

N.B. The catheter may be left in the pelvis to drain a pelviureteric obstruction. In this case withdrawal ureterograms are not possible.

Aftercare　1. Post-anaesthetic observations.
2. Prophylactic antibiotics may be used.

Complications
Due to the anaesthetic

Complications of general anaesthesia.

Due to the contrast medium

1. Contrast medium can be absorbed from the intact renal pelvis, giving rise to adverse reactions. However, the risks are much less than with excretion urography.
2. Chemical pyelitis — if there is stasis of contrast medium.
3. Extravasation due to overdistension of the pelvis. This is usually asymptomatic but may result in pain, fever and rigors.

Due to the technique

1. Introduction of infection.
2. Mucosal damage to the ureter.
3. Perforation of the ureter or pelvis by the catheter.

Further reading　Witten, D.M., Myers, G.H. & Utz, D.C. (1977) Retrograde pyelography. In: Witten, D.M., Myers, G.H. & Utz, D.C. (eds), *Emmett's Clinical Urography*, pp. 58–64. Philadelphia: W.B. Saunders.

Micturating Cystourethrography

Indications	1. Vesicoureteric reflux. 2. Study of the urethra during micturition. 3. Abnormalities of the bladder. 4. Stress incontinence.
Contraindications	Acute urinary tract infection.
Contrast medium	HOCM or LOCM 150.
Equipment	1. Fluoroscopy unit with spot film device and tilting table. 2. Video recorder. 3. Jaques or Foley catheter. In small infants a fine (5–7F) feeding tube is adequate.
Patient preparation	The patient micturates prior to the examination.
Preliminary film	Coned view of the bladder, using the undercouch tube.

Technique

To demonstrate vesicoureteric reflux

1. This indication is almost exclusively confined to children.
2. The patient lies supine on the X-ray table. Using aseptic technique a catheter, lubricated with Hibitane 0.05% in glycerine, is introduced into the bladder. Residual urine is drained. Contrast medium is slowly dripped in and bladder filling is observed by intermittent fluoroscopy.
3. Any reflux is recorded on spot films.
4. The catheter should not be removed until the radiologist is convinced that the patient will micturate or until no more contrast medium will drip into the bladder. The examination is expedited if the catheter remains in situ until micturition commences and then is quickly withdrawn.
5. Older children and adults are given a urine receiver but smaller children should be allowed to micturate onto absorbent pads on which they can lie. Children can lie on the table but adults will probably find it easier to micturate while standing erect.

6. In infants and children with a neuropathic bladder micturition may be accomplished by suprapubic pressure.
7. Spot films are taken during micturition and any reflux recorded. A video recording may be useful. The lower ureter is best seen in the anterior oblique position of that side. Boys should micturate in the LAO position, with right hip and knee flexed, or in the RAO position, with left hip and knee flexed, so that spot films can be taken of the entire urethra.
8. Finally, a full-length view of the abdomen is taken to demonstrate any reflux of contrast medium that might have occurred unnoticed into the kidneys and to record the post-micturition residue.

To demonstrate a vesicovaginal or rectovesical fistula

As above, but films are taken in the lateral position.

To demonstrate stress incontinence

Initially the technique is as for demonstrating vesicoureteric reflux. The catheter is left in situ until the patient is in the erect position.

FILMS
These should include sacrum and symphysis pubis because bony landmarks are used to assess bladder neck descent.
1. Lateral bladder.
2. Lateral bladder, straining.

The catheter is then removed.

3. Lateral bladder during micturition.

Aftercare

No special aftercare is necessary, but patients and parents of children should be warned that dysuria, possibly leading to retention of urine, may be experienced. In such cases a simple analgesic is helpful and children may be helped by allowing them to micturate in a warm bath.

Complications
Due to the contrast medium

1. Adverse reactions may result from absorption of contrast medium by the bladder mucosa.

The risk is small when compared with excretion urography.
2. Contrast medium-induced cystitis.

Due to the technique
1. Acute urinary tract infection.
2. Catheter trauma — may produce dysuria, frequency, haematuria and urinary retention.
3. Complications of bladder filling, e.g. perforation from overdistension — prevented by using a non-retaining catheter, e.g. Jaques.
4. Catheterization of vagina or an ectopic ureteral orifice.
5. Retention of a Foley catheter.

Further reading
Jeffcoate, T.N.A. (1958) Urethrocystography in the female. *J. Fac. Radiol.* **2**, 127–134.
McAlister, W.H., Cacciarelli, A. & Shackelford, G.D. (1974) Complications associated with cystography in children. *Radiology* **111**, 167–172.

Ascending Urethrography in the Male

Indications
1. Strictures.
2. Urethral tears.
3. Congenital abnormalities.
4. Periurethral or prostatic abscess.
5. Fistulae or false passages.

Contraindications
1. Acute urinary tract infection.
2. Recent instrumentation.

Contrast medium
HOCM or LOCM 200–300. 20 ml. Pre-warming the contrast medium will help reduce the incidence of spasm of the external sphincter.

Equipment
1. Tilting radiography table with fluoroscopy unit and spot film device.
2. Foley catheter or penile clamp, e.g. Knutsson's.

Patient preparation
None.

Preliminary film
Coned supine PA of bladder base and urethra.

Technique
1. The patient lies supine on the X-ray table.
2. Using aseptic technique the penile clamp is applied or the tip of the catheter is inserted so that the balloon lies in the fossa navicularis and its balloon is inflated with 1–2 ml of water. Contrast medium is injected under fluoroscopic control and film taken in the following positions:
   (a) 30° LAO, with right leg abducted and knee flexed.
   (b) supine PA
   (c) 30° RAO, with left leg abducted and knee flexed.
3. Ascending urethrography should be followed by micturating cystourethrography or excretory micturating cystourethrography to demonstrate the proximal urethra. Occasionally a urethral fistula or periurethral abscess is seen only on the voiding examination; reflux of contrast medium into dilated prostatic ducts is also better seen during micturition.

Aftercare   None.

Complications
Due to the contrast   Adverse reactions are rare.
medium

Due to the technique   1. Acute urinary tract infection.
2. Urethral trauma.
3. Intravasation of contrast medium, especially if excessive pressure is used to overcome a stricture.

Further reading   McCallum, R.W. (1979) The adult male urethra. Normal anatomy, pathology and method of urethrography. *Radiol. Clin. N. Am.* 17(2), 227–244.

Ultrasound of the Urinary Tract in Adults

Indications
1. Suspected renal mass lesion.
2. Suspected renal parenchymal disease.
3. Possible renal obstruction.
4. Haematuria.
5. Renal cystic disease.
6. Renal size measurement.
7. To facilitate accurate needle placement in interventional procedures.
8. Prostatism.
9. Bladder volume before and after micturition.
10. Bladder tumour.

Contraindications None.

Patient preparation None – unless full bladder is required.

Equipment 3.5–5 MHz transducer.

Technique
1. Patient supine, right and left anterior oblique positions or prone for kidneys. The kidneys are scanned longitudinally and transversely. The right kidney may be scanned through the liver and posteriorly in the right loin. The left kidney is harder to visualize anteriorly unless the spleen is large, but can be visualized from the left loin.
2. The length of the kidney measured by ultrasound is smaller than that measured at excretion urography because there is no geometric magnification and no change in size related to contrast-induced osmotic diuresis. With ultrasound measurement, care must be taken to ensure that the true longitudinal diameter is scanned. The mean length of the normal adult right kidney is 10.7 cm and the left 11.1 cm (range 9–12 cm).
3. The bladder is scanned suprapubically in transverse and longitudinal planes. Measurements taken of three diameters before and after micturition enable an approximate volume to be calculated.

Further reading   Kriegshauser, J.S. & Carroll, B.A. (1991) The urinary tract. In: Rumack, C.M., Wilson, S.R. & Charboneau, J.W. (eds) *Diagnostic ultrasound*, Vol. 1, pp. 210–216. St Louis: Mosby Year Book.
Mittelstaedt, C.A. (1987) *Abdominal Ultrasound*, pp. 226–228. Edinburgh: Churchill Livingstone.

Ultrasound of the Urinary Tract in Children

The availability of high-resolution real-time ultrasound has revolutionized the investigation of paediatric renal disease during the last decade. It demonstrates anatomy without the necessity for adequate renal function but, because it gives no functional information, it is the ideal complement to nuclear medicine imaging. It should be stressed that the technique is only as good as the effort put in to obtain the images.

Indications
(after Lebowitz, 1985)[1]

1. Urinary tract infection — to document scarring, elicit signs of acute upper tract infection and to exclude an underlying structural abnormality[2, 3].
2. An abdominal or pelvic mass. Ultrasonography will demonstrate the relationship of the mass to other organs, its possible site of origin and its characteristics, i.e. solid or cystic and the presence of calcification.
3. Renal failure — to differentiate medical from surgical causes.
4. Abnormal antenatal ultrasound — to confirm or refute an antenatal diagnosis of hydronephrosis or multicystic dysplasia. The role of ultrasound should be to help in the efficient planning of the postnatal management before infection occurs and plasma creatinine rises, rather than to provoke antenatal intervention[4]. It must be remembered that, because urine output falls rapidly after birth when compared with in utero, US on day 1 may show considerably less pelvicalyceal dilatation than was observed on the antenatal scans. Further follow-up scans are mandatory.
5. To determine the site of obstruction when excretion urography or renography have failed to determine the exact level[5].
6. To evaluate a kidney not visualized by other modalities.
7. Conditions associated with a high likelihood of renal abnormalities, e.g. imperforate anus and

genital anomalies. The most frequently found abnormalities are a single or ectopic kidney.

8. Conditions which predispose to renal tumours — Beckwith–Wiedemann syndrome, hemihypertrophy and aniridia. Periodic screening is necessary.

9. Screening of family members for genetically linked renal diseases, e.g. dominant polycystic renal disease.

10. Periodic follow-up of kidneys which are at risk of deterioration, e.g. children with myelomeningocoele or urinary diversion. Patients on chronic dialysis have a high incidence of acquired cystic disease and may develop adenomas or adenocarcinomas.

11. To assess the patency of the IVC in patients with Wilms' tumour.

12. To assess residual bladder volume.

13. To facilitate the accurate placement of needles for renal biopsy, antegrade pyelography, percutaneous nephrostomy, cyst aspiration and drainage of perinephric collections.

When assessing possible renal disease by ultrasonography, a number of normal 'variants' may be confused with disease. These include increased parenchymal echogenicity in the neonatal period, echo-poor papillae which may mimic dilated calyces and persistent fetal lobulation, hepatic and splenic impressions and parenchymal junctional lines which may mimic scarring.

Equipment 3.5–7.5 MHz transducer — dependent on age.

Patient preparation Full bladder. Patients with an indwelling catheter should have this clamped 1 hour before the examination is scheduled.

Technique
1. Begin by examining the bladder, because contact of the transducer and jelly against the skin may promote bladder emptying. You may have only one chance to image the bladder.

2. It may be necessary to examine the uncooperative child while he or she sits on a carer's lap. Otherwise the technique is as for adults.

3. If possible the kidneys are examined in full inspiration or with the child being asked to 'push the tummy out'.

References   1. Lebowitz, R.L. (1985) Pediatric uroradiology. *Pediatr. Clin. N. Am.* **32**, 1353–1362.
2. Kangarloo, H., Gold, R.H., Fine, R.N., et al (1985) Urinary tract infection in infants and children evaluated by ultrasound. *Radiology* **154**, 367–373.
3. Leonidas, J.C., McCauley, R.G.K., Klauber, G.C., & Fretzayas A.M. (1985) Sonography as a substitute for excretory urography in children with urinary tract infection. *Am. J. Roentg.* **144**, 815–819.
4. Lebowitz, R. & Teele, R.L. (1983) Fetal and neonatal hydronephrosis. *Urol. Radiol.* **32**, 1353–1362.
5. Chopra, A. & Teele, R.L. (1983) Hydronephrosis in children: narrowing the differential diagnosis with ultrasound. *J. Clin. Ultrasound* **8**, 473–478.

Static Renal Scintigraphy

Indications
1. Assessment of individual renal function.
2. Assessment of the 'non-functioning' kidney on excretion urography.
3. Demonstration of ectopic renal tissue.
4. Assessment of reflux nephropathy.
5. Acute urinary tract infection.
6. Renal tumour.
7. Demonstration of congenital abnormalities and mass lesions.

Contraindications None.

Radiopharmaceuticals
1. ^{99m}Tc-2,3-dimercaptosuccinic acid (DMSA), 80 MBq max.
   Bound to plasma proteins and cleared by tubular absorption. Retained in the renal cortex, with no significant excretion during the imaging period.
2. ^{99m}Tc-glucoheptonate, 300 MBq max.
   Cleared by glomerular filtration and tubular secretion, with some retention in the renal cortex. Can provide additional information about the urinary tract, but parenchymal images are inferior to DMSA, although there is a lower radiation dose per MBq[1].

Equipment
1. Gamma camera.
2. Low-energy general purpose collimator.
3. Imaging computer.

Patient preparation None.

Technique
1. The radiopharmaceutical is administered i.v.
2. Images are acquired at any time 1–6 hours later. Imaging in the first hour is to be avoided because of free ^{99m}Tc in the urine.

Images
1. *Hard copy*: posterior, right and left posterior oblique views.
2. *Computer, for relative function*: posterior (and anterior — see analysis), 128 × 128 matrix.
3. Zoomed or pinhole views may be useful in children.

Additional image Anterior – in suspected pelvic or horseshoe kidney and severe scoliosis.

Analysis
1. Relative function is best calculated from the geometric mean of posterior and anterior computer images. A single posterior view is often used, but this makes the assumption that the kidneys are at the same depth, unless depth information is available to enable attenuation correction.
2. Absolute uptake can be estimated if required with additional information on patient and kidney size from lateral images.

Additional techniques
1. Tomography.
2. ^{99m}Tc-mercaptoacetyltriglycine(MAG-3) (max. 100 MBq) may be considered as a possible alternative to DMSA; it gives inferior kidney visualization but has the advantage of additional dynamic assessment of excretion in the same study and a lower radiation dose[2, 3].

Aftercare None.

Complications None.

References
1. Blaufox, M.D. (1991) Procedures of choice in renal nuclear medicine. *J. Nucl. Med.* **32**, 1301–1309.
2. Pickworth, F.E., Vivian, G.C., Franklin, K. & Brown, E.F. (1992) ^{99}Tc^m-mercapto acetyl triglycine in paediatric renal tract disease. *Br. J. Radiol.* **65**, 21–29.
3. Gordon, I., Anderson, P.J., Lythgoe, M.F. & Orton, M. (1992) Can technetium-99m-mercaptoacetyltriglycine replace technetium-99m-dimercaptosuccinic acid in the exclusion of a focal renal defect? *J. Nucl. Med.* **33**, 2090–2093.

Further Reading
O'Reilly, P.H., Shields, R.A. & Testa, H.J. (1986) *Nuclear Medicine in Urology and Nephrology*, 2nd edn. London: Butterworths.
Smith, F.W. & Gemmell, H.G. (1989) The urinary tract. In: Sharp, P.F., Gemmell, H.G., & Smith, F.W. (eds) *Practical Nuclear Medicine*, pp. 221–244. Oxford: Oxford University Press.

Dynamic Renal Scintigraphy

Indications

1. Diagnosis of obstructed vs. non-obstructed dilatation.
2. Diagnosis of acute tubular necrosis vs. other causes of renal failure.
3. Differentiation of hydronephrosis from multi-cystic dysplasia.
4. Assessment of renal function following drainage procedures to the urinary tract.
5. Investigation of renovascular hypertension.
6. Detection of renal artery stenosis.
7. Assessment of bladder function.
8. Demonstration of vesicoureteric reflux.
9. Assessment of renal transplantation.
10. Renal trauma.

Contraindications None.

Radiopharma-ceuticals

1. *^{99m}Tc-MAG-3*, 75 MBq typical, 100 MBq max. (400 MBq max. for quantitative haemodynamic imaging).

   Mainly cleared by tubular secretion (mean normal is approx. 370 ml min^{-1}). Fast clearance and greater kidney/background ratio than ^{99m}Tc-diethylene triamine pentacetic acid (DTPA), therefore better for poor renal function, but currently more expensive.

2. *^{99m}Tc-DTPA*. 150 MBq typical, 300 MBq max. (800 MBq max. for quantitative haemodynamic imaging).

   Cleared by glomerular filtration (mean normal is approx. 120 ml min^{-1}). Lower kidney/background ratio than MAG-3 or hippuran. Cheap and widely available.

3. *^{123}I-orthoiodohippurate (hippuran)*. 20 MBq typical (max.).

   Mainly cleared by tubular secretion (mean normal is approx. 500 ml min^{-1}). High kidney/background ratio. Renal function imaging agent of choice, but currently has high cost and limited availability due to ^{123}I being a cyclotron product.

Equipment
1. Gamma camera.
2. Low-energy general purpose collimator.
3. Imaging computer.

Patient preparation
1. The patient should be well hydrated.
2. The bladder should be emptied before injection.

Technique
1. The patient lies supine or sits with the camera posterior.
2. The radiopharmaceutical is injected i.v. and image acquisition is started simultaneously.
3. Image for 20–30 min.
4. If no excretion is seen during this time, a diuretic (frusemide 0.5 mg kg^{-1}) may be administered slowly with further imaging for up to 15 min. (As an alternative, a diuretic may be given 15 min before administration of the radiopharmaceutical[1].)

Images
All posterior.
1. *Hard copy*: 5 to 10-s images over the first minute, then 2 to 3-min images for 20–30 min.
2. *Computer*: 10 to 20-s frames for 20–30 min.

For quantitative haemodynamic investigation of renal artery patency (e.g. in renal artery stenosis or transplant kidney), 1 to 2-s frames over first minute are acquired. A 64 × 64 matrix is usually sufficient for quantitative analysis.

Analysis
The following information can be produced:
1. Kidney time–activity curves.
2. Relative function figures.
3. Perfusion index, especially in renal transplant assessment.
4. Parenchymal and whole kidney transit times.

Additional techniques
1. Pre- and 1 hour post-captopril (25–50 mg) study for evaluation of renovascular disease. The patient should stop diuretic and captopril medication 5 days prior to the test[2, 3].
2. Indirect micturating cystography following renography to demonstrate vesicoureteric reflux. When the kidneys are clear of activity, further dynamic images are acquired during micturition,

with generation of bladder and kidney time–activity curves[4].

3. Glomerular filtration rate (GFR) measurement with DTPA studies by taking blood samples for counting. Similarly, effective renal plasma flow (ERPF) measurement with hippuran and a MAG-3 clearance index may be obtained[5].

4. The images obtained with MAG-3 can be analysed for the presence of renal scarring and there is good correlation with the results obtained with DMSA (MAG-3 is 80% tubular secreted). DMSA remains the 'gold standard' for cortical scarring because of the higher information density and ability to obtain multiple projections, but the radiation dose is higher than with MAG-3[6, 7].

5. With the appropriate computer software and fast-frame acquisition, compressed images may be generated to demonstrate and quantify ureteric peristalsis and show reflux (best with MAG-3 or hippuran)[8].

Aftercare
1. The patient is warned that the effects of diuresis may last a couple of hours. The patient may feel faint because of hypotension when adopting the erect posture at the end of the procedure.

2. After captopril administration, blood pressure monitoring under medical supervision should be carried out for 1 hour.

3. Normal radiation safety precautions (see 'General Notes').

Complications
None, except after captopril, when care must be taken in patients with severe vascular disease to avoid hypotension and renal failure.

References
1. O'Reilly, P.H. (1992) Diuresis renography. Recent advances and recommended protocols. *Br. J. Urol.* **69**, 113–120.

2. Black, H.R. (1992) Captopril renal scintigraphy – a way to distinguish functional from anatomic renal artery stenosis. *J. Nucl. Med.* **33**, 2045–2046.

3. Dondi, M., Fanti, S., De Fabritiis, A. et al (1992) Prognostic value of captopril renal scintigraphy in renovascular hypertension. *J. Nucl. Med.* **33**, 2040–2044.

4. Chapman, S.J., Chantler, C., Haycock, G.B., Maisey,

M.N. & Saxton, H.M. (1988) Radionuclide cystography in vesicoureteric reflux. *Arch. Dis. Child.* **63**, 650–651.

5. Peters, A.M. (1991) Quantification of renal haemodynamics with radionuclides. *Eur. J. Nucl. Med.* **18**, 274–286.

6. Gordon, I., Anderson, P.J., Lythgoe, M.F. & Orton, M. (1992) Can Technetium-99m-mercaptoacetyltriglycine replace technetium-99m-dimercaptosuccinic acid in the exclusion of a focal renal defect? *J. Nucl. Med.* **33**, 2090–2093.

7. Pickworth, F.E., Vivian, G.C., Franklin, K. & Brown, E.F. (1992) [99]Tc[m]-mercapto acetyl triglycine in paediatric renal tract disease. *Br. J. Radiol.* **65**, 21–29.

8. Lepej, J., Kliment, J., Horák, V., Buchanec, J., Marasová, A. & Belákova, S. (1991) A new approach in radionuclide imaging to ureteric peristalsis using [99]Tc[m]-MAG-3 and condensed images. *Nucl. Med. Commun.* **12**, 397–407.

Further reading   Blaufox, M.D. (1991) Procedures of choice in renal nuclear medicine. *J. Nucl. Med.* **32**, 1301–1309.

Cosgriff, P.S., Lawson, R.S. & Nimmon, C.C. (1992) Towards standardisation in gamma camera renography. *Nucl. Med. Commun.* **13**, 580–585.

O'Reilly, P.H., Shields, R.A. & Testa, H.J. (1986) *Nuclear Medicine in Urology and Nephrology*, 2nd edn. London: Butterworths.

Smith, F.W. & Gemmell, H.G. The urinary tract. In: Sharp P.F., Gemmell, H.G. & Smith, F.W. (eds) *Practical Nuclear Medicine*, pp. 221–244. Oxford: Oxford University Press.

Direct Radionuclide Micturating Cystography

Indications Vesicoureteric reflux[1].

Contraindications Acute urinary tract infection.

Radiophar-maceuticals
1. ^{99m}*Tc-colloid.*
2. ^{99m}*Tc-pertechnetate.*

Both 25 MBq max.

Some pertechnetate is absorbed in the urinary tract and gastric activity may be seen. Use of colloid reduces absorption, and refluxed colloid particles tend to be retained for longer in the upper urinary tract[2].

Equipment
1. Gamma camera.
2. Low-energy general purpose collimator.
3. Imaging computer.
4. Sterile saline infusion.
5. Commode or plastic urinal.
6. Screens for patient privacy.

Patient preparation The patient micturates prior to the investigation.

Technique This examination is most frequently performed on children. Direct radionuclide cystography is considered to be at least as sensitive as conventional X-ray micturating cystourethrography (MCU) for the detection of vesicoureteric reflux[1, 3, 4]. It enables continuous imaging and quantification of bladder, ureter and kidney activity to be performed and delivers a much smaller radiation dose than conventional cystography.

The technique requires catheterization and is similar to that for MCU (see pp. 163–165), except that:
1. The radiopharmaceutical is administered using one of two methods:
   (a) diluted in 500 ml sterile saline solution at body temperature and then infused into the bladder via the catheter
   (b) injected directly into the bladder via the

catheter and continuously diluted with sterile saline solution infusion at body temperature.

2. During infusion, the patient lies supine with the gamma camera posterior. Ensure that both kidneys, ureters and bladder are in the field of view for all imaging. Dynamic image acquisition is performed for the duration of bladder filling at 10–20 s per frame with a 64 × 64 or 128 × 128 matrix size to demonstrate any reflux during this phase.

3. When the bladder is as full as tolerable, the infusion is stopped but imaging is continued for a further 30 s. The patient then sits in front of the gamma camera on a commode or child's plastic urinal.

4. Dynamic imaging with 5-s frames is performed during micturition, continuing for 2–5 min after to evaluate bladder re-filling. If the patient is capable, the embarrassment of the procedure may be reduced by giving them a remote control to start computer acquisition just before they micturate, and leaving them in private.

Analysis

1. Time–activity curves are produced from regions over the bladder, kidneys and ureters.

2. If the voided volume is measured, residual and reflux volumes can be calculated[2, 5].

3. Images may be summed to highlight any reflux episodes.

Additional techniques

1. If vesicoureteric reflux is not seen during a single filling and voiding cycle, the sensitivity of the test may be improved by immediately repeating the procedure[6]. The first voiding is performed if possible without removing the catheter, and re-filling is commenced shortly after.

2. Indirect radionuclide cystography may be performed after conventional radionuclide renography[7] (see 'Dynamic Renal Scintigraphy').

3. Intrarenal reflux has been investigated with delayed imaging of radiocolloid reflux at 5 and 20 hours[4].

Aftercare   As for conventional cystography.

Complications   As for conventional cystography.

References

1. Nasrallah, P.F., Nara, S. & Crawford, J. (1982) Clinical applications of nuclear cystography. *J. Urol.* **128**, 550–552.
2. Conway, J.J., Belman, A.B. & King, L.R. (1974) Direct and indirect radionuclide cystography. *Semin. Nucl. Med.* **4**, 197–211.
3. Van den Abbeele, A.D., Treves, S.T., Lebowitz, R.L. et al (1987) Vesicoureteral reflux in asymptomatic siblings of patients with known reflux: Radionuclide cystography. *Pediatrics* **79**, 147–156.
4. Rizzoni, G., Perale, R., Bui, F. et al (1986) Radionuclide voiding cystography in intrarenal reflux detection. *Ann. Radiol.* **29**, 415–420.
5. Gelfand, M.J. (1988) Nuclear cystography. In: Gelfand, M.J. & Thomas, S.R. (eds) *Effective Use of Computers in Nuclear Medicine*, pp. 402–411. New York: McGraw-Hill.
6. Fettich, J.J. & Kenda, R.B. (1992) Cyclic direct radionuclide voiding cystography: Increasing reliability in detecting vesicoureteral reflux in children. *Pediatr. Radiol.* **22**, 337–338.
7. Bower, G., Lovegrove, F.T., Geijsel, H., Van der Schaff, A. & Guelfi, G. (1985) Comparison of 'direct' and 'indirect' radionuclide cystography. *J. Nucl. Med.* **26**, 465–468.

6 Reproductive System

Methods of imaging the female reproductive system

1. Plain abdominal film.
2. Hysterosalpingography.
3. Arteriography.
4. Lymphography.
5. Ultrasound.
6. CT.
7. MRI.

Further reading

Coleman, B.G. (ed) (1992) The Female Pelvis. *Radiol. Clin. N. Am.* **30**(4).

Methods of imaging the scrotum and testes

1. Ultrasound.
2. MRI.
3. Radionuclide imaging.
4. Arteriography.
5. Venography.

Further reading

Clements, R., Griffiths, G.J., Peeling, W.B. & Conn, I.G. (1991) Transrectal ultrasound of the ejaculatory apparatus. *Clin. Radiol.* **44**, 240–244.

Demas, B.E., Hricak, H. & McClure, R.D. (1991) Varicoceles. Radiologic diagnosis and treatment. *Radiol. Clin. N. Am.* **29**, 619–627.

Fowler, R. (1990) Review. Imaging the testis and scrotal structures. *Clin. Radiol.* **41**, 81–85.

Nakielny, R.A., Thomas, W.E.G., Jackson, P., Jones, M. & Davies, E.R. (1984) Radionuclide evaluation of acute scrotal disease. *Clin. Radiol.* **35**, 125–129.

Hysterosalpingography

Indications
1. Infertility.
2. Recurrent miscarriages.
3. Following tubal surgery.

Contraindications
1. Pregnancy
2. A purulent discharge on inspection of the vulva or cervix.
3. Recent dilatation and curettage or abortion, or immediately post-menstruation. This applies only to oily contrast medium because of the risk of intravasation.
   Oily contrast medium is no longer recommended.

Contrast medium
HOCM or LOCM 300. Volume 10–20 ml.
LOCM have no advantage[1] with regard to image quality or side-effects but the nonionic dimer, iotrolan, is associated with a lower incidence and decreased severity of delayed pain[2].

Equipment
1. Fluoroscopy unit with spot film device.
2. Vaginal speculum, vulsellum forceps and uterine cannula or 8F paediatric Foley catheter.

Patient preparation
1. The patient should abstain from intercourse between booking the appointment and the time of the examination unless she uses a reliable method of contraception.
   or
   the examination can be booked between the fourth and tenth days in a patient with a regular 28-day cycle.
2. Apprehensive patients may need premedication.
3. Paracetamol 1 g 1 hour prior to the examination.

Preliminary film
Coned PA view of the pelvic cavity.

Technique
1. The patient lies supine on the table with knees flexed, legs abducted and heels together.
2. Using aseptic technique the operator inserts a speculum and cleans the vagina and cervix with chlorhexidine.

3. The anterior lip of the cervix is steadied with the vulsellum forceps and the cannula is inserted into the cervical canal. If a Foley catheter is used, there is usually no need to grasp the cervix with the vulsellum forceps.

4. Care must be taken to expel all air bubbles from the syringe and cannula, as these would otherwise cause confusion in interpretation. Contrast medium is injected slowly under intermittent fluoroscopic control. Spasm of the uterine cornu may be relieved by inhalation of octyl nitrite.

Films   Using the undercouch tube:

1. As the tubes begin to fill.
2. When peritoneal spill has occurred and with all the instruments removed.

Aftercare   1. It must be ensured that the patient is in no serious discomfort nor has significant bleeding before she leaves.

2. The patient must be advised that she may have bleeding per vaginam for 1–2 days and pain may persist for up to 2 weeks.

Complications
Due to the contrast   1. Allergic phenomenon—especially if contrast
medium   medium is forced into the circulation.

Due to the technique   1. Pain may occur at the following times:
   (a)   using the vulsellum forceps
   (b)   during insertion of the cannula
   (c)   with tubal distension proximal to a block
   (d)   with distension of the uterus if there is tubal spasm
   (e)   with peritoneal irritation during the following day, and up to 2 weeks.

2. Bleeding from trauma to the uterus or cervix.
3. Transient nausea, vomiting and headache.
4. Intravasation of contrast medium into the venous system of the uterus results in a fine lace-like pattern within the uterine wall. When more extensive, intravasation outlines larger veins. It is of little significance when water-soluble contrast media are used. The following factors predispose to intravasation:

     (a) direct trauma to the endometrium
     (b) timing of the procedure near to menstruation
     (c) timing of the procedure within a few days after curettage
     (d) tubal occlusion because of the high pressures generated within the uterine cavity
     (e) uterine abnormalities, e.g. uterine tuberculosis, carcinoma and fibroids.

5. Infection — which may be delayed. Occurs in up to 2% of patients and more likely when there is a previous history of pelvic infection.
6. Abortion. The operator must ensure that the patient is not pregnant.

References

1. Davies, A.C., Keightley, A., Borthwick-Clark, A. & Walters, H.L. (1985) The use of low-osmolarity contrast medium in hysterosalpingography: comparison with a conventional contrast medium. *Clin. Radiol.* **36**, 533–536.
2. Brokensha, C. & Whitehouse, G. (1991) A comparison between iotrolan, a non-ionic dimer, and a hyperosmolar contrast medium, Urografin, in hysterosalpingography. *Br. J. Radiol.* **64**, 587–590.

Ultrasound of the Scrotum

Indications
1. Suspected testicular tumour.
2. Suspected epididymo-orchitis.
3. Hydrocoele.
4. Acute torsion. In boys or young men in whom this clinical diagnosis has been made and emergency surgical exploration is planned, ultrasound should not delay the operation. Although colour Doppler may show an absence of vessels in the ischaemic testis, it is possible that partial untwisting resulting in some blood flow could lead to a false-negative examination.
5. Suspected varicocoele.
6. Scrotal trauma.

Contraindications   None.

Patient preparation   None.

Equipment   5–10 MHz transducer. Linear array for optimum imaging. Stand-off may be helpful in some cases.

Technique
1. Patient supine with legs together. Some operators support the scrotum on a towel draped beneath it or in a gloved hand.
2. Both sides are examined with longitudinal and transverse scans enabling comparison to be made.
3. Real-time scanning enables the optimal oblique planes to be examined.

Further reading   Feld, R. & Middleton, W.D. (1992) Recent advances in sonography of the testis and scrotum. *Radiol. Clin. N. Am.* **30**, 1033–1051.

7 Respiratory System

Methods of imaging the respiratory system

1. Plain films.
2. Tomography.
3. Tracheography.
4. Bronchography.
5. Radionuclide imaging
   - ventilation: ^{81m}Kr, ^{99m}Tc-DTPA, ^{133}Xe, ^{127}Xe, ^{99m}Tc-Technegas
   - perfusion: ^{99m}Tc-macroaggregated albumin (MAA).
6. CT
   - conventional, using 8–10 mm slices
   - high-resolution (HRCT), using 1–2 mm slices and reconstruction with a high spatial frequency algorithm ('bone' algorithm), targetted image reconstruction and, often, a higher kV and mA.
7. Ultrasound.
8. MRI.

Further reading

Gamsu, G. & Klein, J.S. (1989) High resolution computed tomography of diffuse lung disease. *Clin. Radiol.* **40**, 554–556.

Templeton, P.A. & Zerhouni, E.A. (1989) MR Imaging in the management of thoracic malignancies. *Radiol. Clin. N. Am.* **27**, 1099–1111.

Webb, W.R. (1989) High-resolution CT of the lung parenchyma. *Radiol. Clin. N. Am.* **27**, 1085–1097.

Methods of imaging pulmonary embolism

1. *Plain film chest radiograph.* The initial chest radiograph is often normal. Numerous signs have been described in association with pulmonary embolism but, overall, the chest radiograph is neither specific nor sensitive.

2. *Ventilation/perfusion (V/Q) radionuclide scanning.* The technique is described later in this chapter. Interpretation of V/Q images is not clear-cut and there are a number of causes for the typical V/Q mismatch. Diagnostic criteria developed divide results into normal, low-probability, intermediate (or indeterminate) and high-risk groups. Specificity and sensitivity are such that, if the criteria place the images in the normal group, pulmonary embolism is virtually excluded and if the images fit the criteria for high risk it is very likely (85–90%). In the intermediate risk group specificity is poor and pulmonary angiography may be required.

3. *Pulmonary arteriography* (chapter 8) is the 'best' method and will detect most pulmonary emboli.

Further reading

PIOPED Investigators. (1990) Value of ventilation/perfusion scanning in acute pulmonary embolism. *JAMA* **263**, 2753–2759.

Robinson, P.J. (1989) Lung scintigraphy. *Clin. Radiol.* **40**, 557–560.

Bronchography

Indications	1. Bronchiectasis. 2. To demonstrate the site and extent of bronchial obstruction.
Contraindications	1. Acute respiratory infection. 2. Poor respiratory reserve.
Contrast medium	LOCM – most recently new non-ionic dimer agents, e.g. iotrolan 300, have been advocated for the purpose, but iohexol can be used. 2–3 ml iotrolan 300 per lung segment, maximum 25 ml per patient.
Equipment	1. Overcouch tube. 2. Fluoroscopy unit.
Patient preparation	1. Chest physiotherapy. 2. Nothing by mouth for 6 hours. 3. Treat purulent sputum with appropriate antibiotic therapy. 4. Premedication with atropine 0.6 mg and morphine 10 mg. 5. Asthmatics should have steroid prophylaxis and salbutamol preoperatively.
Preliminary films	Chest: 1. PA 2. Lateral
Technique	In the past, using the more viscous contrast agents such as Dionosil, various techniques were described to introduce contrast into the bronchial tree. The low osmolar contrast agents are not so viscous and satisfactory coating is more difficult. The preferred method is direct injection via the bronchoscope.
For children	A catheter may be passed via an endotracheal tube with the child anaesthetized.
Bronchoscopic method	1. The nasopharynx is anaesthetized with local anaesthetic (4 or 10% lignocaine spray).

2. The patient can be sedated with intravenous benzodiazepine (diazemul or midazolam).
3. A fibre-optic bronchoscope is passed via either the nose or the mouth into the trachea.
4. After systematic examination of the bronchial tree, the tip of the bronchoscope is inserted into the appropriate segmental or lobar bronchus and suction carried out to clear any secretions.
5. Contrast medium is injected directly into the suction channel of the bronchoscope under fluoroscopic control.

Films
1. Spot views are taken of the lobe or segment being examined. Timing is critical as the viscosity of the medium is such that any delay will result in inadequate coating.
2. Chest PA at 4 hours to exclude complications.

Aftercare
1. Chest physiotherapy.
2. Nil by mouth until the anaesthetic has worn off.

Complications
1. Slight impairment in respiratory function — drop in Sa_{O_2} during procedure and fall in FEV_1 and FVC at 4 hours.
2. Bronchospasm — well recognized with bronchoscopy alone and particularly in asthmatic individuals.
3. Minor symptoms of headache, nausea, vomiting and a sensation of heat or flushing have been reported.

Further reading
Flower, C.D.R. & Schneerson, J.M. (1984) Bronchography via the fibreoptic bronchoscope. *Thorax* 35, 260–263.
Morcos, S.K., Anderson, P.B., Clout, C., Fairlie, N.C., Baudouin, C. & Warnock, N. (1990) Suitability and tolerance of Iotrolan 300 in bronchography via the fibreoptic bronchoscope. *Thorax* 45, 628–629.

Percutaneous Lung Biopsy

Indications
1. Investigation of a pulmonary opacity when other diagnostic techniques have failed to make a diagnosis.
2. Investigation of a new chest lesion in a patient with a known malignancy.
3. To obtain material for culture when other techniques have failed to identify the causative organism in a patient with persistent consolidation.

N.B. Central lesions are best biopsied transbronchially.

Contraindications
1. Bleeding diathesis, or concurrent administration of anticoagulants.
2. Contralateral pneumonectomy.
3. Presence of bullae.
4. Suspected hydatid disease.
5. Suspected vascular lesion.
6. Seriously impaired respiratory function such that a pneumothorax could not be tolerated.

Equipment
1. Biplane screening or C-arm, if possible.
2. Biopsy needle — there are several types available, e.g.
   (a) hollow aspiration needle
   (b) screw-tipped needle and cannula (Nordenström)
3. Full resuscitation equipment including a chest drain.

Patient preparation
1. Premedication with diazepam. However, the patient must remain co-operative so that a consistent breathing pattern can be maintained during the procedure.
2. The procedure may be performed on an outpatient basis, but a bed should be available in case of complications.
3. Clotting screen.

Preliminary film
1. Chest — PA and lateral.

Technique
1. With posterior lesions the patient lies prone, and if the scapula is obscuring the lesion, the arm can be dangled over the side of the table to move the scapula laterally. If the lesion is anterior, the patient lies supine.
2. Fluoroscopy is used to localize the mass. The puncture site is marked vertically above the lesion.
3. Using the plain films the approximate distance down to the lesion can be measured.
4. With an aseptic technique, local anaesthetic is infiltrated down to the pleura.
5. The needle is inserted under screen control, with suspended respiration, using forceps (or manufacturer's holder, if provided) so that the operator's hand is not irradiated.
6. If a specialized core biopsy needle is used, then the manufacturer's instructions are followed to obtain tissue. With small-bore cell aspiration needles (e.g. 22G spinal) maximum suction is applied with a 20 ml syringe while the needle is rotated and advanced through the lesion. Suction is released prior to withdrawing the needle, to avoid contaminating the sample.

It is extremely helpful if a pathologist can be present to check that there are sufficient cells in the aspirate for diagnostic purposes. If the lesion is necrotic, the most profitable site for biopsy is the margins of the lesion. Up to three passes may be performed to obtain tissue.

Aftercare
1. Chest X-ray in expiration.
2. Patients with pre-existing impairment of respiratory function are best admitted overnight.

Complications
1. Pneumothorax in 15–35%. However, a chest drain is necessary in only a small minority (about 1%). The incidence of pneumothorax is increased if:
   (a) the operator is inexperienced
   (b) larger bore needles are used
   (c) there is an increased number of punctures
   (d) small or central lesions are biopsied.
2. Local pulmonary haemorrhage (10%).

3. Haemoptysis (2–5%).
4. Other complications, such as implantation of malignant cells along the needle track, spread of infection and air embolism, are all extremely rare.

Further reading Allison, D.J. & Hemingway, A.P. (1981) Percutaneous needle biopsy of the lung. *BMJ* **282**, 875–878.

Goddard, P. (1986) *Diagnostic Imaging of the Chest*. Edinburgh: Churchill Livingstone.

Sinner, W.N. (1976) Complications of percutaneous transthoracic needle aspiration biopsy. *Acta Radiol. (Diagn.)* **17**, 813–828.

Radionuclide Lung Ventilation/ Perfusion (V/Q) Imaging

Indications
1. Suspected pulmonary embolism.
2. Assessment of perfusion and ventilation abnormalities, e.g. in congenital cardiac or pulmonary disease.
3. Chronic obstructive airways disease.
4. Assessment of resectability of bullae.
5. Differentiation of primary and secondary pulmonary hypertension (perfusion only).
6. Inhaled foreign body (ventilation only).
7. Assessment of lung permeability (DTPA aerosol).

Contraindications
1. Right-to-left cardiac shunt — because of the risk of cerebral emboli.
2. Severe pulmonary hypertension.

Radiopharmaceuticals

Perfusion: ^{99m}Tc-*macroaggregated albumin (MAA)*, 100 MBq max.

Labelled albumin particles 10–100 μm in diameter which occlude small lung vessels (< 0.5% of total capillary bed).

Ventilation:
1. ^{81m}Kr *(Krypton) gas*, 2000 MBq max.
   Generator-produced agent of choice with a short $T_{1/2}$ of 13 s and a γ-energy of 190 keV. Simultaneous dual isotope ventilation and perfusion imaging is possible because of different γ-energy to ^{99m}Tc. Washin and washout studies are not possible. Expensive and limited availability.
2. ^{99m}Tc-*DTPA*, aerosol, 80 MBq max.
   No simultaneous ventilation and perfusion imaging. Permeability studies are possible. Cheap and readily available alternative to krypton but less preferable in patients with chronic obstructive airways disease or chronic asthma because clumping of aerosol particles is likely.
3. ^{133}Xe *(xenon) gas*, max. 400 MBq diluted in 10 litres and re-breathed for 5 min[1].
   Long $T_{1/2}$ of 5.25 days and a γ-energy of 81 keV.

Ventilation must precede perfusion study because low γ-energy would be swamped by scatter from ^{99m}Tc. Washin and washout studies are possible. β-emission results in higher radiation dose than ^{81m}Kr and discharged gas must be dealt with safely. Poor resolution images, but cheap and widely available.

4. ^{127}*Xe gas*, max. 200 MBq diluted in 10 litres and re-breathed for 5 min.

Long $T_{1/2}$ of 36.4 days and γ-energies of 172, 203 and 375 keV. Higher γ-energy than ^{99m}Tc, so it can be used after perfusion study. Wash-in and washout studies are possible. Radiation dose is higher than ^{81m}Kr but lower than ^{133}Xe. Images are comparable to ^{133}Xe. Discharged gas must be dealt with safely. High-energy collimator required. Expensive and not widely available.

5. ^{99m}*Tc-Technegas*. 20 MBq typical.

Labelled carbon particles, 5–20 nm in size. Longer residence time in lungs than aerosols, so tomography and respiration-gated studies possible. Expensive dispensing system[2].

Equipment
1. Gamma camera.
2. Low-energy general purpose collimator.
3. Gas dispensing system and breathing circuit for ventilation.
4. Foam wedges for oblique positioning.

Patient preparation
1. For ventilation, familiarization with breathing equipment.
2. A current chest X-ray is required to assist with interpretation.

Technique
Perfusion:
1. The injection may be given in the supine, semi-recumbent or sitting position (N.B. MAA particle uptake is affected by gravity).
2. The syringe is shaken to prevent particles settling.
3. A slow i.v. injection is given directly into a vein (particles will stick to a plastic canula) over about 10 s. Avoid drawing blood into the syringe as this can cause clumping.

N.B. MAA must be administered by medically qualified personnel.

4. The patient must remain in position for 2–3 min while the particles become fixed in the lungs.
5. Imaging may begin immediately, preferably in the sitting position.

Ventilation: ^{81m}Kr GAS

This is performed immediately after the perfusion study.

1. The patient is positioned to obtain identical views to the perfusion images.
2. The patient should be asked to breathe normally through the mouthpiece.
3. The air supply attached to the generator is turned on and imaging commenced.
4. Continue until 300–400 kilocounts per view have been collected.

^{99m}Tc-DTPA AEROSOL

This scan is performed before the perfusion study, which may follow immediately unless there is clumping of aerosol particles in the lungs, in which case it is delayed for 1–2 hours.

1. A DTPA kit is made up with approx. 600 MBq ^{99m}Tc per ml (volume dependent upon aerosol equipment).
2. ^{99m}Tc-DTPA is drawn into a 5 ml syringe with 2 ml air.
3. ^{99m}Tc-DTPA is injected into the nebulizer and flushed through with air.
4. The patient is positioned initially with his back to the camera, sitting if possible.
5. The nose-clip is placed on the patient and he is asked to breathe normally through the mouthpiece.
6. The air supply is turned on to deliver a rate of $10 \, \text{l min}^{-1}$.
7. When the count rate reaches 2000 counts s^{-1}, the air supply is turned off.
8. The patient should continue to breathe through the mouthpiece for a further 15 s.
9. The nose-clip is removed and the patient given a mouth wash.
10. Imaging is commenced.

Images   300–400 kilocounts. Anterior, posterior, left and right posterior obliques.

Since perfusion and ventilation images are directly compared, it is important to have identical views for each. Foam wedges between the patient's back and the camera assist accurate oblique positioning.

Aftercare   None.

Complications   Care should be taken when injecting MAA not to induce respiratory failure in patients with severe pulmonary hypertension. In these cases, inject very slowly.

References   1. Buxton-Thomas, M. (1989) The lungs. In: Sharp, P.F., Gemmell, H.G. & Smith, F.W. (eds) *Practical Nuclear Medicine*, pp. 161–177. Oxford: Oxford University Press.
2. James, J.M., Herman, K.J., Lloyd, J.J. et al (1991) Evaluation of ^{99}Tc^m Technegas ventilation scintigraphy in the diagnosis of pulmonary embolism. *Br. J. Radiol.* **64**, 711–719.

Further reading   Miller, R.F. & O'Doherty, M.J. (1992) Pulmonary nuclear medicine. *Eur. J. Nucl. Med.* **19**, 355–368.
White, P.G., Hayward, M.W.J. & Cooper, T. (1991) Ventilation agents – What agents are currently used? *Nucl. Med. Commun.* **12**, 349–352.

8 Heart and Arterial System

Methods of
imaging the
cardiovascular
system

1. Chest radiography.
2. Fluoroscopy.
3. Angiocardiography.
4. Arteriography.
5. Venography.
6. Pulmonary arteriography.
7. Ultrasound.
   - 2-dimensional real-time, Doppler and M-mode.
8. Radionuclide imaging
   - ventriculography
     - gated blood pool study
     - first pass radionuclide angiography
   - myocardial perfusion imaging
     - ^{201}thallium
     - ^{99m}Tc-methoxyisobutylisonitrile (MIBI)
     - ^{99m}Tc-teboroxime
   - acute myocardial infarction imaging
     - ^{99m}Tc-pyrophosphate
     - ^{111}In-antimyosin antibody
   - gastrointestinal tract blood loss imaging (see pp. 96–97).
9. CT.
10. MRI.

Further reading

Meire, H.B. (1990) Editorial. Abdominal Doppler – current status and future potential. *Clin. Radiol.* **41**, 223–224.

Miller, D.D., Elmaleh, D.R., McKusick, K.A., Boucher, C.A., Callahan, R.J. & Strauss H.W. (1985) Radiopharmaceuticals for cardiac imaging. *Radiol. Clin. N. Am.* **23**, 765–781.

Miller, S.W. (1989) Imaging pericardial disease. *Radiol. Clin. N. Am.* **27**, 1113–1125.

Miller, S.W., Brady, T.J., Dinsmore, R.E. et al (1985) Cardiac magnetic resonance imaging: the Massachusetts General Hospital experience. *Radiol. Clin. N. Am.* **23**, 745–764.

Rees, S. (1990) The George Simon Lecture: magnetic resonance studies of the heart. *Clin. Radiol.* **42**, 302–316.

Equipment for an Angiography Room

The following is a list for both angiography and angiocardiography. Only certain items will be needed for individual procedures.

X-ray generator   Three-phase, 12-pulse and at least 1000 mA. For biplane angiography two 1000 mA generators are better than one 2000 mA generator because:
1. A fault in one X-ray generator will not put all the X-ray apparatus out of action.
2. Completely different exposure values can be set for AP and lateral views.

X-ray tube   High-speed, rotating anode with a 0.6 mm^2 focal spot. Two tubes will be needed for biplane angiography and are useful for investigating congenital heart disease. A 0.3 mm^2 focal spot is necessary for macroangiography.

A C- or U-arm device, in which the X-ray tube and intensifier are placed at opposite ends of a C- or U-shaped frame which can be rotated around the patient, has a number of advantages:
1. The patient does not need to be disturbed during the procedure.
2. There is less likelihood of dislodgement of the catheter.
3. Axial views are easier to perform.

It also has the following disadvantages:
1. More space is required.
2. It is expensive.

Fluoroscopy unit   A caesium iodide image intensifier and television.

A biplane screening unit is useful, as is a dual or variable size field of view facility.

A digital unit with subtraction facilities (DSA) is now considered ideal for most of the procedures, and in this chapter guidelines which are given for film acquisition during angiography will not apply to those with digital equipment. With digital units 'hard copy' can be obtained from the computer after the procedure has finished, usually by linkage to a multiformat camera or to a laser imaging system.

Cine radiography 35 mm. Usually 25 frames per s is adequate for most work.

Video recorder Essential for angiocardiography and it enables immediate review of a contrast medium injection.

Cut film A digital subtraction imaging system is preferable, but alternatively a 100 mm camera with the facility to take rapid sequence films is useful. Alternatives which are less ideal, in terms of both cost and radiation exposure to the patient, include the Puck (up to 3 films per s; max. 20 films) and Schonander–Elema AOT (up to 6 films per s; max. 30 films) systems.

Pressure injector There are two basic types:
1. An electric motor injector using a computation of injection rate after setting catheter variables, e.g. a Cordis pump.
2. An electric motor injector which uses a feedback mechanism to monitor the injection rate, e.g. Medrad, Contrac and Simtrac pumps.

X-ray table The angiocardiography table should have a floating top.

For arteriography of the lower aorta and lower limb arteries a moving table top is desirable. The timing of movements may be controlled electronically and films obtained by either a stepping table top function or bolus chasing, allowing a full sequence of films following a single injection. Less ideal is multiple injections at a static site.

Pressure monitoring equipment Necessary for cardiac catheter studies and for aortoiliac angioplasty.

ECG monitor Essential if a catheter is to be passed into or through the heart.

Resuscitation equipment Including a defibrillator, endotracheal tubes, ventilation bag and appropriate drugs.

Introduction to Catheter Techniques

The basic technique of arterial catheterisation is applicable to veins also.

Patient preparation
1. The patient will need to be admitted to hospital as careful preparation before and observation after the procedure will be required. With the introduction of smaller diameter catheters, day case admission may be all that is needed for routine peripheral angiography using 3–5F catheters and some simple angioplasty cases.
2. If the patient is taking anticoagulants, he should be monitored to ensure that they are within their therapeutic 'window'.
3. The radiologist should see the patient on the ward prior to the examination in order to:
   (a) explain the procedure
   (b) obtain informed consent
   (c) examine the patient, with special reference to blood pressure and peripheral pulses as a baseline for post-arteriographic problems.
4. The puncture site is shaved.

Puncture sites
1. Femoral artery — most frequently used.
2. Brachial artery — a high approach is preferable (see p. 206). The Sones technique for coronary arteriography uses a brachial arteriotomy.
3. Axillary artery.
4. Aorta — by using a Teflon-sleeved needle for translumbar aortography the sleeve can be directed antegradely or retrogradely in the aorta[1].

Equipment for the Seldinger technique

Needles
The technique of catheter insertion via double-wall needle puncture and guide-wire is known as the Seldinger technique[2]. The original Seldinger needle consisted of three parts:
1. An outer thin-walled blunt cannula.
2. An inner needle.
3. A stilette.

Many radiologists now prefer to use modified needles:
1. Double-wall puncture with a two-piece needle consisting of a bevelled central stilette and an outer tube.
2. Single-wall puncture with a simple sharp needle (without a stilette) with a bore just wide enough to accommodate the guide-wire.

Guide-wires These consist of two central cores of straight wire around which is wound a tightly coiled wire spring (Figure 8.1). The ends are sealed with solder. One of the central core wires is secured at both ends — a safety feature in case of fracturing. The other is anchored in solder at one end, but terminates 5 cm from the other end, leaving a soft flexible tip. Some guide-wires have a movable central core so that the tip can be flexible or stiff. Others have a J-shaped tip which is useful for negotiating tortuous vessels and selectively catheterizing vessels. The size of the J-curve is denoted by its radius in millimetres. Guide-wires are polyethylene coated but may be coated with a thin film of Teflon to reduce friction. Teflon, however, also increases their thrombogenicity, though this can be countered by using heparin-bonded

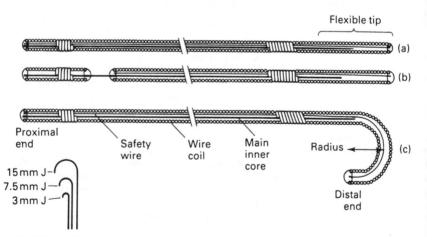

Fig. 8.1　Guide-wire construction. (a) Fixed core, straight. (b) Movable core, straight. (c) Fixed core, J-curve.

Teflon[3]. The most common sizes are 0.035 and 0.038 inches diameter. A more recent development is hydrophilic wires. These are very slippery with excellent torque and are useful in negotiating narrow tortuous vessels. They require constant lubrication with saline.

Catheters

Most catheters are manufactured commercially, complete with end hole, side holes, preformed curves and Luer Lok connection. They are made of Dacron, Teflon, polyurethane or polyethylene. Details of the specific catheter types are given with the appropriate technique.

Some straight catheters may be shaped for specific purposes by immersion in hot sterile water until they become malleable, forming the desired shape and then fixing the shape by cooling in cold sterile water.

For the average adult a 100 cm catheter with a 145 cm guide-wire is suitable for reaching the aortic branches from a femoral puncture.

The introduction of a catheter over a guide-wire is facilitated by dilatation of the track with a dilator (short length of graded tubing).

Taps and connectors

These should have a large internal diameter that will not increase resistence to flow and Luer Loks which will not come apart during a pressure injection.

References

1. Stocks, L.O., Halpern, M. & Turner, A.F. (1969) Complete translumbar aortography. The Teflon sleeve technique. *Am. J. Roentg.* **107**, 835–839.
2. Seldinger, S. (1953) Catheter replacement of needle in percutaneous arteriography: new technique. *Acta Radiol.* **39**, 368–376.
3. Roberts, G.M. Roberts, E.E., Davies, R.Ll. & Lawrie, B.W. (1977) Thrombogenicity of arterial catheters and guide wires. *Br J. Radiol.* **50**, 415–418.

FEMORAL ARTERY PUNCTURE

This is the most frequently used puncture site providing access to the left ventricle, aorta and all its branches. It also has the lowest complication rate of the peripheral sites.

Relative 1. Blood dyscrasias.
contraindications 2. Femoral artery aneurysm.
3. Marked tortuosity of the iliac vessels may prevent further advancement of the guide-wire or catheter. In such a case, high brachial artery puncture or intravenous DSA may be necessary.

Technique 1. The patient lies supine on the X-ray table. Both
(Figure 8.2) femoral arteries are palpated and if pulsations are of similar strength the side opposite to the symptoms is chosen. The reasoning for this is that this leaves the symptomatic groin untouched so that future surgery in this region is not made more hazardous. If all else is equal, then the right side is technically easier (for right handed operators.)
2. Before beginning, the appropriate catheter and guide-wire are selected and their compatibility

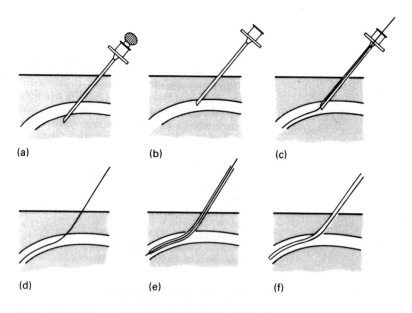

(a)   (b)   (c)

(d)   (e)   (f)

Fig. 8.2 Seldinger technique. (a) Both walls of vessel punctured. (b) Stillette removed. Needle withdrawn so that bevel is within the lumen of the vessel and blood flows from the hub. (c) Guide-wire inserted through needle. (d) Needle withdrawn, leaving guide-wire in situ. (e) Catheter threaded over wire. (f) Guide-wire withdrawn.

checked by passing the guide-wire through the catheter and needle.

3. Using aseptic technique, local anaesthetic is infiltrated either side of the artery down to the periosteum. A 5 mm transverse incision is made over the artery to avoid binding of soft tissues on the catheter. In thin patients the artery may be very superficial and, to avoid injury to it, a position is chosen and the skin reflected laterally before making the incision.

4. The actual point of puncture of the femoral artery must be considered. The femoral artery arches medially and posteriorly as it becomes the external iliac artery. Attempts to puncture the artery cephalad to the apex of the arch will result in either failure to puncture the artery or puncture of the artery deep in the pelvis at a point where haemostasis cannot be secured by pressure. Correct puncture is made at the apex of the arch with the needle directed 45° to the skin surface and slightly medially.

5. The artery is immobilized by placing the index and middle fingers of the left hand on either side of the artery, and the needle is held in the right hand. The needle is advanced through the soft tissues until transmitted pulsations are felt. Both walls of the artery are punctured with a stab (single-wall puncture increases the risk of intimal disection). The stilette is removed, and the needle hub is depressed so that it runs more parallel to the skin and then withdrawn until pulsatile blood flow indicates a satisfactory puncture. Poor flow may be due to:
   (a) femoral vein puncture
   (b) the end of the needle lying sub-intimally
   (c) hypotension — due to vasovagal reaction during the puncture
   (d) atherosclerosis.

6. When good flow is obtained the guide-wire is inserted through the needle and advanced gently up the artery whilst screening. When it is in the descending aorta the needle is withdrawn over the guide-wire, keeping firm pressure on the puncture site to prevent bleeding. The guide-wire is then wiped clean with a wet sponge and the catheter

threaded over it. For 5F and greater diameter catheters, particularly those which are curved, a dilator is recomended of a size matched to the catheter. The catheter is advanced up the descending aorta, under fluoroscopic control, and when in a satisfactory position the guide-wire is withdrawn.

7. The catheter is connected via a two-way tap to a syringe of heparinized saline (2500 units in 500 ml of 0.9% saline), and flushed. Flushing should be done rapidly otherwise the more distal catheter holes will remain unflushed. Flushing should be performed regularly throughout the procedure or alternatively a continuous flushing technique with a bag of heparinized saline may be used.

8. At the end of the procedure the catheter is withdrawn and compression of the puncture site should be maintained for 5 min. If continued bleeding becomes a concern, consideration should be given to neutralizing the effects of heparin by giving protamine sulphate, 1 mg for each 100 units of heparin.

Aftercare
1. Bed rest — if a 5F system (or less) is used on a day-case basis, then this should be for at least 4 hours. Larger catheters require longer bed rest and observation.
2. Careful observation of the puncture site.
3. Pulse and blood pressure observation half-hourly for 4 hours and then 4-hourly for the remainder of 24 hours, if the larger catheter systems are used.

HIGH BRACHIAL ARTERY PUNCTURE

Indications
As for femoral artery puncture, but as this approach is associated with a higher incidence of complications, it should only be used if femoral artery puncture is not possible.

Contraindications
1. Atherosclerosis of the axillary or subclavian arteries.
2. Subclavian artery aneurysm.

Technique
Good accounts are given by Gaines and Reidy[1] and Watkinson and Hartnell[2].

1. The patient lies on the X-ray table with his arm in supination. The peripheral pulses are palpated and the brachial artery localized approx. 10 cm above the elbow.
2. A small incision is made in the skin, 1–2 cm distal to the selected point of arterial puncture.
3. A single-wall puncture needle is used, with an acute angle of entry into the artery.
4. A straight, soft-tipped guide-wire is introduced when good pulsatile flow is obtained.
5. A 5F pigtail catheter is introduced over the guide-wire and its pigtail formed in the aorta.
6. At the end of the procedure the catheter tip is straightened using the guide-wire and then removed. This reduces the risk of intimal damage and flap formation during withdrawal of the catheter.

AXILLARY ARTERY PUNCTURE

Indications
As for femoral artery puncture, but this approach is associated with a higher incidence of complications and should only be used if femoral or high bracial artery puncture is not possible. (Intravenous DSA may be more appropriate in diagnostic studies; see below.)

Contraindications
1. Atherosclerosis of the axillary or subclavian arteries.
2. Subclavian artery aneurysm.

Technique
1. The patient lies supine on the X-ray table with his arm fully abducted. The puncture point is just distal to the axillary fold, which is infiltrated with local anaesthetic.
2. A small incision is made in the skin, 1–2 cm distal to the point of the arterial puncture.
3. The needle is directed more horizontally than the femoral approach and along the line of the humerus.
4. Following satisfactory puncture the remainder of the technique is as for femoral artery catheterization.

INTRAVENOUS DIGITAL SUBTRACTION ANGIOGRAPHY (DSA)

Indications
1. Where femoral artery catheterization is not possible and fine arterial detail is not required.
2. Postoperative graft follow-up.

Contraindications
1. Borderline cardiac failure (because of the sudden bolus load directly to the right heart).
2. Where detailed anatomical information is required.

Technique
1. The patient is positioned supine on the X-ray table.
2. The antecubital fossae of the patient are inspected and a suitable basilic vein is chosen and the skin prepared.
   In many patients the femoral vein can be punctured by palpating a non-pulsatile femoral artery and aiming medial to it. Where this is possible the problems of arm vein spasm are not encountered.
3. Using a single-wall puncture needle, the vein is entered at an oblique angle, and a straight, soft-tipped guide-wire introduced.
4. The vessel is then dilated and a 5F pigtail catheter introduced over the guide-wire. The catheter tip is manoeuvred to lie in the right atrium or superior vena cava (SVC). The right atrial position is the preferable site[3].
5. The catheter is kept well flushed with heparinized saline, as always.
6. If the abdominal vessels are to be imaged then the patient is given Buscopan 20 mg i.v., to reduce subtraction errors due to movement of bowel gas. Abdominal compression may also be applied.
7. Each projection requires a separate injection of contrast medium (due to the need for mask acquisition at each position). A suitable rate is 35 ml at 20 ml s^{-1}, using full strength LOCM (e.g. 350 mg I ml^{-1}).
8. At the end of the procedure the catheter is straightened with the guide-wire and removed. Firm pressure is applied over the puncture site to achieve haemostasis.

References

1. Gaines, P.A. & Reidy, J.F. (1986) Percutaneous high brachial aortography: a safe alternative to the translumbar approach. *Clin. Radiol.* **37**, 595–597.
2. Watkinson, A.F. & Hartnell, G.G. (1991) Complications of direct brachial artery puncture for arteriography: a comparison of techniques. *Clin. Radiol.* **44**, 189–191.
3. Pinto, R.S., Manuell, M. & Kricheff, I.I. (1984) Complications of digital iv angiography. *AJR* **143**, 1295–1299.

General Complications of Catheter Techniques

An excellent review is provided by Herlinger[1].

Due to the anaesthetic

See p. 9.

Due to the contrast medium

ALLERGIC AND IDIOSYNCRATIC
Non-fatal reactions are much less common with intra-arterial injections than with intravenous injections[2].

TOXIC
In addition to those mentioned in Chapter 2, the following points are important:

1. *Hot feeling.* This is localized to the region supplied by the injected artery. Injection of conventional contrast media may cause severe pain – typically when injected into the arm, the atherosclerotic lower limb or the external carotid artery. Symptoms are due to the high osmolality and it is for this reason that the new LOCM are preferred[3]. They are, however, expensive.

2. A large dose delivered to a specific organ may have a *chemotoxic effect.*
   (a) Coronary arteries. Pure sodium or meglumine salts produce impaired myocardial contractility and ECG changes[4]. Addition of calcium to the contrast medium (the Isopaque series) improves contractility but also increases the subjective feeling of warmth.
   (b) *Cerebral arteries.* Sodium salts are more neurotoxic than meglumine salts.
   (c) *Spinal cord.* Direct injection into a lumbar or intercostal artery which feeds the artery of Adamkiewicz, or diversion of contrast medium into the spinal vascular bed in low aortic obstruction, can result in spinal cord damage. Tonic and clonic leg movements with a positive Babinski response may progress to paraplegia, or paraplegia may be the first sign.

The treatment proposed by Mishkin et al[5] is to replace CSF with N-saline in 10 ml aliquots. Improvement accompanies a lowering of CSF iodine.

(d) *Kidneys.* Acute renal failure is a rare complication and is more likely in association with:
(i) pre-existing renal disease, diabetes or myelomatosis
(ii) decreased renal perfusion (hypotension, dehydration, low-output cardiac failure)
(iii) large volumes of contrast medium
(iv) recent administration of nephrotoxic drugs.

Treatment is as for acute renal failure of any cause.

Due to the technique

LOCAL
1. *Haemorrhage/haematoma.*
2. *Arterial thrombus.* May be due to:
(a) stripping of thrombus from the catheter wall as it is withdrawn
(b) trauma to the vessel wall.

Factors implicated in increased thrombus formation are:
(a) large catheters
(b) excessive time in the artery
(c) many catheter changes
(d) inexperience of the radiologist
(e) polyurethane catheters, because of their rough surface.

The incidence is decreased by the use of:
(a) heparin-bonded catheters
(b) heparin-bonded guide-wires
(c) flushing with heparinized saline.

3. *Infection at the puncture site.*
4. *Damage to local structures,* especially the brachial plexus during axillary artery puncture.
5. *False aneurysm.* Rare. Presents as a pulsatile mass at the puncture site, usually 1–2 weeks after arteriography and is due to communication between the lumen of the artery and a cavity

within an organized haematoma. Treatment is surgical.

6. *Arteriovenous fistula*. Rare. More frequent with direct vertebral puncture than femoral puncture.

DISTANT

1. *Peripheral embolus* from the stripped catheter thrombus. Emboli to small digital arteries will resolve spontaneously; emboli to large arteries may need surgical embolectomy.

2. *Atheroembolism*. More likely in old people. J-shaped guide-wires are less likely to dislodge atheromatous plaques.

3. *Air embolus*. May be fatal in a coronary or cerebral artery. It is prevented by:
   (a) ensuring that all taps and connectors are tight
   (b) always sucking back when a new syringe is connected
   (c) ensuring that all bubbles are excluded from the syringe before injecting
   (d) keeping the syringe vertical, plunger up, when injecting.

4. *Cotton fibre embolus*[6]. Occurs when syringes are filled from a bowl containing swabs. Prevented by:
   (a) separate bowls of saline for flushing and wet swabs, or
   (b) a closed system of perfusion.

5. *Artery dissection*, due to entry of the catheter, guide-wire or contrast medium into the subintimal space. It is recognized by resistance to movement of the guide-wire or catheter or increased resistance to injection of contrast medium. The risk of serious dissection is reduced by:
   (a) floppy J-shaped guide-wires
   (b) pigtail catheters
   (c) a test injection prior to a pump injection
   (d) careful and gentle manipulation of catheters.

6. *Catheter knotting*. More likely during the investigation of complex congenital heart disease. Non-surgical reduction of catheter knots is discussed by Thomas and Sievers.[7]

7. *Catheter impaction*
   (a) In a coronary artery produces cardiac ischaemic pain.

(b) In a mesenteric artery produces abdominal pain.

There should be rapid wash-out of contrast medium after a selective injection.

8. *Guide-wire breakage.* More common in the past and tended to occur 5 cm from the tip, where a single central core terminates.

9. *Bacteraemia/septicaemia.*

References

1. Herlinger, H. (1976) Aortography and peripheral arteriography. In: Ansell, G. (ed). *Complications in Diagnostic Radiology*, pp. 42–75. Oxford: Blackwell Scientific.

2. Shehadi, W.H. (1975) Adverse reactions to intravascularly administered contrast media. *Am. J. Roentg.* **124**, 145–152.

3. Holm, M. & Praestholm, J. (1979) Ioxaglate, a new low osmolar contrast medium used in femoral angiography. *Br. J. Radiol.* **52**, 169–172.

4. Gensini, G.G. & di Giorgi, S. (1964) Myocardial toxicity of contrast agents used in angiography. *Radiology* **82**, 24–34.

5. Mishkin, M.M., Baum, S. & di Chiro, G. (1973) Emergency treatment of angiography induced paraplegia and tetraplegia and tetraplegia. *New Engl. J. Med.* **288**, 1184–1185.

6. Adams, D.F., Olin, T.B. & Kosek, J. (1965) Cotton fibre embolisation during angiography. *Radiology* **84**, 678–681.

7. Thomas, H.A. & Sievers, R.E. (1979) Nonsurgical reduction of arterial catheter knots. *Am J. Roentg.* **132**, 1018–1019.

Head and Neck Arteriography

N.B. In this and the following arteriography procedures the omission of subheadings for 'contra-indications', 'patient preparation' and 'complications' implies that there are none specific to that procedure over and above those pertaining to the Seldinger technique already discussed in the introductory section of this chapter.

Indications
1. Vascular disease, e.g. the investigation of patients with cerebral ischaemia or intracranial haemorrhage.
2. Further investigation of tumours. The primary diagnostic tools are now CT or MRI.
3. Interventional procedures e.g. embolization.

Contrast medium
LOCM 240.
Common carotid injection 7 ml ⎫ over
Internal carotid injection 6 ml ⎬ 1.5 s.
Vertebral artery injection 6 ml ⎭

Aorta 40 ml over 2 s

Equipment
1. Fluoroscopy unit, preferably with digital subtraction facilities.
2. Serial film changer (if DSA is not available).
3. Pump injector.

Methods
Via a percutaneous femoral artery catheter
1. Aortogram — pigtail catheter (see Figure 8.7)
2. Selective carotid or vertebral injection — headhunter (Figure 8.3), sidewinder (Figure 8.4) or Newton's catheters.

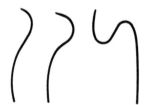

Fig. 8.3 Headhunter catheters.

end holes: 1   side holes: 0

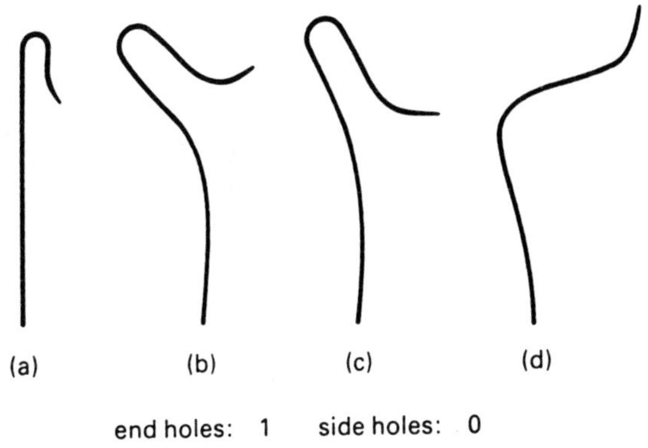

Fig. 8.4 Simmons (sidewinder) catheters. (a) For narrow aorta. (b) For moderately narrow aorta. (c) For wide aorta. (d) For elongated aorta.

(a)   (b)   (c)   (d)

end holes: 1   side holes: 0

ADVANTAGES
1. Selective and superselective injections are possible from one arterial puncture.
2. The position of the catheter tip is easily maintained.
3. Radiographic positioning is easier.
4. If performed under local anaesthesia, it is much less unpleasant for the patient.
5. Because the radiologist is manipulating the catheter at the groin, the radiation dose to his hands is much less.

DISADVANTAGES
1. More sophisticated X-ray equipment and more expensive materials are necessary.
2. The technique may be more difficult in older patients with atheromatous and tortuous arteries.
3. A higher level of technical skill is necessary.

Direct puncture of a carotid or vertebral artery

The carotid artery is punctured with a needle and cannula.

The vertebral artery is punctured with a specifically designed needle with a closed end and a single side hole (Lindgren's needle).

INDICATIONS
1. Failed catheterization.
2. Expected difficulty in negotiating atheromatous vessels.

ADVANTAGES
It is not technically difficult.

DISADVANTAGES
1. Separate puncture is needed for each artery.
2. Selective injections are difficult.
3. The proximal common carotid and vertebral arteries are not visualized.
4. Damage to the vessels.
5. Damage to other structures, e.g. the sympathetic plexus with a resulting Horner's syndrome.
6. Atheroma at the carotid bifurcation may be dislodged.
7. Pressure on the carotid sinus may result in bradycardia and hypotension, even if atropine premedication has been given.
8. The needle tip may be dislodged.
9. The vertebral artery may be too small to accommodate the needle.
10. The radiologist's hands are nearer the primary beam.

Technique   The catheter method will be described, as it is the most frequently used. The catheter is introduced into the femoral artery, using the Seldinger technique, and advanced to the aortic arch.

Aortography   This is performed when disease at the origins of the head and neck vessels is suspected. A pigtail catheter is advanced into the ascending aorta. The patient is positioned 45° RPO, with the head 10° off lateral. The beam is centred and collimated to show the aortic arch and arteries in the neck.

The extracerebral   When patients are being investigated because of
vessels   ischaemic cerebrovascular disease, coned views of the extracerebral arteries in the neck are taken to identify a possible source of emboli. Arteries are selectively catheterized[1]:
1. Right subclavian artery — to include the origin of the right vertebral artery.
2. Right common carotid artery — at least two views are necessary to demonstrate small atheromatous plaques and stenoses. The beam is centred on the carotid bifurcation.

3. Left common carotid artery — as for the right.
4. Left subclavian artery — as for the right.
5. The intracerebral arteries — both internal carotids and one vertebral artery are catheterized in turn. (Injection of contrast medium into one vertebral artery is sufficient to demonstrate the basilar artery and its branches.) For convenience each artery is examined after its respective extracerebral continuation, e.g. the right internal carotid is catheterized after the right common carotid artery injection. Hard-copy films are taken from the subtraction unit to demonstrate the arterial, capillary and venous phases.

Views of the internal carotid injections are taken from the 20° fronto-occipital and lateral positions. The vertebral artery injections are viewed from the 30° fronto-occipital (centred 2 cm above the glabella) and lateral (centred 3 cm below the external auditory meatus) positions.

ADDITIONAL FILMS
1. For aneurysms. An additional view to profile the neck of the aneurysm is necessary and this series of films should be taken during all examinations performed for subarachnoid haemorrhage, even if an aneurysm has not been demonstrated on the initial films. The head is rotated 25° away from the side of injection and films are taken during the arterial phase only, with the vertical tube.
2. For the superior sagittal sinus. This is usually well shown on the lateral run, but narrowings and occlusions may be confirmed with the 20° fronto-occipital run repeated with the head turned 10° away from the side of the injection. This will separate the anterior and the posterior ends of the sinus.
3. For patency of the anterior communicating artery. A carotid injection is made while the opposite carotid is compressed in the neck (cross compression view). The anterior communicating artery is patent if contrast medium flows into the arteries of both hemispheres. Films are taken in the 20° fronto-occipital position.
4. Macroradiography. This is useful for:

(a) defining the relationship of the neck of an aneurysm to adjacent small vessels
(b) detecting small vessel disease
(c) resolving individual small vessels in the vascular blush of tumours[2].

Aftercare In addition to the routine post-catheterization observations, facial movements and muscle power in the upper limbs should be assessed.

Complications As for the general complications of arteriography, but the risk of cerebral embolus is higher. Overall mortality should be < 0.1% and morbidity < 1%. Transient cortical blindness may also occur after injection of contrast onto the vertebral vessels.

References
1. Jeans, W.D., MacKenzie, S. & Baird, R.N. (1986) Angiography in transient cerebral ischaemia using three views of the carotid bifurcation. *Br. J. Radiol.* **59**, 135–142.
2. Kendall, B. (1984) Angiography of the head. In: du Boulay, G.H. (ed.) *A Textbook of Radiological Diagnosis*, Vol. 1, 5th edn, pp. 79–152. London: H.K. Lewis.

Further reading
Hincke, V.C., Judkins, M.P. & Paxton, H.D. (1967) Simplified selective femorocerebral angiography. *Radiology* **89**, 1048–1052.
Molyneux, A.J. & Sheldon, P.W.E. (1982) A randomised blind trial of iopamidol and meglumine calcium metrizoate (Triosil 280, Isopaque cerebral) in cerebral angiography. *Br. J. Radiol.* **55**, 117–119.
Molyneux, A.J., Sheldon, P.W.E. & Yates, D.A. (1982) A comparative trial of sodium meglumine ioxaglate (Hexabrix) and iopamidol (Niopam) for cerebral angiography. *Br. J. Radiol.* **55**, 881–884.
Simmons, C.R., Tsao, E.C. & Thompson, J.R. (1973) Angiographic approach to the difficult aortic arch: a new technique for transfemoral cerebral angiography in the aged. *Am. J. Roentg.* **119**, 605–610.

Angiocardiography

Usually performed simultaneously with cardiac catheterization, in which pressures and oximetry are measured in the cardiac chambers and vessels that are under investigations. The right heart, left heart and great vessels are examined together or alone, depending on the clinical problem.

Indications
1. Congenital heart disease and anomalies of the great vessels.
2. Valve disease.
3. Myocardial disease and ventricular function.

Contrast medium   LOCM 370 (see Table 8.1).

Table 8.1   Volumes of contrast media in angiocardiography.

| | Injection site | |
	Ventricle	Aorta or pulmonary artery
ADULT	1 ml kg^{-1} at 18–20 ml s^{-1}	0.75 ml kg^{-1} at 18–20 ml s^{-1} (max. 40 ml)
CHILD First year 2–4 years 5 years	1.5 ml kg^{-1} ⎫ injected 1.2 ml kg^{-1} ⎬ over 1.0 ml kg^{-1} ⎭ 1–2 s	75% of the ventricular volume

In general, hypoplastic or obstructed chambers require smaller volumes and flow rates and large shunts require greater volumes and flow rates of contrast medium.

Equipment
1. Biplane fluoroscopy.
2. Biplane cineradiography or biplane serial changer (preferable with C-arms to facilitate axial projections).
3. Pressure recording device.
4. ECG monitor.
5. Blood oxygen analyser.
6. Catheter
   (a) For pressure measurements and blood sampling: Cournand (Figure 8.5), 4F–7F
   (b) For angiocardiography: NIH (Figure 8.6) or pigtail (Figure 8.7), 5F–8F.

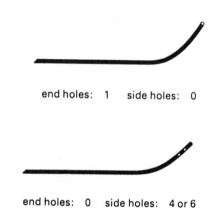

Fig. 8.5   Cournand catheter.

end holes: 1   side holes: 0

Fig. 8.6   NIH catheter.

end holes: 0   side holes: 4 or 6

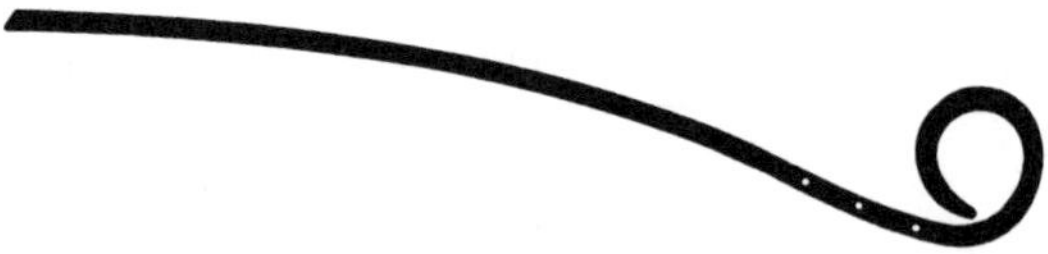

Fig. 8.7   Pigtail catheter.

end holes: 1   side holes: 12

Technique

1. Right-sided cardiac structures and pulmonary arteries are examined by introducing a catheter into a peripheral vein. In babies the femoral vein may be the only vein large enough to take the catheter. If an atrial septal defect is suspected, the femoral vein approach offers the best chance of passing the catheter into the left atrium through the defect.

2. In adults the right antecubital or basilic vein may be used. The cephalic vein should not be used because it can be difficult to pass the catheter past the site where the vein pierces the clavipectoral fascia to join the axillary vein. The catheter, or introducer, is introduced using the Seldinger technique. (The NIH catheter must be introduced via an introducer as there is no end hole for a guide-wire.)

3. In children it is usually possible to examine the left heart and occasionally the aorta by manipulating a venous catheter through a patent foramen ovale.

In adults the aorta and left ventricle are studied via a catheter passed retrogradely from the femoral artery.

4. The catheter is manipulated into the appropriate positions for recording pressures and sampling blood for oxygen saturation. Following this, angiography is performed.

Films 1. The recording of cardiac images is now most commonly performed using cine at 25–80 frames per s. Up to 200 frames per s is possible, but there is no significant increase in the amount of information gained.

Pulmonary arteriography for peripheral lung lesions and arch aortography for aortic or great vessel disease are most commonly performed using rapid cut film because of the improved detail that is possible (see later).

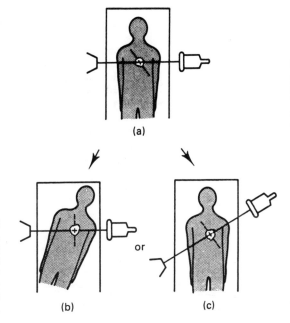

Fig. 8.8 Principles of axial angiography. Alignment of the heart perpendicular to the X-ray beam (b) by moving the patient, or (c) by moving the equipment.

2. Until recently angiocardiographic diagnosis depended on frontal (vertical tube) and lateral (horizontal tube) projections. It is now recognized that angled views that place the pathological lesion at right-angles to the X-ray beam increase diagnostic accuracy in angiocardiography. The first principle of axial cineangiography is axial alignment of the heart, i.e. placing the long axis of the heart perpendicular to the X-ray beam (Figure 8.8). The second principle involves rotation of the heart on this long axis so as to profile those areas of heart under examination.

3. Depending on the equipment that is available, axial alignment can be accomplished in one of three ways:
   (a) rotation of the patient in relation to fixed AP and lateral tubes (Figure 8.8b)
   (b) movement of equipment alone (Figure 8.8c)
   (c) movement of both equipment and patient.

4. Three angled views have been found to be most useful:
   (a) *40° caudal-cranial (sitting up) view.* This is obtained by placing a 45° wedge under the patient's shoulders and filming with a vertical X-ray beam or by keeping the patient supine and angling the tube (Figure 8.9). This manoeuvre places the pulmonary trunk and its bifurcation perpendicular to the X-ray beam. Because these structures are no longer foreshortened, this projection is ideal for demonstrating the pulmonary trunk, pulmonary valve, annulus and bifurcation into right and left pulmonary arteries.
   (b) *40° cranial/40° LAO (hepatoclavicular or four-chamber) view.* This projection can be obtained by elevating the patient's thorax

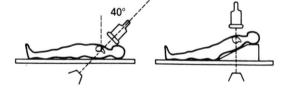

Fig. 8.9 The 40° caudal cranial view (sitting-up view).

40°, elevating the left shoulder 40° and using the vertical X-ray tube. With a C-arm intensifier the arm is moved to the left and tilted cranially. This view places the vertical tube perpendicular to the long axis of the heart and aligns the atrial septum and posterior interventricular septum parallel to the beam. When filming biplane the patient is slanted 20° feet to the right side of the table in the horizontal plane so that the long axis of the heart is perpendicular to the horizontal X-ray beam. Alternatively a horizontal C-arm can be rotated 20° (Figure 8.8). The defects and structures best seen in this projection are listed in Table 8.2.

(c) *Long axial 20° RAO (long axial oblique) view.* With a C-arm arrangement, the lateral tube and image intensifier is angled 25–30° cranially, to align with the long axis of the heart, and 20° RAO. Alternatively, when there is only a fixed horizontal tube, the long axis of the body can be slanted 30° away from the line of the X-ray beam and the right shoulder elevated 20°. Because it is not possible to slant an adult 30° across the table, the latter method is suitable only for children.

The complementary biplane view to the long axial oblique is an RAO view using the vertical AP tube rotated 30–45° to the right. The structures seen in the long axial oblique view are listed in Table 8.2.

Reference   1. Kelley, M.J., Jaffe, C.C. & Kleinman, C.S. (1982) *Cardiac Imaging in infants and Children*. Philadelphia: W.B. Saunders.

Further reading   Elliot, L.P., Bargeron Jr, L.M., Soto, B. & Bream P.R. (1980) Axial cineangiography in congenital heart disease. *Radiol. Clin. N. Am.* **18**(3), 515–546.

Verel, D. & Grainger, R.G. (1978) *Cardiac Catheterization and Angiography*, 3rd edn. Edinburgh: Churchill Livingstone.

Table 8.2 Anatomy depicted in axial views.

Anatomy	Defects identified
Four-chamber view — vertical tube	
LV injection	
Posterior interventricular septum	Endocardial cushion defects
LV outflow tract	Subvalvar aortic stenosis; membranous and supracristal VSDs
LV/RA region	LV/RA shunts
Mitral valve/aortic valve relationship	Double outlet right ventricle
Aortic arch	PDA
Aortic valve region and coronary arteries	Sinus of Valsalva aneurysm; anomalous coronary origin (esp. LAD from RCA)
Pulmonary valve, trunk and bifurcation	d-TGA; tetralogy of Fallot
LA injection	
Left atrium	Sinus venosus ASD; cor triatriatum
Right upper lobe pulmonary vein injection	
Atrial septum	ASD
RV injection	
Ventricular septum	VSD in a right-to-left shunt
Pulmonary trunk	Bifurcation
Four-chamber view — horizontal tube	
LV injection	
Mitral valve; posterior papillary muscles; LV outflow tract; aortic valve	Supracristal VSDs
RV injection	
Ostium of RV infundibulum, pulmonary valve and origin of right pulmonary artery	Tetralogy of Fallot
Tricuspid valve	Ebstein's malformation

Table 8.2 contd.

Anatomy	Defects identified
Long axial oblique view – horizontal tube	
LV injection	
Anterior ventricular septum	Membranous, supracristal and muscular VSDs; relationship of aorta to anterior interventricular septum
LV outflow tract	IHSS; subvalvar aortic stenosis
Mitral valve – LV outflow	IHSS; prolapse of anterior leaflet of mitral valve
RV injection	
Anterior ventricular septum	VSD in tetralogy of Fallot
Left pulmonary artery	Origin in tetralogy of Fallot
Long axial oblique view – vertical tube	
LV injection	
Atrioventricular part of cardiac septum	Common atrioventricular canal; mitral valve incompetence
RV injection	
	Tetralogy of Fallot

Modified from Kelley et al [1].

ASD	Atrial septal defect		PDA	Patent ductus arteriosus
IHSS	Idiopathic hypertrophic subaortic stenosis		RA	Right atrium
			RCA	Right coronary artery
LA	Left atrium		RV	Right ventricle
LAD	Left anterior descending artery		TGA	Transposition of great arteries
LV	Left ventricle		VSD	Ventricular septal defect

Pulmonary Arteriography

Indication Demonstration of pulmonary emboli and other peripheral abnormalities, e.g. arteriovenous malformations.

Contrast medium As for ascending aortography (see Table 8.1).

Equipment
1. Fluoroscopy unit on a C- or U-arm, with digital subtraction facilities if possible.
2. Pump injector.
3. Rapid serial film changer (if DSA is not available).
4. Catheter:
   (a) pigtail (coiled end, end hole and 12 side holes; Figure 8.7), or
   (b) NIH (no end hole, six side holes; Figure 8.6).

Technique Seldinger technique via the right femoral vein. The NIH catheter is introduced via an introducer sheath. The catheter tip is sited, under fluoroscopic control, to lie 1–3 cm above the pulmonary valve.

Films
1. Three per s for 3 s, and
2. One per s for 4 s.

To cover the arterial, capillary and venous phases.

Additional techniques
1. If the entire chest cannot be accommodated on one field of view, the examination can be repeated by examining each lung. The catheter is advanced to lie in each main pulmonary artery in turn. For the right lung the patient, or the tube, is turned 10° LPO and for the left lung 10° RPO.
2. Sitting-up view or 40° caudal-cranial view. This view is optimal for the visualization of the bifurcation of the right and left pulmonary arteries, the pulmonary valve, annulus and trunk. With this manoeuvre the pulmonary trunk is no longer foreshortened and is not superimposed over its bifurcation.

   The view can be obtained by either tube angulation or by propping the patient to a 45° sitting position (see Figure 8.9).

Coronary Arteriography

Indications
1. Diagnosis of the presence and extent of ischaemic heart disease.
2. After revascularization procedures.
3. Congenital heart lesions.

Contrast medium
LOCM 370. 8–10 ml given as a hand injection for each projection.

Equipment
1. C-arm or rotating cradle.
2. Cineradiography and video recorder.
3. Pressure recording device and ECG monitor.
4. Catheters:
   (a) Judkins
       – designed for a femoral approach; the left and right coronary artery catheters are of different shape[1] (Figure 8.10)
   (b) Amplatz left and right catheters also differ (Figure 8.11)
   (c) Sones
       – One catheter is suitable for both coronary arteries and although originally designed for use via a brachial artery cutdown, femoral artery catheterization is possible[2].

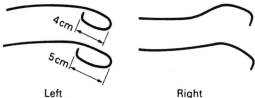

Left   Right

end holes: 1 side holes: 0

Fig. 8.10 Judkins' coronary artery catheters.

4 cm : normal aortic arch
5 cm : unfolded aortic arch

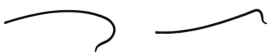

Fig. 8.11 Amplatz coronary artery catheters.

Left   Right

end holes: 1 side holes: 0

Patient preparation   1. As for routine arteriography.
2. β-blockers are stopped 48 hours prior to the procedure.

Preliminary films   Chest:
1. PA.
2. Left lateral.

Technique   The catheter is introduced using the Seldinger technique and advanced until its tip lies in the ostium of the coronary artery. The technique using the Judkins' catheters is illustrated diagrammatically in Figure 8.12.

Films   Cine-angiography (32 films per s) is performed in the following positions:

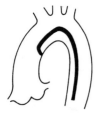
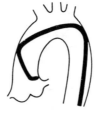
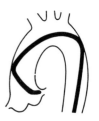

Left: push only

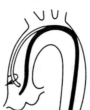
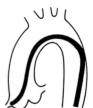

Right: push – rotate – push

Fig. 8.12 Catheter manipulation for engagement of the coronary ostia using Judkins' catheters.

Right coronary artery	1. 60° LAO. 2. 30° RAO. 3. Right lateral.

Left coronary artery	1. 30° RAO. 2. 60° LAO. 3. Left lateral.

Additional film

The left main stem coronary artery may appear foreshortened in the above three projections. If so, the 40° caudal-cranial view should be performed (Figure 8.9).

Coronary arteriography is usually preceded by left ventricular angiography, in the 30° RAO position, to assess left ventricular function.

Complications

In addition to the general complications discussed on p. 210, patients undergoing coronary arteriography are particularly liable to:
1. Sudden death.
2. Myocardial infarction.
3. Arrhythmias.

A review of recent experiences is to be found in the *British Medical Journal*[3].

References

1. Judkins, M.P. (1967) Selective coronary arteriography. Part I: a percutaneous transfemoral technic. *Radiology* **89**, 815–824.
2. Sones, F.M. & Shirey, E.K. (1962) Cine coronary arteriography. *Mod. Concepts Cardiovasc. Dis.* **31**, 735–738.
3. Leading Article (1980) *BMJ* **281**, 627–628.

Ascending Aortography

Indications
1. Aortic aneurysm or dissection (echocardiography, CT with intravenous contrast enhancement, and MRI can also be used to demonstrate a dissection).
2. Atheroma at the origin of the major vessels.
3. Aortic regurgitation (echocardiography is more sensitive and less invasive if available).
4. Congenital heart disease — particularly the demonstration of congenital or iatrogenic aortopulmonary shunts and coarctation.
5. Aortic trauma.

Contrast medium
LOCM 370, 0.75 ml kg^{-1} (max. 40 ml). Inject at 18–20 ml s^{-1}. See Table 8.1.

Equipment
1. Fluoroscopy unit, preferably with DSA.
2. Pump injector.
3. Catheter:
   (a) pigtail (see Figure 8.7), or
   (b) Gensini (Figure 8.13), or
   (c) NIH (see Figure 8.6).

Technique
1. The catheter is introduced using the Seldinger technique via the femoral artery, and its tip sited 1–3 cm above the aortic valve.
2. The patient is positioned 45° RPO to open out the aortic arch, and to show the aortic valve and the left ventricle to best advantage.
3. A test injection is performed to ensure that:
   (a) the catheter is correctly placed in relation to the aortic valve (which is particularly important in the hyperkinetic heart)
   (b) the catheter tip is not in a coronary artery.

Films
Two per s for 6 s or cine at 25 frames per s.

ADDITIONAL FILMS
If, on the original run, the right common carotid artery overlies the right innominate artery or an aneurysm is present on the anterior aspect of the ascending aorta, the injection is repeated with the patient positioned LPO.

Fig. 8.13 Gensini catheter. Note tapered end.

end holes: 1   side holes: 6

Translumbar Aortography

This procedure is rarely performed nowadays in departments which utilize modern catheter techniques and equipment.

Indications   Investigation of the abdominal aorta and its branches when other access is not possible.

Contraindications
1. Severe hypertension.
2. Aneurysm (relative contraindication) — requires a high puncture.
3. Bleeding diathesis or anticoagulant treatment.

Contrast medium   LOCM 320. 10 ml is used for the test injections, 35 ml for the definitive aortic injection.

Equipment
1. Fluoroscopy unit, with digital facility if possible.
2. Moving table top.
3. Rapid serial film changer.
4. Aortogram needle (15G − 15, 18 or 25 cm).

Patient preparation   As for a general anaesthetic.

Methods
1. Needle puncture at L3 level, i.e. below the renal arteries.
2. High needle puncture at T12/L1 level.
3. Using a Teflon-sheathed needle.

Technique
Needle puncture
(Figure 8.14)
1. Using aseptic technique the skin is punctured just above the level of the iliac crest, one hand's breadth to the left of the spine. The aim is to puncture the aorta at the L3 level.
2. If the needle hits a vertebral body, it is withdrawn and re-inserted with an increased forward angle of entry. Pulsations may be felt through the needle when it rests against the aortic wall.
3. The aorta is punctured and the stilette withdrawn. Pulsatile blood flow indicates arterial puncture. The needle is connected via a length of extension tubing to a syringe and intermittently flushed with heparinized saline. A test injection of contrast is given and, if this shows the tip of the needle to lie

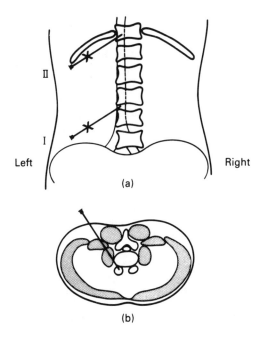

Fig. 8.14 Technique of translumbar aortography. (a) Diagrammatic representation with the patient lying prone. Low (I) and high (II) puncture points indicated by x. (b) Transverse section through the abdomen at the level of a low puncture.

in the aortic lumen (as opposed to an aortic branch), the main injection should follow.
4. Hand injection of contrast.
5. The contrast medium is followed down the legs taking films at 1 per s if a 100 mm camera is used.

ADDITIONAL FILMS
Patient 30° LAO or RAO to demonstrate overlapping vessels.

High needle puncture   Indicated when there is an abdominal aortic aneurysm or bilateral absent femoral pulses. In the latter situation, when both femoral arteries are impalpable, there is a high likelihood that the distal aorta will be occluded. The needle is introduced just below and following the line of the twelfth rib. The remainder of the procedure is as described above.

Catheter technique[1]　Has the advantage of less likelihood of dislodgement out of the aorta.

The Teflon-sleeved needle is inserted as described above. When in a satisfactory position the needle is removed, leaving the sheath in place. If required, it can be directed downstream using a tip-deflector guide-wire.

Aftercare
1. Bed rest for 24 hours.
2. Pulse and blood pressure quarter-hourly for 4 hours and then 4-hourly for 24 hours.
3. Temperature and respiration 4-hourly for 24 hours.

Complications

Due to anaesthetic　See p. 9.

Due to the contrast medium
1. Hypersensitivity reactions.
2. Injection into named vessels:
   (a) lumbar artery
   (b) renal artery
   (c) coeliac/mesenteric artery.

Prevented by a test injection (thus the test injection must not be omitted, even if there is good pulsatile flow through the needle).

Due to technique
1. Haemorrhage/haematoma. Occurs in all patients and is worse with high puncture.
2. Puncture of other structures:
   (a) pancreas, producing pancreatitis
   (b) pleura, producing pneumothorax
   (c) heart, producing cardiac tamponade
   (d) thoracic duct, producing chylothorax, or cysterna chyli, producing chylous ascites
   (e) spinal cord.
3. Emboli.
4. Lumbar osteitis. There is narrowing of the inter-vertebral disc space and boney sclerosis, usually within 6 months. The aetiology is uncertain.

Reference   1. Stocks, L.O., Halpern, M. & Turner, A.F. (1969) Complete translumbar aortography. The Teflon sleeve technique. *Am. J. Roentg.* **107**, 835–839.

Arteriography of the Lower Limb

Indications
1. Arterial ischaemia.
2. Trauma.
3. Investigation of a mass.
4. Arteriovenous malformation.

Methods

Both lower limbs
1. Catheter angiography — using a pigtail catheter introduced into the femoral artery and sited proximal to the aortic bifurcation.
2. Intravenous DSA.
3. Brachial or axillary puncture.
4. Translumbar aortography (see previous section).

One lower limb
1. Using a femoral artery catheter:
   (a) introduced retrogradely and sited in the ipsilateral common iliac artery
   (b) introduced retrogradely from the contralateral side and sited in the common iliac, external iliac or femoral artery (Sidewinder catheter)
   (c) introduced antegradely.
2. Direct injection through a Potts or Sutton needle in the femoral artery. The syringe is connected to the needle via a short length of polythene tubing (rarely, if ever, used now).

Contrast medium
With the exception of translumbar aortography, all of these techniques can be performed under local anaesthesia. It is, therefore, more comfortable for the patient if a low osmolar contrast medium is used. 10–20 ml of 300 mg I ml^{-1} concentration is suitable for the examination of one limb. 50 ml of 350 mg I ml^{-1}, at a rate of 12–15 ml s^{-1}, is suitable for the catheter aortogram.

Further reading
Fletcher, E.W.L. (1982) A comparison of iopamidol and diatrizoate in peripheral angiography. *Br. J. Radiol.* 55, 36–38.

Whitehouse, G.H. & Snowdon, S.L. (1982) An assessment of iopamidol, a non-ionic contrast medium in aorto-femoral angiography. *Clin. Radiol.* 33, 231–234.

Coeliac Axis, Superior Mesenteric and Inferior Mesenteric Arteriography

Indications
1. Gastrointestinal haemorrhage.
2. Staging tumours prior to intervention (surgical or radiological).
3. Gastrointestinal ischaemia.
4. Portal venography.

Contrast medium   LOCM 370.

Equipment
1. Fluoroscopy unit, preferably with digital subtraction facilities.
2. Rapid serial film changer.
3. Pump injector.
4. Catheter — selective femorovisceral or cobra catheter (Figures 8.15 and 8.16).

Technique   Femoral artery puncture.

Bowel movement causing subtraction artefact can be reduced by using a smooth muscle relaxant (e.g. Buscopan 10–20 mg) and abdominal compression.

Fig. 8.15 Selective femorovisceral catheters. (a) For coeliac and superior mesenteric arteries in larger patients. (b) For coeliac and superior mesenteric arteries in smaller patients. (c) For inferior mesenteric artery.

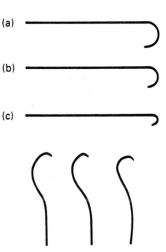

(a)

(b)

(c)

Fig. 8.16 Cobra catheters.

end holes: 1   side holes: 0

When performed for gastrointestinal bleeding, provided that the patient is bleeding at the time, a blood loss of 0.5–0.6 ml min^{-1} can be demonstrated. The site of active bleeding is revealed by extravasated contrast medium remaining in the bowel on the late films, when intravascular contrast has cleared. Vascular malformations, tumours and varices may be demonstrated.

Coeliac axis   Patient supine. 36 ml contrast medium at 6 ml s^{-1}.

FILMS
Two per s for 5 s. One per s for 16 s.

Or similar on digital equipment, with appropriate hard copy.

(Angiography of the pancreas is best achieved by selective injection into the splenic, dorsal pancreatic and gastroduodenal arteries.)

Superior mesenteric   Patient supine. 42 ml contrast medium at 7 ml s^{-1}.
artery

FILMS
As for coeliac artery.

Late phase visceral   Patient slightly PRO.
arteriography
When selective catheterization of the coeliac or SMA has been achieved, delayed venous phase films will show the portal vein. (Opacification of the superior mesenteric and portal veins may be increased by the use of phentolamine, 10 mg, immediately prior to the contrast injection.)

N.B. If splenic vein opacification is required, then a late phase coeliac arteriogram is necessary.

Inferior mesenteric   If the inferior mesenteric artery is to be examined as
artery   part of a procedure which will examine the superior mesenteric artery or coeliac axis as well, e.g. to find the source of gastrointestinal bleeding, then the inferior mesenteric artery should be examined first so that contrast medium in the bladder will not obscure its terminal branches.

Patient 30° LPO (to open the sigmoid loop).

Hand injection of 10 ml of contrast medium.

FILMS
As for coeliac artery.

Further reading   Allison, D.J. (1980) Gastrointestinal bleeding. Radiological
diagnosis. *Br. J. Hosp. Med.* **23**, 358–365.
Herlinger, H. (1978) Arterioportography. *Clin. Radiol.* **29**,
255–275.

Renal Arteriography

Indications
1. Renal artery stenosis.
2. Renal tumour prior to embolization or rarely for diagnosis.
3. Kidney donor.
4. Haematuria of unknown cause.

Contrast medium
Selective renal artery injection

LOCM 300. 10 ml at 5 ml s^{-1}, or by hand injection.

Flush aortic

LOCM 370. 50 ml at injection 12 ml s^{-1}.

Equipment
1. Fluoroscopy unit, with DSA facilities if possible.
2. Rapid serial film changer.
3. Pump injector.
4. Catheters
   (a) selective injection – Sidewinder or Cobra
   (b) flush aortic injection – pigtail (see Figure 8.7).

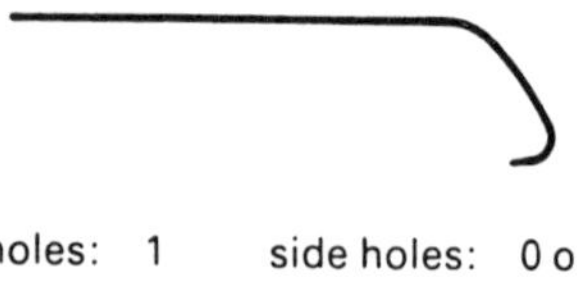

Fig. 8.17 Selective renal artery catheter.

end holes: 1   side holes: 0 or 2

Films

If DSA is available, appropriate hard copy is obtained at the end of the procedure. If not then films at two per s for 3 s and one per s for 4 s are appropriate.

Technique
Flush aortography

Femoral artery puncture. The catheter is placed proximal to the renal vessels (i.e. approx. T12) and AP and oblique (10° raise on the side of interest) runs are performed (the oblique run demonstrating the renal origins). Selective catheterization may overlook a stenosis at the origin of the renal artery or convert a stenosis into an occlusion, but is occasionally required to define better the renal vasculature.

Renal tumours

Selective catheterization more accurately defines the

anatomy and tumour vessels may be shown better after the administration of 5 µg of adrenaline. The adrenaline is injected into the renal artery over 30 s, the catheter is then quickly flushed with saline and 10 ml of contrast medium is injected by hand[1].

Donor kidneys A flush aortogram is performed to count the number of renal vessels and to ensure normality of the contralateral kidney. Selective injection may occasionally be required to accurately number the renal arteries.

Reference 1. Ekelund, L., Gerlock Jr, J. & Goncharenko, V. (1978) The epinephrine effect in renal angiography revisited. *Clin. Radiol.* **29**, 387–392.

Vascular Dilatation

(Also known as percutaneous transluminal angio-plasty or balloon dilatation.)

Indications
1. Dilatation of localized vascular stenoses, mainly of the renal, iliac, lower limb and coronary arteries.
2. Dilatation of occluded segments of vessels in selected cases.

Dilatation procedures are often combined with preparatory diagnostic angiography in the same session; the majority are done under local anaesthetic.

The procedure is often needed after lysis of arterial thrombus: this is outlined below.

Equipment
1. Fluoroscopy unit with moving table top.
2. Image recording facilities – digital subtraction, 105 mm or rapid large film changer.
3. Arterial pressure measuring equipment (optional).
4. Catheters
   (a) Gruntzig double-lumen dilatation catheters (these vary in length of catheter from 80 to 120 cm, in balloon length from 2 to 10 cm and in balloon diameter from 2 to 10 mm: they may also be straight, curved or of the 'sidewinder' type, and are chosen in relation to the particular lesion to be treated)
   (b) van Andel dilatation catheter (a tapered, straight Teflon catheter, occasionally useful)
   (c) straight Teflon or polyethylene catheters, 7F.
5. Guide-wires
   (a) 0.035 or 0.038 inch diameter wires, 145 cm long (straight), with 2, 3 and 15 mm J-shapes; a Terumo Teflon coated wire may be helpful for crossing tight stenoses
   (b) 250 cm exchange guide-wire.
6. Streptokinase may be infused into recently throm-bosed vessels, prior to dilatation. This is diluted and used with a pressure injector to infuse 5000 units per hour. Recombinent tissue plasminogen activator (rTPA) may be used as an alternative, in which case 0.5 mg per hour is used. Heparin, 500

units per hour, may also be infused to prevent catheter thrombosis.

Technique
Principles

1. Adequate angiograms must be available before any dilatation is attempted.
2. Dilatation is always performed with the guide-wire remaining across the stenosis or occlusion until the procedure is completed.
3. Adequate vascular surgical assistance must be readily available before attempting dilatation.
4. If the history suggests that a thrombosis has occurred within the previous 3 weeks, strepto-kinase (or rTPA) lysis may be helpful.
5. The patient should be anticoagulated during the procedure, using 3000–5000 units of heparin.
6. The balloon diameter is selected by reference to the measured size of the normal artery on the preceding angiogram, allowing for magnification. Usually the iliac arteries take a 7 mm and the superficial femoral artery a 5 mm balloon.

Renal arteries

1. A J-guide-wire is positioned in the renal artery distal to the stenosis, from either the femoral or high brachial artery approach.
2. A balloon catheter of suitable diameter is positioned across the stenosis and distended (approx. 7 atmospheres, for 1 min), after injecting 3000 units of heparin. A post-dilatation angiogram is then taken. If a residual stenosis remains, further dila-tations may be necessary.

Iliac arteries

1. These are preferably dilated retrogradely from a femoral puncture on the side of the lesion.
2. If the femoral pulse is absent or difficult to feel, it may be located using a portable Doppler scanner and its position marked. The artery can then be found and fixed with a fine needle attached to a syringe. The fine needle can then be used as a guide for the Seldinger needle. (Alternatively a sidewinder catheter can be introduced from the opposite groin and a guide-wire directed over the aortic bifurcation and across the lesion.)
3. If possible, a femoral artery pressure should be measured immediately after introducing the

catheter, and before a guide-wire is passed through the lesion. This is to assess the severity of the pressure gradient before and after angioplasty.

4. A 3 mm J-guide-wire is then advanced carefully through the lesion. If the lesion is eccentrically situated, it may be preferable to advance using a headhunter catheter, to inject contrast medium to position the catheter, and then to advance through the patent lumen, so avoiding possible dissection from below. If the lesion is particularly tight, a Terumo wire may be useful to negotiate the lesion.

5. A catheter is passed over the guide-wire and into the distal aorta.

6. No heparin need be injected.

7. The guide-wire is removed, to allow a pressure measurement in the aorta. It is then replaced and the catheter exchanged for a balloon catheter. After dilating the lesion, an angiogram is performed and the pressures checked to ensure that a gradient no longer exists.

Femoral arteries (common, and origins of SFA and profunda)

1. These cannot be approached by a puncture on the side of the lesion, since there is not enough room for manoeuvre.

2. The contralateral femoral artery is catheterized using a sidewinder catheter. The tip of this is positioned in the iliac artery ipsilateral to the lesion and a heavy-duty exchange guide-wire advanced down through the lesion. The catheter is then exchanged for a balloon catheter and, after injecting heparin 3000 units, the lesion is dilated and a check angiogram performed.

Superficial femoral and popliteal arteries

1. An antegrade puncture is performed (i.e. needle angled towards the feet) on the side of the lesion, the puncture site being about 2 cm higher than normal (the highest point at which the artery can be felt).

2. A 15 mm J-guide-wire is used to select the required branch, usually the superficial femoral artery.

3. The guide-wire is advanced almost down to the lesion, and a straight Teflon or polyethylene catheter is inserted over the guide-wire to the same point. The guide-wire is then gently passed across the lesion with the catheter following. A van

Andel dilatation catheter may be useful once the lesion has been traversed.

4. If the catheter becomes impacted in an occlusion, the guide-wire is removed and a little dilute contrast medium is injected. If the catheter is still in the lumen, immediate venous filling is seen. Ten ml of heparinized saline should be injected, the guide-wire reintroduced, and passage of the occlusion attempted. Usually the saline will have acted as a hydrostatic dilator, and a pathway will be obtained.

If the dilute contrast medium runs down parallel to the expected lumen, dissection has occurred. The catheter should be withdrawn into the patent lumen, and the operator should wait 5 min before trying again.

5. When the lesion has been passed the catheter is exchanged for a balloon catheter (usually 5 mm diameter), 3000 units of heparin are injected, and dilatation is performed. The distal 'run-off' should be carefully assessed on the post-dilatation films, since success is related to the adequacy of 'run-off' and it is also necessary to ensure that there has been no distal embolization.

Streptokinase lysis

1. A 5F catheter is advanced to the site of occlusion. If possible, a guide-wire is passed across the occlusion and the catheter advanced through the thrombus, its tip being placed in the distal part of the thrombus. If this is not possible, the tip of the catheter is embedded in the proximal thrombus. The catheter is connected to a pressure injector and securely fixed to the skin to prevent accidental movement.

2. A solution of streptokinase is run in at a rate of 5000 units per hour. To this solution may be added heparin, 500 units per hour to prevent catheter thrombosis.

3. The patient is returned to the ward, and brought back in about 4 hours for assessment, which is done by injecting a few millilitres of contrast medium, by hand, to see if lysis is taking place.

4. If lysis is seen, the catheter is withdrawn back into the remaining thrombus. If the catheter had ori-

ginally been embedded in the proximal thrombus, then the external part of the catheter is cleaned and its tip advanced once again into the thrombus. This process is repéated for up to 24 hours, unless no progress is seen, or unless bleeding occurs around the catheter, in which case the procedure is terminated.

5. If a stenosis is shown after the thrombus has lysed, a guide-wire is passed across the lesion and it is dilated.

N.B. Streptokinase is antigenic and so may cause allergic reactions including anaphylaxis. Thus previous allergic reactions to streptokinase or therapy, from 5 days to 6 months previously, are a contraindication to its use[1]. A useful, if more expensive, alternative is rTPA.

Aftercare

1. The pulses distal to the artery that has been dilated and the colour of the toes should be observed half-hourly for 4 hours.
2. Aspirin 150 mg daily (for life, unless there is a contraindication).
3. Reinforcement of the need to stop smoking.

Complications
Due to technique

1. Perforation of iliac artery leading to retroperitoneal haemorrhage.
2. Embolization of clot or atheroma distally, down either leg. This may be removed by suction thromboembolectomy or by surgical embolectomy[2].
3. Occlusion of main artery.
4. Occlusion of collateral artery.
5. Major haematoma formation, which may suddenly develop several hours after the procedure is completed.
6. Increased risk of false aneurysm formation at the puncture site.

References

1. *British National Formulary* (1992) London: British Medical Association and The Pharmaceutical Press.
2. Dorros, G., Jamnadas, P., Lewin, R.F. & Sachdev, N. (1989) Percutaneous aspiration of a thromboembolus. *Catheterization and Cardiovascular diagnosis* 17(4), 202–206.

Further reading   Auster, M., Kadir, S., Mitchell, S.E., Williams, G.M., Perler, B.A., Chang, R. & White, R.I. (1984) Iliac artery occlusion: management with intrathrombus streptokinase infusion and angioplasty. *Radiology* **153**, 365–388.

Cumberland, D.C. (1982) Percutaneous transluminal angioplasty: experience in balloon dilatation of peripheral, coronary and renal arteries. *Br. J. Radiol.* **55**, 330–337.

Gruntzig, A. & Kumpe, D.A. (1979) Technique of percutaneous transluminal angioplasty with the Gruntzig balloon catheter. *Am. J. Roentg.* **132**, 547–552.

Levin, D.C., Harrington, D.P., Bettmann, M.A., Garnic, J.D., Torman, H., Murray, P., Boxt, L.M. & Geller, S.C. (1984) Equipment choices, technical aspects and pitfalls of percutaneous transluminal angioplasty. *Cardiovasc. Intervent. Radiol.* **7**, 1–10.

Zeitler, E., Richter, E.O., Roth, F.J. & Schoop, W. (1983) Results of percutaneous transluminal angioplasty. *Radiology* **146**, 57–60.

Vascular Embolization

Indications
1. To control bleeding — from the gastrointestinal and genitourinary tracts, from the lungs and after trauma.
2. To infarct or reduce the blood supply to tumours or organs.
3. To reduce or stop blood flow through arteriovenous malformations, aneurysms, fistulae or varicoceles.
4. To reduce the blood flow in priapism.

Equipment
1. Fluoroscopy unit, preferably with multidirectional angulation, digital subtraction and 'road mapping' facilities.
2. Image recording — digital subtraction, 105 mm or large film.
3. Catheters; end hole only. Size and shape will depend on the particular problem.

   Balloon occlusion catheters and co-axial catheters may also be useful.

4. Embolic materials
   (a) Liquid — 50% dextrose alcohol, quick-setting glues.
   (b) Particulate — gel-foam, polyvinyl-alcohol.
   (c) Solid — Gianturco steel coils, detachable balloons.

   The material used depends on the lesion, its site, and the duration of the occlusion required. Other materials than those listed have been reported.

Patient preparation
1. As for arteriogram.
2. Some procedures and materials are painful and sedation may be needed.

Technique
Principles
1. All therapeutic occlusions are potentially dangerous: the expected gain must justify the risk.
2. Adequate angiograms must be available before commencing.
3. The operator must be an experienced angiographer.

4. The lesion must be selectively catheterized. When permanent occlusion is required, the centre of the lesion should be filled with non-absorbable material (e.g. silicone spheres, polyvinyl-alcohol) before the supplying blood vessels are occluded.
5. Reflux of embolic material is likely to occur as the blood flow slows down; injection of emboli should be done slowly with intermittent gentle injections of contrast medium to assess flow and progress.
6. It is safer to come back another day than to continue for too long.

Aftercare
1. Infarction of tissue often causes pain, and adequate pain relief should be provided.
2. Arterial clotting may be progressive, and observations on the tissues distal to the occluded vessel should be maintained for 24 hours.
3. Many patients have fever for up to 10 days. However infarcted tissue may become infected, and so antibiotics should be used with care.

Complications
1. Misplacement of emboli: this may occur without the operator being aware that it has happened.
2. There may be propagation of thrombus, with embolization to the lungs or elsewhere.
3. The infarcted tissue may become infected.

Further reading

Allison, D.J., Jordan, H., & Hennessy, O. (1985) Therapeutic embolisation of the hepatic artery: a review of 75 procedures. *Lancet* iii, 595–599.

Berenstein, A. & Kricheff, I. (1979) Catheter and material selection for transarterial embolisation: technical considerations. II. Materials. *Radiology* 132, 631–639.

Chuang, V.P., Wallace, S. & Gianturco, C. (1980) A new improved coil for tapered-tip catheter for arterial occlusion. *Radiology* 135, 507–509.

MacErlean, D.P., McDermott, E. & Kelly, D.G. (1982) Priapism: successful management by arterial embolisation. *Br. J. Radiol.* 55, 924–926.

White, R.I. (1984) Embolotherapy in vascular disease. *Am. J. Roentg.* 142, 27–30.

Radionuclide Ventriculography

Indications

Gated blood-pool study

1. Evaluation of ventricular function, particularly left ventricular ejection fraction (LVEF).
2. Assessment of myocardial reserve in coronary artery disease.
3. Aneurysm.
4. Valvar regurgitation and stenosis.
5. Cardiomyopathy, including the effects of cardio-toxic drugs.

First pass radionuclide angiography

1. Evaluation of right ventricular ejection fraction (RVEF).
2. Detection and quantification of intracardiac shunts.
3. Primary hypertension.
4. Right-sided infarction.
5. Cor pulmonale.

Contraindications

1. Gross arrhythmias may make gated blood-pool imaging impossible.
2. Contraindications to exercise are given in 'Radionuclide Myocardial Perfusion Imaging'.

Radiopharmaceuticals

^{99m}Tc-in-vivo-*labelled red blood cells*, 800 MBq max.

Before radiolabelling with ^{99m}Tc-pertechnetate, the red blood cells are 'primed' with an injection of stannous pyrophosphate. The stannous ions reduce the pertechnetate and allow it to bind to the pyrophosphate which adsorbs on to the red blood cells.

Equipment

1. Gamma camera, mobile if patient cannot be moved from coronary care unit.
2. Low-energy general purpose collimator.
3. Imaging computer with multi-gated acquisition (MUGA) and preferably list-mode acquisition for first pass studies.
4. ECG monitor with gating pulse output.

Patient preparation

1. Give i.v. injection of 'cold' stannous pyrophosphate ($20 \mu g \ kg^{-1}$) directly into a vein 20–30 min

before the pertechnetate injection. (Injection via a plastic cannula will result in a poor label.)

2. Place three ECG electrodes in standard positions to give a gating signal.

Technique
Gated blood-pool study

1. The patient lies supine.
2. Give i.v. injection of ^{99m}Tc-pertechnetate.
3. Allow 1 min for the bolus to equilibrate, then commence multi-gated computer acquisition (see 'Images' below).

The start of an acquisition cycle is usually triggered by the R wave of the patient's ECG. A series of 16–32 fast frames are then recorded before the next R wave occurs. Each of these has very few counts in from a single cycle, so every time the R wave trigger arrives, another set of frames is recorded and summed with the first. The sequence continues until 100–200 kilocounts per frame have been acquired in about 4–7 min.

First pass radionuclide angiography

This can provide additional information on right ventricular function and intracardiac shunts, although only from one view unless a multi-headed camera or biplanar collimator is available.

1. The patient lies supine with the camera against the chest in the RAO 30° position for best visualization of the right atrium and ventricle, or the LAO 45° position for best separation of the ventricles. A caudal tilt of 15–30° may improve separation.
2. The validity of the first pass study is critically dependent on a tight bolus injection. Inject the ^{99m}Tc-pertechnetate i.v. using the Oldendorf or similar technique (see 'General Notes').
3. Start computer acquisition (list-mode or short-frame dynamic — see 'Images' below) an instant before the cuff is released.
4. Follow with gated blood-pool study as above.

Images   All images are acquired on computer.

Gated blood-pool study   A number of views may be recorded, depending on the clinical problem:

1. LAO 35–45° with a 15–30° caudal tilt, chosen to give best separation between left and right ventricles. Patient supine. This view is sufficient if only LVEF is required.
2. Anterior, patient supine.
3. LPO, chosen to give best separation between atria and ventricles. Patient in right lateral decubitus position.

FILMS
See analysis below.

First-pass study   The choice of list-mode or short-frame dynamic acquisition will depend largely on the available computer system and analysis software. Dynamic acquisition should be at a rate of 20 frames s^{-1} or faster, with a 64×64 matrix size. Although the first pass usually takes only 10–15 s, it is advisable for data acquisition to continue for at least 50 s.

FILMS
See analysis below.

Analysis
Gated blood-pool study
1. The LVEF is calculated.
2. Systolic, diastolic, phase and amplitude images are generated.
3. The frames can be displayed in cine mode to give good visualization of wall motion.

First pass study
1. The RVEF can be calculated.
2. Serial images can be produced showing the sequence of chamber filling.
3. A time–activity curve from the pulmonary region can be used for quantitative assessment of a shunt.
4. LVEF may be calculated, although the gated study provides a more reliable method.
5. Chamber transit times may be calculated.

Additional techniques
1. Gated blood-pool imaging can be carried out during controlled exercise with appropriate precautions to assess ventricular functional reserve. Leg exercise using a bed-mounted bicycle ergometer is the method of choice. Shoulder restraints and hand grips help to reduce upper body movement during imaging[1].

For patients unable to exercise effectively, stress with dobutamine infusion may be useful[2]. Dobutamine increases cardiac contractility by stimulating the β_1 receptors. Under continuous monitoring, incrementally increase dose from 5 to 20 μg kg^{-1} min^{-1}, infusing each dose for 8 min. Terminate infusion on S-T segment depression of > 3 mm, any ventricular arrhythmia, systolic blood pressure > 220 mmHg, attainment of maximum heart rate, or any side-effects.

An alternative method of stress is with ventricular pacing, gradually increasing the rate up to maximum predicted heart rate.

2. With new technetium cardiac agents such as ^{99m}Tc-sestamibi (see 'Radionuclide Myocardial Perfusion Imaging'), it is now possible to combine ventriculography and perfusion scans in a single study[3].

Aftercare
1. Monitor recovery from exercise.
2. Normal radiation safety precautions (see 'General Notes').

Complications
Exercise test
1. Induction of angina.
2. Cardiac arrhythmias.
3. Cardiac arrest.

References
1. Tamaki, N., Fischman, A.J. & Strauss, H.W. (1991) Radionuclide imaging of the heart. In: Maisey, M.N., Britton, K.E. & Gilday, D.L. (eds) *Clinical Nuclear Medicine*, 2nd edn, pp. 1–40. London: Chapman & Hall.
2. Konishi, T., Koyama, T., Aoki, T., et al (1990) Radionuclide assessment of left ventricular function during dobutamine infusion in patients with coronary artery disease: Comparison with ergometer exercise. *Clin. Cardiol.* **13**, 183–188.
3. Borges-Neto, S., Coleman, R.E., Potts, J.M. & Jones, R.H. (1991) Combined exercise radionuclide angiocardiography and single photon emission computed tomography perfusion studies for assessment of coronary artery disease. *Semin. Nucl. Med.* **21**, 223–229.

Further reading Adam, W.E., Clausen, M., Hellwig, D., Henze, E. & Bitter, F. (1988) Radionuclide ventriculography (equilibrium gated blood pool scanning) – its present clinical position and recent developments. *Eur. J. Nucl. Med.* **13**, 637–647.

Feiglin, D. (1989) The cardiovascular system. In: Sharp, P.F., Gemmell, H.G. & Smith, F.W. (eds) *Practical Nuclear Medicine*, pp. 137–159. Oxford: Oxford University Press.

Radionuclide Myocardial Perfusion Imaging

Indications
1. Diagnosis and assessment of extent of coronary artery disease.
2. Evaluation of effects of angioplasty and bypass surgery on myocardial perfusion with pre- and post-intervention imaging.
3. Confirmation or exclusion of old myocardial infarction (rest test only).

Contraindications
Exercise test and dipyridamole stress test
1. Unstable angina.
2. Frequent ventricular arrhythmias at rest.
3. Second- or third-degree heart block.
4. Uncontrolled hypertension.
5. Severe valvular disease, especially aortic valve stenosis.
6. Heart failure (New York Heart Association, NYHA, class III or IV).
7. Hypersensitivity and other contraindications for dipyridamole.

Radiopharmaceuticals
1. ^{201}Tl-*thallous chloride*, 80 MBq max.[1-3].

Thallium is a potassium analogue with initial rapid myocardial uptake in near proportion to coronary blood flow, and subsequent washout and redistribution. Still the most widely used myocardial perfusion agent, although with principal photon energies of 68–72 and 167 keV and $T_{1/2}$ of 73 hours, it is not ideal for imaging and gives a higher radiation dose than the newer ^{99m}Tc alternatives (see below). Same-day stress and rest redistribution studies can be performed with a single injection.

2. ^{99m}Tc-*methoxyisobutylisonitrile (MIBI or sestamibi)*[1-4], 300 MBq max. for planar imaging, 400 MBq max. for tomography (or 1000 MBq max. for the total of 2 injections in single day rest–exercise protocols).

Cationic complex with similar myocardial uptake to ^{201}Tl but minimal redistribution. Better physical characteristics for imaging, but separate injections required for stress/rest studies.

3. ^{99m}Tc-teboroxime[2-4].

Neutral lipophilic complex with higher initial myocardial uptake than other agents, but very fast washout so potentially good for rapid repeat studies. A promising new agent not yet widely used.

Equipment

1. Gamma camera, preferably tomographic.
2. Low-energy general purpose collimator.
3. Imaging computer.
4. Exercise equipment, e.g. bicycle ergometer or treadmill.
5. 12-lead ECG monitor.
6. Resuscitation facilities including defibrillator.
7. Aminophylline to reverse possible severe side-effects after dipyridamole infusion.
8. Medical supervision during stress study.

Patient preparation

1. Nil by mouth or light breakfast 4–6 hours prior to test.
2. Cessation of cardiac medication on the day of the test if possible, particularly β-blockers.

Technique

^{201}Tl *stress/rest test*

The study consists of a single injection under stress conditions followed by imaging. Ischaemic and infarcted myocardium should appear as cold areas. A second set of images taken at rest 3–4 hours later should show redistribution of thallium into ischaemic but not infarcted tissue.

1. Position an i.v. line in a forearm vein.
2. Exercise patient using a standard regime. Raising heart rate above 85% of maximum is widely used as an end point, although if higher rates can be achieved, this will produce better images. Observe clinical indications which may require premature termination of exercise[5]. For patients incapable of substantial exercise, pharmacological stress can be used. A popular agent is the potent coronary vasodilator, dipyridamole[6] (i.v. infusion over 4 min of 0.56 mg kg^{-1} diluted in 50 ml glucose 5%).
3. Administer i.v. bolus of ^{201}Tl and continue maximal exercise for approximately 1 min. If stress with dipyridamole has been used, inject ^{201}Tl 2–4

minutes after infusion ceases, with the patient upright to reduce splanchnic flow. If some low level of exercise can be performed at this time, the image quality will be improved.

4. Commence imaging after 5 min and monitor recovery with ECG and blood pressure recording.

5. Image at rest 3–4 hours later with accurate repositioning to facilitate comparison with stress images.

6. If fixed defects are present in exercise and rest images in a patient with no history of myocardial infarction, either:
   (a) image again at 18–24 hours, or
   (b) administer a second smaller dose of ^{201}Tl (40 MBq typical) and image immediately. If defects still persist, image again at 18–24 hours.

A significant number (around 30%) of fixed defects at 3–4 hours will show reversibility, probably more likely after re-injection[7]. It is very important to identify reversible defects since they indicate ischaemic but viable myocardium to which revascularization may completely restore perfusion.

^{99m}Tc-MIBI rest/stress test

Because MIBI has minimal redistribution, separate injections are needed for stress and rest studies. 2-day protocols are optimal, but it is usually more convenient to perform both studies on the same day. A number of groups have shown that this is possible without degrading the results, most effectively when the resting study is performed first[4, 8]. For example[8]:

1. Administer 250 MBq MIBI i.v.

2. Image at rest 60 min later.

3. 2 hours after first injection, exercise patient or give dipyridamole infusion and administer 750 MBq MIBI i.v. at peak exercise as for thallium. (If a longer period is available between injections, the activity of the second injection may be reduced.)

4. Image 60 min later.

MIBI is significantly excreted via the hepatobiliary route. A drink of milk or fatty meal 30–60 min after injection will facilitate this clearance.

^{201}Tl or ^{99m}Tc-MIBI
rest test

1. Administer radiopharmaceutical i.v.
2. Image after 10 min for ^{201}Tl or after 60 min for ^{99m}Tc-MIBI.

Images

Planar or tomographic images may be taken. Tomography is considered to improve the diagnostic quality of the test by improving contrast between lesions and normal tissue and permitting image reconstruction in long- and short-axis planes. Tomographic images may be severely degraded by patient movement, so attention should be paid to anxious or uncomfortable post-exercise patients when considering which imaging mode to adopt, since planar views are much quicker to repeat than tomography.

Planar images

Hard copy and 128 × 128 computer images:
1. Anterior, patient supine.
2. LAO 45°, patient supine.
3. LAO 70° or left lateral. Patient supine unless inferior wall of heart is obscured by diaphragm, in which case image in right lateral decubitus position.

Tomographic images

1. 180° orbit from LPO 45° to RAO 45°, elliptical if possible.
2. Matrix size and zoom to give a pixel size of 3–4 mm.
3. 45–90 projections, clockwise and anticlockwise rotations if possible, with a total imaging time of about 30 min.

Analysis
Planar

1. Background-subtracted images.
2. Circumferential profiles.

Tomography

1. Short- and long-axis slice reconstruction.
2. 2-dimensional polar 'bull's-eye' views may be generated[9].

Additional techniques

Gated imaging has been used to improve specificity in patients with atypical chest pain and a low pre-test probability of coronary artery disease[10], although this may result in unacceptably long acquisition times.

Aftercare   1. Monitoring of patient post-exercise.
2. Normal radiation safety precautions (see 'General Notes').

Complications   1. Induction of angina.
2. Cardiac arrhythmias.
3. Cardiac arrest.
4. Common dipyridamole side-effects: transient headache, dizziness, hypotension, facial flushing, nausea and angina. Aminophylline may be administered to reverse severe dipyridamole side-effects (i.v. 75–100 mg given slowly, then up to 250 mg if symptoms persist)[6].

References   1. Bonow, R.O., Dilsizian, V. (1992) Thallium-201 and technetium-99m-sestamibi for assessing viable myocardium. *J. Nucl. Med.* **33**, 815–818.
2. Taillefer, R., Lambert, R., Essiambre, R., Phaneuf, D.C. & Léveillé, J. (1992) Comparison between thallium-201, technetium-99m-sestamibi and technetium-99m-teboroxime planar myocardial perfusion imaging in detection of coronary artery disease. *J. Nucl. Med.* **33**, 1091–1098.
3. Berman, D.S. (ed.) (1991) Cardiovascular nuclear medicine: an update. *Semin. Nucl. Med.* **21**(3).
4. Leppo, J.A., DePuey, E.G. & Johnson, L.L. (1991) A review of cardiac imaging with sestamibi and teboroxime. *J. Nucl. Med.* **32**, 2012–2022.
5. Brennand-Roper, D.A. (1991) Exercise electrocardiogram testing and thallium scintigraphy. In: Maisey, M.N., Britton, K.E. & Gilday, D.L. (eds) *Clinical Nuclear Medicine*, 2nd edn, pp. 41–46. London: Chapman & Hall.
6. Botvinick, E.H. & Dae, M.W. (1991) Dipyridamole perfusion scintigraphy. *Semin. Nucl. Med.* **21**, 242–265.
7. Pieri, P., Abraham, S.A., Katayama, H. & Yasuda, T. (1990) Thallium-201 myocardial scintigraphy: single injection, re-injection, or 24-hour delayed imaging? *J. Nucl. Med.* **31**, 1390–1396.
8. Borges-Neto, S., Coleman, R.E. & Jones, R.H. (1990) Perfusion and function at rest and treadmill exercise using technetium-99m-sestamibi: comparison of one- and two day protocols in normal volunteers. *J. Nucl. Med.* **31**, 1128–1132.
9. Garcia, E.V., Van Train, K., Maddahi, J. et al (1985) Quantification of rotational thallium-201 myocardial tomography. *J. Nucl. Med.* **26**, 17–26.

10. Handler, C.E., Ardley, R.G. & Maisey, M.N. (1985) Gated thallium tomography – potential for improved accuracy in the detection of coronary artery disease. *Br. J. Radiol.* **58**, 107–110.

Further reading

McKillop, J.H. (1989) The clinical role of myocardial perfusion imaging. *Nucl. Med. Commun.* **10**, 311–313.

Feiglin, D. (1989) The cardiovascular system. In: Sharp P.F., Gemmell, H.G. & Smith, F.W. (eds) *Practical Nuclear Medicine*, pp. 137–159. Oxford: Oxford University Press.

Acute Myocardial Infarction Imaging

Indications	Differentiation of viable and necrosed myocardium in recent infarcts.
Contraindications	*111In-antimyosin*. Adverse reaction to skin test (see 'Patient Preparation').

Radiopharmaceuticals

1. *99mTc-pyrophosphate*, 600 MBq max.
   Considered to form a complex with calcium in damaged myocardium. Localizes quickly after administration in 0.5- to 6-day-old infarcts, so early imaging is possible. There is greater uptake in the ischaemic area around the margins of an infarct than in the infarct itself, producing a 'doughnut' shape in large regions of infarction. Good radionuclide for imaging, but also localizes in bone, so rib uptake interferes with planar images.
2. *111In-antimyosin antibody*, 75 MBq typical.
   Accumulates on myosin exposed by damaged cell membranes in acute infarcts within 48–72 hours of administration. Significant uptake occurs with administration for up to 4 weeks after onset of infarction. Better localization in necrotic infarct centres than pyrophosphate and no bone uptake. Need to wait 48 hours before imaging. Not widely available. Sub-optimal radionuclide for imaging and radiation dose, although to address these deficiencies antimyosin labelled with *99mTc* has recently been assessed in animal studies[1].

Equipment

1. Gamma camera, mobile if patient cannot be moved from coronary care unit.
2. Low-energy general purpose collimator for *99mTc*, medium-energy collimator for *111In*.

Patient preparation

111In-antimyosin. Intradermal skin test with DTPA–antimyosin for sensitivity reactions.

Technique

99mTc-pyrophosphate

1. Give i.v. injection 1–3 days after suspected infarction.
2. Image 3 hours later.

¹¹¹In-antimyosin

Correction: ^{111}In-antimyosin

1. Give i.v. injection slowly over 30–60 s up to 2 weeks after suspected infarction.
2. Image 48 hours later.

Images

Patient supine, 300–500 kilocounts (approx. 5–7 min) per view:
1. Anterior.
2. LAO 45°.
3. Left lateral or LAO 70°.

Additional technique

Tomography may improve sensitivity and localization of infarcts, in particular by removing overlying bone uptake of pyrophosphate.

Aftercare

Normal radiation safety precautions (see 'General Notes').

Complications

Antimyosin antibody may cause a hypersensitivity reaction on repeated dosage.

Reference

1. Pak, K.Y., Nedelman, M.A., Kanke, M. et al (1992) An instant kit method for labeling antimyosin Fab' with technetium-99m: evaluation in an experimental myocardial infarct model. *J. Nucl. Med.* **33**, 144–149.

Further reading

Botvinick, E.H. (1990) "Hot spot" imaging agents for acute myocardial infarction. *J. Nucl. Med.* **31**, 143–146.

Tamaki, N., Yamada, T., Matsumori, A. et al (1990) Indium-111-antimyosin antibody imaging for detecting different stages of myocardial infarction: comparison with technetium-99m-pyrophosphate imaging. *J. Nucl. Med.* **31**, 136–142.

9 Venous System

Methods of imaging the venous system

1. Contrast medium venography.
2. Ultrasound.
3. Radionuclide imaging.
   - ^{125}I-fibrinogen.
   - ^{99m}Tc-macroaggregates.
   - ^{99m}Tc-plasmin.
   - ^{99m}Tc-urokinase.
   - ^{111}In-platelets.
   - ^{111}In white blood cells.
4. CT can show inferior vena cava involvement and renal vein involvement in renal cell carcinoma and Wilms' tumour.
5. MRI will show presence or absence of flowing blood. In addition MRI can be used to 'age' thrombus and differentiate acute from chronic clot.

Further reading

Whitehouse, G.H. (1990) Editorial. Venous thrombosis and thromboembolism. *Clin. Radiol.* **41**, 77–80.

Peripheral Venography

LOWER LIMB

Methods
1. Intravenous venography
2. Intrasseous venography (this technique is rarely performed today and will not be dealt with further — for further information refer to Schobinger[1]).

Indications
1. Deep venous thrombosis.
2. To demonstrate incompetent perforating veins.
3. Oedema of unknown cause.
4. Congenital abnormality of the venous system (rare).

Contraindications Local sepsis.

Contrast medium LOCM 240.

Equipment
1. Fluoroscopy unit with spot film device.
2. Tilting radiography table.

Patient preparation Elevated leg overnight if oedema is severe.

Preliminary films Using the undercouch tube to assess exposure factors:
1. PA knee.
2. PA ankle.

Technique
For intravenous venography
1. The patient is supine and tilted 40° head up, to delay the transit time of the contrast medium.
2. A tourniquet is applied tightly just above the ankle to occlude the superficial venous system. It is important to remember that this may also occlude the anterior tibial vein, and so its absence should not automatically be interpreted as due to a venous thrombosis.
3. A 19G butterfly needle (smaller if necessary) is inserted into a distal vein on the dorsum of the foot. If the needle is too proximal, the contrast medium may bypass the deep veins and so give the impression of a deep venous occlusion.
4. 40 ml of contrast medium is injected by hand. The first series of spot films is then taken.

5. A further 20 ml of contrast are injected quickly whilst the patient performs a Valsalva manoeuvre to delay the transit of contrast medium into the proximal and pelvic veins. The patient is tilted quickly into a slightly head down position and the Valsalva manoeuvre is relaxed. Alternatively, if the patient is unable to Valsalva, direct manual pressure over the femoral vein whilst the table is being tilted into the head-down position will delay transit of contrast medium proximally. Films are taken 2–3 s after releasing pressure.

FILMS
AP collimated to include common femoral and iliac veins.

6. At the end of the procedure the needle should be flushed with 0.9% saline to avoid the risk of phlebitis due to stasis of contrast medium.

Aftercare The limb should be exercised.

Complications

Due to the contrast medium
1. As for the general complications of intravascular contrast media (see p. 24).
2. Thrombophlebitis.
3. Tissue necrosis due to extravasation of contrast medium. This is rare, but may occur in patients with peripheral ischaemia, and can be severe[2].
4. Cardiac arrhythmia — more likely if the patient has pulmonary hypertension.

Due to the technique
1. Haematoma.
2. Pulmonary embolus — due to dislodged clot or air.

References
1. Schobinger, R.A. (1960) *Intraosseus Venography*. New York: Grune & Stratton.
2. Berge, T., Bergquist, D., Efsing, H. & Hallbook, T. (1978) Local complications of ascending phlebography. *Clin. Radiol.* **29**, 691–696.

UPPER LIMB

Methods
1. Intravenous venography.
2. Intraosseous venography (see above)

Indications
1. Oedema.
2. To demonstrate the site of a venous obstruction.

Contrast medium   LOCM 300.

Equipment   Fluoroscopy unit with spot film device.

Patient preparation   None.

Preliminary film   PA shoulder.

Technique
For intravenous venography
1. The patient is supine.
2. An 18G butterfly needle is inserted into the median cubital vein at the elbow. The cephalic vein is not used, as this bypasses the axillary vein.
3. Spot films are taken of the region of interest during a hand injection of 30 ml of contrast medium.

Aftercare   None.

Complications
Due to the contrast medium
See p. 24.

Peripheral Varicography

Indications
1. To demonstrate distribution of varicose veins.
2. To demonstrate sites of communication with deep venous system.
3. Assessment of recurrent varicosity.

Contraindications   Local sepsis.

Contrast medium   LOCM 240. Volume depends on extent and volume of varicosities.

Equipment
1. Fluoroscopy unit with spot film device or 100 mm camera.
2. Tilting radiography table.

Patient preparation   None

Technique
1. The patient lies supine and tilted 40° head up to delay washout of contrast.
2. A 19G butterfly needle is inserted into a suitable varix below the knee.
3. 40–50 ml of contrast are injected by hand under fluoroscopic control.
4. A series of spot films is taken.

   FILMS
   (a) AP calf and 2 obliques
   (b) lateral knee – to assess the short saphenopopliteal junction.

5. If contrast filling above the knee is adequate, then further views of the thigh can be taken to demonstrate the extent of long saphenous varicosity.
6. Due to the large volume of varicose veins, it may be necessary to re-site the needle in a suitable varix above the knee to obtain adequate contrast filling of the entire system.
7. A further 40 ml of contrast are then injected and spot films taken.

   FILMS
   (a) AP thigh and oblique – particular attention should be given to the potential sites of communication, e.g. midthigh perforator

(b) AP and oblique of groin — views to demonstrate the saphenofemoral junction are particularly necessary in assessing recurrent varicosity even if there has been previous saphenofemoral ligation, as recurrence at this site is common.

8. After injection and imaging is complete the veins should be flushed with saline to prevent contrast stasis and the risk of phlebitis.

9. The needles are removed and pressure applied to ensure haemostasis.

Aftercare   The limb should be exercised gently to washout any remaining contrast.

Complications   As for peripheral venography.

Central Venography

SUPERIOR VENA CAVOGRAPHY

Indications
1. To demonstrate the site of a venous obstruction.
2. Congenital abnormality of the venous system, e.g. left-sided superior vena cava,

Contrast medium LOCM 370. 60 ml.

Equipment Rapid serial radiography unit.

Patient preparation Nil orally for 5 hours prior to the procedure.

Preliminary films PA film of upper chest and lower neck.

Technique
1. The patient is supine.
2. 18C butterfly needles are inserted into the median antecubital vein of both arms.
3. Hand injections of contrast medium 30 ml per side, are made simultaneously, as rapidly as possible by two operators. The injection is recorded by rapid serial radiography (see 'Films' below). The film sequence is commenced after about two-thirds of the contrast medium has been injected.

N.B. If the study is to demonstrate a congenital abnormality, or on the rare occasion that the opacification obtained by the above method is too poor, a 5F catheter with side holes, introduced by the Seldinger technique, may be used.

Films Rapid serial radiography is performed: one film per s for 10 s.

Aftercare None unless a catheter is used.

Complications
Due to the contrast medium See p. 24.

INFERIOR VENA CAVOGRAPHY

Indications
1. To demonstrate the site of a venous obstruction, displacement or infiltration.
2. Congenital abnormality of the venous system.

Contrast medium LOCM 370. 40 ml.

Equipment
1. Rapid serial radiography unit.
2. Catheter (5F) with side holes.
3. Pump injector.

Preliminary film Centred to the region of interest.

Technique
1. With the patient supine, the catheter is inserted into the femoral vein using the Seldinger technique. A Valsalva manoeuvre may facilitate venepuncture by dilating the veins.
2. An injection of 40 ml of contrast medium is made in 2 s by the pump injector, and recorded by rapid serial radiography (see 'Films' below).

N.B. It is possible to obtain an inferior vena cavogram in children undergoing excretion urography for the investigation of a renal mass by taking an abdominal film during a hand injection of contrast medium into a dorsal pedal vein. If the child is crying, the contrast medium may be forced into the ascending lumbar veins, resulting in non-opacification of the inferior vena cava. This must be borne in mind when the film is interpreted.

Films Rapid serial radiography is performed: one film per s for 10 s.

Aftercare
1. Pressure at venepuncture site.
2. Routine observations for 2 hours.

Complications
Due to the contrast medium See p. 24.

Due to the technique See p. 210 — complications of catheter technique.

PELVIC VENOGRAPHY

Indications   To demonstrate the site of a venous obstruction.

Contrast medium   LOCM 300.

Equipment
1. Fluorosocopy unit with spot film device.
2. Two catheters (5F) with side holes (or two 16G needles).

Patient preparation   Nil orally for 5 hours prior to the procedure.

Preliminary film   Spot film of the pelvis.

Technique
1. The patient is supine.
2. Bilateral catheterization of the femoral veins is performed using the Seldinger technique (alternatively direct puncture with the 16G needles may be used).
3. Injections of contrast medium, 20 ml per side, are made simultaneously by hand, and recorded by a spot film of the pelvis.
4. The injections may be repeated with the patient in an oblique position.

Films
Aftercare   }   As for superior vena cavography.
Complications

Portal Venography

Methods	1. Trans-splenic approach (discussed below).
	2. Transhepatic approach (see p. 275).
	3. Late-phase superior mesenteric angiography (see p. 237).
	4. Paraumbilical vein catheterization.
	5. Transjugular approach[1].

Indications
1. To demonstrate prior to operation the anatomy of the portal system in patients with portal hypertension.
2. To check the patency of a portosystemic anastomosis.

Contrast medium LOCM 370, 50 ml.

Equipment
1. Rapid serial radiography unit.
2. 10 cm needle (20G) with stilette and outer plastic sheath, e.g. Longdwell.

Patient preparation
1. Admission to hospital. A surgeon should be informed in case complications of procedure arise.
2. Clotting factors are checked.
3. Severe ascites is drained.
4. Nil orally for 5 hours prior to the procedure.
5. Premedication, e.g. diazepam 10 mg orally.

Preliminary film Plain abdominal film using a soft-tissue exposure to assess the position of the spleen.

Technique
For trans-splenic approach
1. With the patient supine, the position of the spleen is percussed. The access point is as low as possible in the midaxillary line, usually at the level of the tenth or eleventh intercostal space.
2. The region is anaesthetized using a sterile procedure.
3. The patient is asked to hold his breath in mid-inspiration, and the needle is then inserted inwards and upwards into the spleen (about three-quarters of the length of the needle is inserted, i.e. 7.5 cm). The needle and stilette are then withdrawn, leaving the plastic cannula in situ.

Blood will flow back easily if the cannula is correctly sited. The patient is then asked to breathe as shallowly as possible to avoid trauma to the spleen from excessive movement of the cannula.

4. A test injection of a small volume of contrast medium under screening control can be made to ensure correct siting of the cannula. If it is sited outside the spleen, simple withdrawal into the body of the spleen is not acceptable, as any contrast medium subsequently injected would follow the track created by the withdrawal. Complete repuncture is necessary.

5. When the cannula is in a satisfactory position, the splenic pulp pressure may be measured with a sterile manometer. (It is normally 10–15 cmH$_2$O.)

6. A hand injection of 50 ml of contrast medium is made in 5 s, and recorded by rapid serial radiography. The cannula should be removed as soon as possible after the injection to minimize trauma to the spleen.

7. Occasionally a patent portal vein will fail to opacify, owing to major portosystemic collaterals causing reversed flow in the portal vein. The final arbiter of portal vein patency is direct mesenteric venography performed at operation. The maximum width of a normal portal vein is said to be 2 cm.

Films
Rapid serial radiography:
One film per s for 10 s.

Aftercare
1. Blood pressure and pulse initially quarter-hourly, subsequently 4-hourly.
2. The patient must remain in hospital overnight.

Complications

Due to the contrast medium
See p. 24.

Due to the technique
1. Haemorrhage.
2. Subcapsular injection.
3. Perforation of adjacent structures (e.g. pleura, colon).
4. Splenic rupture.

5. Infection.
6. Pain (especially with an extracapsular injection).

Reference   1. Rosch, J., Antonovic, R & Dotter, C.T. (1975) Trans-jugular approach to the liver, biliary system, and portal circulation. *Am. J. Roentg.*, **125**, 602–608.

Further reading   Frimann-Dahl, J. (1970) Percutaneous splenoportography. In: McLaren, J.W. (ed.) *Modern Trends in Diagnostic Radiology*, Vol. 4, pp. 175–189. London: Butterworths.

Transhepatic Portal Venous Catheterization

Indications
1. To localize pancreatic hormone-secreting tumours before operation.
2. To perform portal venography.
3. To occlude oesophageal varices. (This is now rarely needed since the introduction of direct endoscopic injection of varices.)

Contraindications
None specific to the technique. Ascites and hepatic cirrhosis make the procedure more difficult.

Contrast medium
LOCM 370, to demonstrate anatomy and position of catheter.

Equipment
1. Fluoroscopy unit.
2. Real-time ultrasound scanner.
3. Image recording — rapid serial film changer, 105 mm film or digital subtraction facilities.
4. Pump injector.
5. 25 cm sheathed needle (Lunderquist).
6. Guide-wires — 15 mm J movable core.
7. 5F polyethylene catheters.
8. Heparinized bottles for blood samples. (Prior arrangements should be made with the pathology laboratory.)

Patient preparation
1. Nil by mouth for 4 hours prior to the procedure.
2. Valium 10 mg by mouth 1.5 hours prior to the procedure.
3. Pethidine or similar analgesic i.v. during the procedure if painful.

Technique
1. Using the real-time ultrasound scanner the portal vein is localized from the side and from the front, so that the entry height and depth of needle penetration required are known. The portal vein lies posteriorly just in front of the inferior vena cava, and is best approached laterally from the upper part of the liver just below the costophrenic angle, with the needle horizontal and angled towards the umbilicus. The selected points are

marked with an indelible pen, and the skin cleaned.

2. The entry point and liver capsule are anaesthetized with 1% lignocaine, and a small skin incision made.

3. The sheathed needle is inserted along the line previously determined, the needle is withdrawn and suction is applied with a syringe, whilst the sheath is slowly withdrawn. When blood is aspirated contrast medium is injected to discover which vessel has been entered. Contrast medium in hepatic veins flows upwards and medially; in the portal vein it flows peripherally.

4. When a portal vein is entered the 15 mm J guidewire is passed through the sheath into the splenic vein. The sheath is then withdrawn and with the patient holding his breath the catheter is advanced over the wire, which is then removed.

To demonstrate the portal venous system and pancreatic veins

1. The tip of the catheter is positioned in the splenic vein, and the X-ray beam is centred 2.5 cm to the right of the midline, halfway between the xiphisternum and umbilicus and coned to approximately 15 cm deep and 20 cm wide.

2. An initial film is taken for subtraction and 40 ml of contrast medium is injected at a rate of 10 ml per s, with films at one per s for 8 s.

To localize hormonesecreting pancreatic tumours

1. 5 ml samples of blood are taken at points along the splenic vein, superior mesenteric vein and first part of the portal vein. The samples are numbered sequentially, and the site from which each was taken is marked on a sketch map of the portal drainage system. Simultaneous peripheral blood samples should be obtained at the same time as each portal sample to assess changing blood levels.

2. The accuracy of sampling can be improved by selective catheterization of pancreative veins using varying shapes of catheter[1].

To occlude the coronary and short gastric veins in patients with bleeding gastrooesophageal varices

This technique may be useful in controlling haemorrhage for a time, so that an elective rather than an emergency portocaval shunt may be performed. In most cases endoscopic injection of oesophageal varices is the preferred technique.

1. Transhepatic portocavography is performed.
2. The coronary vein is selectively catheterized. Small pieces of gel-foam soaked in contrast medium are injected, with frequent injections of contrast medium to assess flow. When this decreases occlusion may be completed by positioning a Gianturco coil in the vein.
3. A further portocavogram is performed: if there is filling of varices through the short gastric veins, these should also be occluded.

After all these procedures a plug of gel-foam should be placed in the catheter track near the liver edge during withdrawal of the catheter, to reduce the chance of blood or bile leakage into the peritoneum. A small dressing is placed on the skin wound.

Aftercare Temperature, pulse and blood pressure — quarter-hourly for 1 hour, then half-hourly for 3 hours.

Complications
1. Intraperitoneal bleeding and irritation.
2. Bacteraemia and septicaemia.
3. Renal failure from overdosage with contrast medium.

Reference
1. Reichardt, W. & Ingemansson, S. (1980) Selective vein catheterization for hormone assay in endocrine tumours of the pancreas. Technique and Results. *Acta Radiol. (Diagn.)* **21**, 177–187.

Further reading
Cho, K.J., Vinik, A.I., Thompson, N.W., Shields, J.J., Porter, D.J., Brady, T.M., Cadavid, G. & Fajans, S.S. (1982) Localization of the source of hyperinsulinism: percutaneous transhepatic portal and pancreatic vein catheterization with hormone assay. *Am. J. Roentg.* **132**, 237–245.

Lunderquist, A. & Vang, J. (1974) Transhepatic catheterization and obliteration of the coronary vein in patients with portal hypertension and oesophageal varices. *New Engl. J. Med.* **291**, 646–649.

Pereiras, R., Schiff, E., Barkin, J. & Hutson, D. (1979) The role of interventional radiology in diseases of the hepatobiliary system and the pancreas. *Radiol. Clin. N. Am.* **17** 555–605.

Viamonte, M., Le Page, J., Lunderquist, A., Pereiras, R., Russell, E., Viamonte, M. & Camacho, M. (1975)

Selective catheterization of the portal vein and its tributaries. *Radiology* 114, 457–460.

Viamonte, M., Pereiras, R., Russell, E., Le Page, J. & Meier, W. L. (1977) Pitfalls in transhepatic portography. *Radiology* 124, 325–329.

Ultrasound Venography

Indications   1. Suspected deep vein thrombosis.
2. Follow-up of known deep vein thrombosis.

Contraindications   None.

Patient preparation   None.

Equipment   5–7.5 MHz transducer.

Technique   1. Patient supine with foot-down tilt. The popliteal and calf veins can be easily examined with the patient sitting with legs dependent or lying on a tilted couch with flexed knees and externally rotated hips. The femoral veins and external iliac veins are examined supine and popliteal veins may be examined with the patient prone.
2. Longitudinal and transverse scans for external iliac, femoral and popliteal veins. For tibial and peroneal veins, these may be supplemented by oblique coronal scans.
3. Each vein may be identified by real-time scanning and colour Doppler. If in any doubt it may be confirmed as a vein by the spectral Doppler tracing. A normally patent vein can be completely occluded on real time scanning by transducer pressure. This is not always possible for a superficial femoral vein in the adducter canal.
4. The normal venous signal is phasic and in the larger veins varies with respiration. Flow can be stopped by a Valsalva manoeuvre and is augmented by distal compression of the foot or calf. Acute thrombus may be non-echogenic but the vein should not fill with colour Doppler and should not be compressible. The thrombus tends to become echogenic after a few days.
5. Although this technique is less well established for the exclusion of thrombus in the calf vessels, it has been shown to have a sensitivity and specificity close to that of venography. Cannulation of a vein and injection of contrast medium can thus be avoided.

Further reading   Baxter, G.M. & Duffy, P. (1992) Calf vein anatomy and flow: implications for colour Doppler imaging. *Clin. Radiol.* **46**, 84–87.

Baxter, G.M., McKeckney, S. & Duffy, P. (1990) Colour Doppler ultrasound in deep venous thrombosis. A comparison with venography. *Clin Radiol.* **42**, 32–36.

Dorfman, G.S. & Cronan, J.J. (1992) Venous ultrasonography. *Radiol. Clin. N. Am.* **30**, 879–894.

Rose, S.C., Zwiebell, W.J., Nelson, B.D. et al. (1990) Symptomatic lower extremity deep venous thrombosis: accuracy, limitations, and role of colour Duplex flow imaging in diagnosis. *Radiology* **174**: 639–644.

Imaging of deep venous thrombosis (DVT)

Ultrasound   Veins can be systematically examined using a combination of continuous wave, B-mode, pulsed Doppler and colour Doppler systems. With increasing experience it is likely that ultrasound will become the method of choice for examining for DVT and that the former 'gold' standard of venography will be used less.

Continuous wave   Continuous wave Doppler assesses movement, it is difficult to be sure which vein is being examined and incomplete venous thrombus can be missed. Its overall sensitivity and specificity are not sufficiently satisfactory for it to be used in isolation.

Duplex   Duplex scanning uses a combination of direct visualization using B-mode and pulsed Doppler. Expansion and filling of the normal echo-free lumen can be identified but slow moving blood may be misinterpreted for thrombus. Valsalva manoeuvre will cause expansion in the normal vein but is not a totally reliable sign. Pulsed Doppler assesses flow, and enhancement due to respiratory excursion and distal venous compression suggest patency. The most reliable sign is compressibility. Direct pressure with the ultrasound probe over the vein will cause the normal vein to collapse. If thrombus is present, this will not occur.

Colour Doppler   Colour Doppler examination gives the added advantage of assessing more accurately the veins in the calf which may be difficult to examine with B-mode alone. Once identified the veins are examined for thrombus in the manner above.

Contrast venography   This technique provides an image of the venous system. There are disadvantages. It is an invasive procedure requiring intravenous injection of contrast medium, with the attendant risks that this entails. Failure to cannulate veins occurs with swollen limbs. False-negative results do occur.

Radioisotopes   A number of radioisotopes have been proposed to image thrombus:
1. ^{125}I-fibrinogen
2. ^{99m}Tc-plasmin
3. ^{99m}Tc-urokinase
4. ^{111}In-platelets
5. ^{111}In white blood cells
6. ^{99m}Tc-anti-fibrinogen antibodies.

None of these techniques have been widely accepted for the accurate diagnosis of deep vein thrombosis. Fibrinogen scanning, for example, has disadvantages. It takes 24–48 hours to obtain images. It is not sensitive for proximal veins. False-positive results occur in trauma, inflammation and swelling. ^{125}I crosses the placenta and enters breast milk. Tracer must be given before thrombus forms. It is best kept for screening high-risk patients rather than assessing the acute situation.

Impedance plethysmography   This technique depends on the principle of the capacity of the veins to fill and empty in response to temporary obstruction to venous outflow by occlusion of the thigh veins with a pneumatic cuff. Changes in calf volume produce changes in impedance measured by electrodes applied to the calf. The technique is demanding and requires skilled personnel. Clinical states that impair venous return, such as cardiac failure and pelvic pathology and also arterial insufficiency, produce abnormal results.

Magnetic resonance   In some series, MRI has been shown to be as sensitive as ultrasound and venography. Using surface coils to obtain high resolution, popliteal and femoral thrombus are easy to detect but the small vessels in the calf may not be seen with certainty. A number of imaging sequences are advocated, including standard T1- and T2-weighted images and more accurately gradient-recalled acquisition in the steady state (GRASS). Recently MRI has been advocated as a method of 'ageing' thrombus.

Further reading   Cronan, J. (1991) Contemporary venous imaging. *Cardiovasc. Intervent. Radiol.* **14**, 87–97

10 Lymph Glands and Lymphatics

Methods of imaging lymph glands

1. *Plain films*, may show:
   - (a) a soft tissue mass, e.g. hilar lymph glands
   - (b) calcification, e.g. mesenteric glands and tuberculous glands.
2. *Indirect evidence from displacement of normal structures*, e.g. displacement of ureters seen during excretion urography or displacement of the inferior vena cava during inferior vena cavography.
3. *Lymphography* (p. 285)
   Advantages:
   - (a) can detect tumour within normal-size lymph glands
   - (b) can distinguish reactive lymph glands from tumour-containing lymph glands
   - (c) enables surveillance of residually opacified glands over several months.

   Disadvantages:
   - (a) does not image internal iliac, mesenteric retrocrural, splenic and renal hilar nodes
   - (b) the liver and spleen are not visualized
   - (c) uncomfortable and technical skill needed for cannulation.

4. *Computed tomography*
   Advantages:
   - (a) can image all intra-abdominal glands (intra-pelvic glands can be difficult to assess owing to variation in the course of adjacent vascular structures)
   - (b) technically easier to perform.

   Disadvantages:
   - (a) internal structure of glands is not seen
   - (b) retroperitoneal glands are difficult to define if there is a paucity of retroperitoneal fat.

5. *Ultrasound*
   Advantage:
   (a) non-invasive and without risk to the patient.

   Disadvantages:
   (a) highly operator-dependent
   (b) intestinal gas is a major factor in poor visualization
   (c) the internal structure of lymph glands is not seen.

6. *Radioisotopes*
   See p. 291.

Further reading

Dixon, A.K. (1985) The current practice of lymphography: a survey in the age of computed tomography. *Clin. Radiol.* **36**, 287–290.

Kinmouth, J.B. (1972) The lymphatics. Diseases, lymphography and surgery. In: Kinmonth, J.B., *Methods of Lymphography*, pp. 1–19. London: Edward Arnold.

Paterson, A.H.G. & McCready, V.R. (1975) Review article. Tumour imaging radiopharmaceuticals. *Br. J. Radiol.* **48**, 520–531.

Lymphography

Indications

1. Staging of lymphomas, and assessment of their response to treatment (contrast medium will remain in affected glands for up to 2 years).
2. Assessment of spread form other tumours: testicular, prostate, female genital tract, kidney, bladder, melanoma.
3. Primary lymphoedema: due to lymphatic hypoplasia or aplasia, and lymphangiectasis.
4. Miscellaneous: thoracic duct injury, chyluria, elephantiasis.

Contraindications

1. Local sepsis, or active thrombophlebitis.
2. Severe respiratory disease.
3. Right-to-left cardiac shunt, or arteriovenous malformation in the lungs (owing to the risk of systemic emboli).
4. Within 3 weeks of radiotherapy or cytoxic treatment (see 'complications' p. 289).
5. Iodine sensitivity.

N.B. In patients with moderate dyspnoea, lymphography may be performed on the right side alone. A smaller volume of contrast medium must be used. The right side is chosen as there is a greater incidence of right-to-left cross-over of lymphatics, than vice versa[1], so allowing a degree of visualization of both sides. However, if adequate cross-over of contrast medium does not occur, an interval of at least 1 week must elapse before the other side is injected, to allow contrast medium trapped in the lungs from the first injection to disperse.

Contrast medium
Oily   Lipiodol ultrafluid.

Glands and lymphatic vessels are opacified. Volume used:
(a) maximum 7 ml per side for the lower limb of a 70 kg adult (4 ml per side for the upper limb).
(b) 10 ml into the right lower limb only if moderately dyspnoeic.
(c) 1 ml per side for a baby aged 1 year.

Water-soluble	LOCM 240. 10 ml. Only lymphatic vessels are opacified.

Equipment
1. McCarthy disposable lymphogram needles (30G).
2. Motor-driven or gravity pump injector.

Patient preparation
1. If leg oedema is present, the leg must be elevated for 24 hours prior to the procedure, and severe cases may require a compression bandage so that the lymphatic may be cannulated more easily.
2. Children under 10 may require a general anaesthetic.
3. The patient micturates prior to the procedure.
4. It should be explained to the patient that the urine and skin may be blue for a few days after the investigation.

Preliminary films
1. PA chest (to ensure that there is no evidence of respiratory disease).
2. Supine abdomen.

Technique
Sites of injection: foot, hand, spermatic cord (depending on the region under investigation).

Foot injection
1. 2 ml of 1 % lignocaine is mixed with 2 ml of 2.5 % patent blue dye. 0.5 ml of the mixture is injected subcutaneously into each of the medial two web spaces of both feet.
2. The feet are exercised for half an hour until the lymphatics are visible on the dorsum of the feet.
3. The patient lies supine on the X-ray table, and is made comfortable, as this may be a long procedure.
4. Using a sterile technique, the skin overlying the lymphatic is anaesthetized. A transverse incision is made to expose the lymphatic, which is then dissected out. All the loose fascia must be removed as its presence interferes with accurate cannulation. A small triangle of sterile cardboard (e.g. from lymphogram cannulation packaging) is placed beneath the lymphatic, which is then elevated to give good visualization. The distal lymphatic in the web space is massaged to increase the distension of the vessel, thus facilitating easier cannulations.

5. The McCarthy cannulation set is flushed with saline to check patency and exclude air. The lymphatic is cannulated and the needle secured with silk ties. If cannulation is unsuccessful, the skin incision can be extended to expose a second lymphatic.

6. Prior to the injection of oily contrast medium, it is important that the following checks are made:
   (a) that the vessel cannulated is not a vein, by attempting aspiration; alternatively, if the needle is correctly sited, the trial injection of a small volume of water-soluble contrast medium will produce a characteristic painful sensation which ascends the leg
   (b) that there is no leakage, by injecting saline.

7. The same procedure is performed on the other side.

8. The contrast medium is delivered over 45 min (approx 0.2 ml min^{-1}) by the pump injector. If any pain is experienced this may be due to:
   (a) extravasation — remedied by decreasing the rate of injection
   (b) dermal backflow — the injection must be terminated.

9. The injection is terminated before the full amount of contrast medium has been injected if the film series (see below) shows that contrast medium has reached the level of L3.

10. The needles are removed and the wounds sutured.

Films

Initial series

1. 10 min — AP ankle.
2. 15 min — AP knees.
3. 20 min — AP thighs.

Intermittent fluoroscopy may replace these initial three films in order to reduce the radiation dose.

4. 30 min — AP pelvis and upper femora.
5. 40 min — supine abdomen.

The above films are taken for the following reasons:
(a) to assess the progress of the contrast medium
(b) to exclude a venous injection — the oily con-

trast medium will appear as multiple small globules if within a vein (caviar sign)
  (c) to exclude extravasation
  (d) to exclude an abnormal lymphaticovenous connection.

6. Supine abdomen every 15 min thereafter until contrast medium has reached L3 or the injection is completed.
7. 2 hours post-injection:
  (a) PA chest (the thoracic duct can usually be seen)
  (b) supine abdomen
  (c) AP pelvis and upper femora.

24 hour series

1. PA chest.
2. Supine abdomen.
3. AP pelvis and upper femora, (45° posterior oblique views may be required to separate superimposed glands.)
4. Excretion urography may also be performed at this time. Walker et al[2] suggest the following as indications:
  (a) an abnormal lymphogram
  (b) failure to visualize the position of the kidneys on the plain film prior to radiotherapy
  (c) when clinically indicated, e.g. carcinoma of the cervix or bladder.

N.B. The lymph glands are better visualized after 24 hours because they will contain more contrast medium and any overlying lymphatic vessels will have emptied.

Delayed series

1. Supine abdomen.
2. AP pelvis and upper femora.

These are taken at 2, 4 and 8 weeks. The response to treatment is assessed on these films and clarification of an equivocal lymphogram may be obtained.

Aftercare

1. Admission overnight.
2. No general anaesthetic, radiotherapy or cytotoxic treatment should be given for at least 1 week after the procedure.
3. Stitches out at 10 days.

Complications

Due to the dye and the contrast medium

PATENT BLUE DYE
Allergic reactions – seldom severe.

OILY CONTRAST MEDIUM
1. *Allergic reactions.*
2. *Pulmonary oil emboli.* Small pulmonary emboli producing fine, pin-point opacities on the 24-hour chest radiograph are commonly seen and are asymptomatic. Ventilatory function is unaffected but carbon monoxide diffusion capacity (T_{CO}) is diminished. This effect is maximal 37 hours after the injection[3]. However, if a larger than normal volume of oily contrast medium reaches the pulmonary circulation, a dangerous number of pulmonary oil emboli may occur. Certain predisposing factors are:
   (a) a large volume of contrast medium, e.g. 10–15 ml per side
   (b) lymphatic obstruction, since this may cause abnormal lymphaticovenous communications; this is commonly with the inferior vena cava at the level of the renal veins
   (c) radiotherapy or cytotoxic treatment within 1 week of the procedure, as this may damage the architecture of the lymph glands, so allowing more oily contrast medium into the venous circulation.
3. *Systemic oil emboli.* Cerebral emboli are the most important. Predisposing factors are:
   (a) a right-to-left cardiac shunt
   (b) radiotherapy to the lung fields within 3 weeks of the procedure, as this can disrupt the architecture and so allow oily contrast medium to pass through into the systemic circulation.
4. *Hepatic oil emboli.* These occur when there is lymphatic obstruction and lymphaticoportal venous communication[4].

Due to the technique
1. Extravasation – occurs in approx. 5%.
2. Infection – occurs in approx. 1%.
3. Lymphangitis – occurs in approx. 0.1%.
4. Dermal backflow i.e. visualization of fine dermal lymphatics owing to obstruction of the deeper lymphatics. This is always abnormal.

References   1. Jackson, B.T. & Kinmonth, J.B. (1974) Lumbar lymphatic cross-over. *Clin. Radiol.* **25**, 187–203.
2. Walker, T.M., Davies, E.R. & Roylance, J. (1977) The value of urography following lymphography in malignant disease. *Br. J. Radiol.* **50**, 93–96.
3. Gold, W.M., Youker, J., Anderson, S. & Nadel, J.A. (1965) Pulmonary function abnormalities after lymphangiography. *New Engl. J. Med.* **273**, 519–524.
4. Ngan, H. & James, K.W. (1978) Hepatic oil embolism following lymphography. *Br. J. Radiol.* **51**, 788–792.

Lymphoscintigraphy

Lymphoscintigraphy provides a more physiological and less invasive alternative to lymphography if high-resolution anatomical detail is not required.

Indications
1. Differentiation of lymphoedema from venous oedema.
2. Assessment of lymphatic flow in lymphoedema.
3. Confirmation and assessment of lymph node metastases.

Contraindications
1. Complete blockage of the lymphatic system (because of the local radiation dose at the injection sites).
2. Nanocolloidal albumin is contraindicated if there is a history of hypersensitivity to human albumin products.

Radiopharmaceuticals
1. *99mTc-nanocolloidal albumin.* Particle size < 80 nm.
2. *99mTc-antimony sulphide colloid.* Particle size 3–30 nm. Currently unavailable in the UK.

40 MBq max. total for all injections.

These colloids are injected subcutaneously and cleared from the interstitial space by lymphatic drainage. Antimony sulphide colloid is slightly acidic and causes more pain on injection than nanocolloid, which has an approximately neutral pH. A number of other radiopharmaceuticals have been used for lymphoscintigraphy[1].

Equipment
1. Gamma camera.
2. High-resolution general purpose collimator.
3. Imaging computer for quantitative studies.

Patient preparation
Clean injection sites, especially on feet.

Technique
1. The patient lies supine for lower limb investigation, in the lithotomy position for ischiorectal injection and sitting for other sites.
2. 99mTc-colloid in 0.1–0.3 ml volume is injected

subcutaneously at sites depending upon the area to be studied:

(a) Nodes below diaphragm and lower limb drainage — 1 or 2 equal injections in each foot in the first and second interdigital webbed spaces for drainage into lymphatics following the long saphenous vein, or over the lateral dorsum of the foot for lymphatics following the short saphenous vein[1-3].

(b) Axillary nodes and upper limb drainage, e.g. in breast cancer — 1 or 2 equal injections in each hand in the second and third interdigital webbed spaces[4].

(c) Internal mammary chains — separate studies for each side if required because of the possibility of cross-over drainage patterns. A variety of injection sites have been used including the periosteum of the ribs, the posterior rectus sheath beside the xiphisternum and the sub-areolar region[5].

(d) Ileopelvic lymphatic network — bilateral injections into the ischiorectal fossae adjacent to the anal margin[6].

(e) Drainage routes from a particular region, e.g. in cutaneous malignant melanoma — a ring of small injections around the site of interest[7].

Check that the needle is not sited in a blood vessel by aspirating before injection. If any blood appears, another site should be chosen.

3. Static images are taken of the injection site(s) immediately, followed by injection site, drainage route and liver images at intervals, e.g. 15, 30, 60, and 180 min, continuing up to 24 hours or until the liver is seen. Visualization of the liver indicates patency of at least one lymphatic channel (except early liver activity within 15 min, which implies some colloid entry into blood vessels).

Analysis If more frequent imaging or a long dynamic study is performed, time–activity curves for regions along the drainage route can be plotted and used to quantify flow impairment[8].

Aftercare None.

Complications Rarely, an anaphylactic reaction.

References
1. Kramer, E.L. (1990) Lymphoscintigraphy: radiopharmaceutical selection and methods. *Nucl. Med. Biol. Int. J. Radiat. Appl. Instrum. Part B* 17, 57–63.
2. Rijke, A.M., Croft, B.Y., Johnson, R.A., De Jongste, A.B. & Camps, J.A.J. (1990) Lymphoscintigraphy and lymphedema of the lower extremities. *J. Nucl. Med.* 31, 990–998.
3. Proby, C.M., Gane, J.N., Joseph, A.E.A. & Mortimer, P.S. (1990) Investigation of the swollen limb with isotope lymphography. *Br. J. Dermatol.* 123, 29–37.
4. Hayes, D.F. (1990) Axillary lymphoscintigraphy for breast cancer: should we do it? Can we do it? *J. Nucl. Med.* 31, 1835–1838.
5. Terui, S. & Yamamoto, H. (1989) New simplified lymphoscintigraphic technique in patients with breast cancer *J. Nucl. Med.* 30, 1198–1204.
6. Ege, G.N. & Cummings, B.J. (1980) Interstitial radiocolloid iliopelvic lymphoscintigraphy: technique, anatomy and clinical application. *Int. J. Radiat. Oncol. Biol. Phys.* 6, 1483–1490.
7. Wanebo, H.J., Harpole, D. & Teates, C.D. (1985) Radionuclide lymphoscintigraphy with technetium 99m antimony sulfide colloid to identify lymphatic drainage of cutaneous melanoma at ambiguous sites in the head and neck and trunk. *Cancer* 55, 1403–1413.
8. Weissleder, H. & Weissleder, R. (1988) Lymphedema: evaluation of qualitative and quantitative lymphoscintigraphy in 238 patients. *Radiology* 167, 729–735.

Further reading Jewkes, R.F. (1991) Lymph node scanning. In: Maisey, M.N., Britton, K.E. & Gilday, D.L. (eds) *Clinical Nuclear Medicine*, pp. 503–508, 2nd edn. London: Chapman & Hall.

Radionuclide Imaging of Infection and Inflammation

Indications Diagnosis and localization of infection and inflammation in soft tissue and bone.

Contraindications None.

Radiopharmaceuticals 1. *[111]In-labelled leucocytes,* 20 MBq max.

[111]In-oxine, tropolonate and acetylacetonate are highly lipophilic complexes that will label leucocytes, erythrocytes and platelets. In plasma, ^{111}In will dissociate from the complex and bind to plasma proteins. Hence the leucocytes have to be separated from these other components in a patient's blood sample by a lengthy procedure and labelled in vitro under aseptic conditions. The labelled cell suspension is then reinjected[1,2]. ABO/Rh-matched donor leucocytes can be used with neutropenic patients or to reduce infection hazard in HIV positive patients[3]. [111]In has a $T_{1/2}$ of 67 hours and principal γ-emissions at 171 and 245 keV.

2. *[99m]Tc-hexamethylpropyleneamineoxime (HMPAO)-labelled leucocytes,* 200 MBq max.

HMPAO is also a highly lipophilic complex which preferentially labels granulocytes. The cell-labelling technique is similar to that for [111]In[1,2], but HMPAO has the advantage that kits can be stocked and used at short notice. There is more bowel uptake than with ^{111}In-labelled leucocytes, so images must be taken earlier than 4 hours post-injection for diagnosis of abdominal infection[4,5]. The ^{99m}Tc label delivers a lower radiation dose than ^{111}In-labelled leucocytes and has better imaging resolution, which can, for example, help identify inflammation in small bowel[6].

3. *[67]Ga-gallium citrate,* 150 MBq max.

Localizes in inflammatory sites. Considered to be superior to labelled leucocytes in chronic infection[1]. There is significant bowel activity up to 72 hours, so delayed imaging may be necessary for suspected abdominal infection. [67]Ga, with a $T_{1/2}$ of 78 hours and principal γ-emissions at 93,

185 and 300 keV, delivers a higher radiation dose than ^{99m}Tc-HMPAO- and ^{111}In-labelled leucocytes, but it has the advantage of requiring no special preparation.

4. A number of newer agents are under investigation, for example anti-granulocyte antibodies for *in vivo* labelling, but they are not yet widely used in the UK[7].

Equipment

1. Gamma camera, preferably with whole body imaging facility.
2. Low-energy high-resolution collimator for ^{99m}Tc, medium-energy for ^{111}In, medium- or high-energy for [67]Ga.
3. Imaging computer if comparison with other radionuclide scans by image subtraction is required (see 'Additional techniques').

Patient preparation   None.

Technique

1. The radiopharmaceutical is administered i.v.
2. Image timing depends upon the radiopharmaceutical used and the suspected source of infection. Whole-body imaging may be employed for all of the radiopharmaceuticals.
   (a) *[111]In-labelled white cells.* Static images are acquired at 3 and 24 hours post-injection at sites determined by the clinical history. Further imaging at 48 hours may prove helpful.
   (b) *[99m]Tc-HMPAO-labelled white cells.* For suspected abdominal infections, image at 0.5 and 2 hours, i.e. before significant normal bowel activity is seen[4]. For other sites, image at 1, 2 and 4 hours. Additional 24 hour images may be useful.
   (c) *[67]Ga-citrate.* Images are acquired at 48 and 72 hours for regions where normal bowel, urinary and blood pool activity may obscure abnormal collection sites. Later images may prove helpful in non-urgent cases. Extremities and urgent cases may be imaged from as early as 6 hours. Laxatives, given for 48 hours post-injection, will help to clear bowel activity, although frequently they may not be clinically appropriate.

Additional techniques

1. The diagnosis of bone infection may be improved by combination with three-phase radioisotope bone scanning[8, 9] or radiocolloid bone marrow imaging[8, 10].

2. A radiocolloid scan may help to discriminate between infection in the region of the liver or spleen and normal uptake in these organs.

Aftercare   Normal radiation safety precautions (see Chapter 1).

Complications   None.

References

1. Peters, A.M. (1989) Infection. In: Sharp, P.F., Gemmell, H.G. & Smith, F.W. (eds) *Practical Nuclear Medicine*, pp. 299–327. Oxford: Oxford University Press.

2. Danpure, H.J. & Osman, S. (1988) A review of methods of separating and radiolabelling human leucocytes. *Nucl. Med. Commun.* 9, 681–685.

3. O'Doherty, M.J., Revell, P., Page, C.J., Lee, S., Mountford, P.J. & Nunan, T.O. (1990) Donor leucocyte imaging in patients with AIDS: a preliminary report. *Eur. J. Nucl. Med.* 17, 327–333.

4. Lantto, E.H., Lantto, T.J. & Vorne, M. (1991) Fast diagnosis of abdominal infections and inflammations with technetium-99m-HMPAO labeled leukocytes. *J. Nucl. Med.* 32, 2029–2034.

5. Mountford, P.J., Kettle, A.G., O'Doherty, M.J. & Coakley, A.J. (1990) Comparison of technetium-99m-HM-PAO leukocytes with indium-111-oxine leukocytes for localizing intraabdominal sepsis. *J. Nucl. Med.* 31, 311–315.

6. Peters, A.M. & Lavender, J.P. (1991) Editorial. Imaging inflammation with radiolabelled white cells; $^{99}Tc^{m}$-HMPAO or ^{111}In? *Nucl. Med. Commun.* 12, 923–925.

7. Pike, M.C. (1991) Editorial. Imaging of inflammatory sites in the 1990s: new horizons. *J. Nucl. Med.* 32, 2034–2036.

8. Peters, A.M. & Lavender, J.P. (1990) Editorial. Diagnosis of bone infection. *Nucl. Med. Commun.* 11, 463–467.

9. Copping, C., Dalgliesh, S.M., Dudley, N.J. et al (1992) The role of $^{99}Tc^{m}$-HMPAO white cell imaging in suspected orthopaedic infection. *Br. J. Radiol.* 65, 309–312.

10. King, A.D., Peters, A.M., Stuttle, A.W.J. & Lavender, J.P. Imaging of bone infection with labelled white blood cells: role of contemporaneous bone marrow imaging. *Eur. J. Nucl. Med.* 17, 148–151.

Further reading   Peters, A.M. (1992) Imaging inflammation: current role of labeled autologous leukocytes. *J. Nucl. Med.* **33**, 65–67.

Cerqueira, M.D. (1992) Editorial. Detection of cardio-vascular infections with radiolabeled leukocytes. *J. Nucl. Med.* **33**, 1493–1495.

Alazraki, N.P. (1990) Editorial. Diagnosing prosthetic joint infection. *J. Nucl. Med.* **31**, 1955–1957.

Baldwin, J.E. & Wraight, E.P. (1990) Indium labelled leucocyte scintigraphy in occult infection: a comparison with ultrasound and computed tomography. *Clin. Radiol.* **42**, 199–202.

Wegener, W.A. & Alavi, A. (1991) Diagnostic imaging of musculoskeletal infection: roentgenography; gallium, indium-labeled white blood cell, gammaglobulin, bone scintigraphy; and MRI. *Orthop. Clin. N. Am.* **22**, 401–418.

Coakley, A.J. & Mountford, P.J. (1986) Indium-111 leuco-cyte scanning – underused? *BMJ* **293**, 973–974.

Gallium Radionuclide Tumour Imaging

Indications
1. Staging of lymphomas, assessment and prediction of their response to therapy and detection of early relapse[1-3].
2. Gallium imaging has been used with variable success in a variety of other tumours, e.g. hepatoma[4], bronchial carcinoma[5], multiple myeloma[6] and sarcoma[7].

Contraindications None.

Radiopharmaceutical ^{67}Ga-Gallium citrate. 150 MBq max.

Highly protein-bound in plasma, mainly to transferrin. Normal accumulation is seen in the liver, bone marrow and nasal sinuses and variably in the spleen, salivary and lacrimal glands. There is significant excretion via the gut and some via the kidneys. Gallium is also taken up by inflammatory sites, metabolically active bone and non-specifically by a variety of tumours.

^{67}Ga has a $T_{1/2}$ of 78 hours and principal γ-emissions at 93, 185 and 300 keV.

Equipment
1. Gamma camera, preferably with whole body and tomographic facilities.
2. Medium- or high-energy collimator.
3. Imaging computer if comparison with other radionuclide scans by image subtraction is required (see 'Additional techniques').

Patient preparation If the abdomen is being investigated, laxatives may be given (if not contraindicated) for 2 days after injection of ^{67}Ga-citrate to clear bowel activity. Additionally, an enema or suppository may be given on the day of imaging.

Technique
1. ^{67}Ga-citrate is administered i.v.
2. Acquire delayed images as below with energy windows about the lower two or all three of the main photopeaks.

Images

1. 48 and 72 hours. Whole-body, spot views and tomography as appropriate. Tomography can increase the sensitivity and specificity of the investigation[3].

2. Non-specific bowel activity can be discriminated by imaging on two separate occasions. Activity in bowel contents should move between scans and abnormal areas of accumulation will be stationary. If there is still any doubt at 72 hours, later images at up to 7 days may prove helpful.

Additional techniques

1. A radionuclide bone scan may be performed prior to gallium imaging.

2. A radiocolloid scan may help to discriminate between lesions in the region of the liver or spleen and normal uptake in these organs. If both scans are acquired on computer, image subtraction techniques may be used.

Aftercare   None.

Complications   None.

References

1. McLaughlin, A.F., Magee, M.A., Greenough, R. et al (1990) Current role of gallium scanning in the management of lymphoma. *Eur. J. Nucl. Med.* **16**, 755–771.

2. Front, D., Ben Haim, S., Israel, O. et al (1992) Lymphoma: Predictive value of Ga-67 scintigraphy after treatment. *Radiology* **182**, 359–363.

3. Tumeh, S.S., Rosenthal, D.S., Kaplan, W.D., English, R.J. & Holman, B.L. (1987) Lymphoma: evaluation with Ga-67 SPECT. *Radiology* **164**, 111–114.

4. Suzuki, T., Honjo, I. & Hamamoto, K. (1971) Positive scintophotography of cancer of the liver with 67 gallium citrate. *Am. J. Roentg. Rad. Therapy. Nucl. Med.* **113**, 92–103.

5. Bekerman, C., Caride, V.J., Hoffer, P.B. & Boles, C.A. (1990) Noninvasive staging of lung cancer. Indications and limitations of gallium-67 citrate imaging. *Radiol. Clin. N. Am.* **28**, 497–510.

6. Waxman, A.D., Siemsen, J.K., Levine, A.M. et al (1981) Radiographic and radionuclide imaging in multiple myeloma: the role of gallium scintigraphy: concise communication. *J. Nucl. Med.* **22**, 232–236.

7. Southee, A.E., Kaplan, W.D., Jochelson, M.S. et al (1992) Gallium imaging in metastatic and recurrent soft-tissue sarcoma. *J. Nucl. Med.* **33**, 1594–1599.

Further reading　Bekerman,C., Hoffer, P.B. & Bitran, J.D. (1984) The role of gallium-67 in the clinical evaluation of cancer. *Semin. Nucl. Med.* **14**, 296–323.

Clarke, S.E.M. (1991) Tumour imaging. In: Maisey, M.N., Britton, K.E. & Gilday, D.L. (eds) *Clinical Nuclear Medicine*, pp. 426–459, 2nd edn. London: Chapman & Hall.

Radioiodine MIBG Scan

Indications
1. Neuroblastoma[1-4].
2. Phaeochromocytoma[5,6].
3. Carcinoid tumours[7,8].
4. Medullary thyroid carcinoma[9,10].
5. Other tumours deriving from the neural crest[11].

Contraindications None.

Radiopharmaceuticals *Metaiodobenzylguanidine (MIBG)* radiolabelled with:
(a) ^{123}I (250 MBq typical, 400 MBq max.)
(b) ^{131}I (20 MBq max.).

MIBG has a similar structure to noradrenaline, and localizes in the storage vesicles of catecholamine-secreting tumours. ^{123}I-MIBG has better physical imaging properties and delivers a smaller radiation dose per MBq than ^{131}I-MIBG, but is more expensive and less available because ^{123}I is a short-lived cyclotron product ($T_{1/2}$ of 13 hours compared to 8 days for ^{131}I). The longer $T_{1/2}$ of ^{131}I permits later imaging.

Equipment
1. Gamma camera, preferably with whole-body imaging and tomographic capabilities.
2. Low-energy general purpose collimator for ^{123}I, high-energy general purpose for ^{131}I.

Patient preparation
1. Stop tricyclic antidepressants, labetalol, decongestants containing pseudoephedrine, phenylpropanolamine and phenylephrine (many are available over the counter) and other medications that interfere with MIBG uptake[12].
2. Thyroid blockade, continuing for 1 day after MIBG injection for ^{123}I or 5 days for ^{131}I:
   (a) *Adults* — either oral potassium perchlorate (400 mg 0.5–1 hour before MIBG injection, then 200 mg every 6 hours) or oral potassium iodate (85 mg twice daily starting 24 hours before MIBG injection).
   (b) *Children* — Lugol's iodine 0.1–0.2 ml diluted with water or milk three times a day starting 48 hours before MIBG injection. Potassium

iodate is more palatable–the tablets need splitting for paediatric dosage.

3. Children with neuroblastoma should also have a radionuclide bone scan or approximately 10% of skeletal metastases will be missed[1].

Technique

1. Slowly administer MIBG i.v. over 1–2 min (a fast injection may cause adrenergic side effects).
2. Image at 4 and 24 hours for ^{123}I or 24 and 48 hours for [131]I. Later imaging with ^{131}I at up to 7 days may be necessary, e.g. for detection of liver metastases, when normal urinary and hepato-biliary excretion have reduced liver uptake and blood background significantly.

Images

1. Anterior and posterior abdomen, 10–20 min per view.
2. Whole-body imaging for comprehensive search for metastases.
3. Tomography may help to localize lesions, par-ticularly in thorax and abdomen.

Aftercare Normal radiation safety precautions (see Chapter 1).

Complications None.

References

1. Gilday, D.L. & Greenberg, M. (1990) Editorial. The controversy about the nuclear medicine investigation of neuroblastoma. *J. Nucl. Med.* **31**, 135.
2. Jacobs, A., Delree, M., Desprechins, B. et al (1990) Consolidating the role of *I-MIBG-scintigraphy in childhood neuroblastoma: five years of clinical experience. *Paediatr. Radiol.* **20**, 157–159.
3. Troncone, L., Rufini, V., Danza, F.M. et al (1990) Radioiodinated metaiodobenzylguanidine (*I-MIBG) scintigraphy in neuroblastoma: a review of 160 studies. *J. Nucl. Med. Allied Sci.* **34**, 279–288.
4. Gordon, I., Peters, A.M., Gutman, A., Morony, S., Dicks-Mireaux, C. & Pritchard, J. (1990) Skeletal assessment in neuroblastoma — the pitfalls of iodine-123-MIBG scans. *J. Nucl. Med.* **31**, 129–134.
5. Warren, M.J., Shepstone, B.J. & Soper, N. (1989) Iodine-131 metaiodobenzylguanidine (^{131}I-MIBG) for the localization of suspected phaeochromocytoma. *Nucl. Med. Commun.* **10**, 467–475.
6. Hanson, M.W., Feldman, J.M., Beam, C.A., Leight, G.S. & Coleman, R.E. (1991) Iodine 131-labeled

metaiodobenzylguanidine scintigraphy and biochemical analyses in suspected pheochromocytoma. *Arch. Intern. Med.* **151**, 1397–1402.

7. Hoefnagel, C.A., Den Hartog Jager, F.C.A., Taal, B.G., Abeling, N.G.G.M. & Engelsman, E.E. (1987) The role of I-131-MIBG in the diagnosis and therapy of carcinoids. *Eur. J. Nucl. Med.* **13**, 187–191.

8. Bomanji, J., Ur, E., Mather, S. et al (1992) A scintigraphic comparison of iodine-123-metaiodobenzylguanidine and an iodine-labeled somatostatin analog (Tyr-3-octreotide) in metastatic carcinoid tumors. *J. Nucl. Med.* **33**, 1121–1124.

9. Guerra, U.P., Pizzocaro, C., Terzi, A. et al (1989) New tracers for the imaging of the medullary thyroid carcinoma. *Nucl. Med. Commun.* **10**, 285–295.

10. Clarke, S.E.M., Lazarus, C.R., Edwards, S. et al (1987) Scintigraphy and treatment of medullary carcinoma of the thyroid with iodine-131 metaiodobenzylguanidine. *J. Nucl. Med.* **28**, 1820–1825.

11. Von Moll, L., McEwan, A.J., Shapiro, B. et al (1987) Iodine-131 MIBG scintigraphy of neuroendocrine tumors other than pheochromocytoma and neuroblastoma. *J. Nucl. Med.* **28**, 979–988.

12. Solanki, K.K., Bomanji, J., Moyes, J., Mather, S.J., Trainer, P.J. & Britton, K.E. (1992) A pharmacological guide to medicines which interfere with the biodistribution of radiolabelled meta-iodobenzylguanidine (MIBG). *Nucl. Med. Commun.* **13**, 513–521.

Further reading

Troncone, L., Rufini, V., Montemaggi, P., Danza, F.M., Lasorella, A. & Mastrangelo, R. (1990) The diagnostic and therapeutic utility of radioiodinated metaiodobenzylguanidine (MIBG): 5 years of experience. *Eur. J. Nucl. Med.* **16**, 325–335.

11 Bones and Joints

Methods of imaging joints
1. Plain films.
2. Tomography.
3. Arthrography.
4. Radionuclide imaging
   $-$ ^{99m}Tc methylene diphosphonate
   $-$ ^{67}gallium citrate.
5. Ultrasound.
6. CT.
7. MRI.

Further reading
McDowell Anderson Jr, T. (1981). Arthrography. *Radiol. Clin. N. Am.* 19(2).
Freiberger, R. & Kaye, J. (1979) *Arthrography*. New York: Appleton-Century-Crofts.

General Points

1. The plain films should always be reviewed prior to the procedure, as it may be necessary to take further views to demonstrate fully an abnormality that would otherwise be obscured by the presence of contrast medium.

2. Aspiration of an effusion should always be performed before contrast medium is injected. This is because an effusion will dilute the contrast medium, and can also lead to a 'foamy' appearance on the radiographs.

   The aspirate should be sent, where appropriate, for:
   (a) microscopy, culture (aerobic and anaerobic) and sensitivity
   (b) crystal analysis
   (c) cytology
   (d) biochemistry.

3. Although meglumine salts can be used safely for arthrography, LOCM are generally diluted more slowly and allow more time for the examination. In addition the large molecular size of ioxaglate delays absorption further than other low osmolar agents (e.g. iohexol). This is of particular benefit in those investigations that may take some time, e.g. knee arthrography or CT arthrography of the shoulder or ankle.

4. If a needle is correctly sited within a joint space, a test injection of a small volume of contrast medium will stream around the joint. However, if it is incorrectly sited, the contrast medium will remain in a diffuse cloud around the tip of the needle.

5. In the investigation of a suspected loose body, delayed films should be taken after an interval of half an hour. These may show adsorption of contrast medium onto a cartilaginous loose body.

6. The positive contrast medium is absorbed from the joint and excreted from the body in a few hours. However, the air may take up to 4 days to be completely absorbed from the joint space.

Double Contrast Knee Arthrography

Indications
1. Cartilage, capsular or ligamentous injuries.
2. Loose body.
3. Popliteal cyst.

Contraindications   Local sepsis

Contrast medium
1. LOCM 320.
2. Air 40 ml.

Equipment
1. Fluoroscopy unit with spot film device and fine focal spot (0.3 mm^2).
2. Overcouch tube.

Patient preparation   None

Preliminary films   Knee:
1. AP.
2. Lateral.

ADDITIONAL FILMS
1. Axial view of the patella (skyline).
2. Intercondylar view (tunnel).

Technique
1. The patient lies supine; either a medial or a lateral approach can be used and it is as well to be familiar with both.
2. Using a sterile technique, the skin and underlying soft tissue are anaesthetized at a point 1–2 cm posterior to the mid-point of the patella.
3. A 21G needle is advanced into the joint space from this point by angling it slightly anteriorly so the tip comes to lie against the posterior surface of the patella. By virtue of the anatomy, the tip of the needle must be within the joint space (Figure 11.1). A more horizontal approach may result in the needle penetrating the infrapatellar fat pad, resulting in an extra-articular injection of contrast
4. Any effusion is aspirated. If there is any doubt about the position of the needle, the injection of a few millilitres of air will encounter little resistance if the needle is correctly sited. If incorrectly sited, then resistance will be met, and as soon as pressure

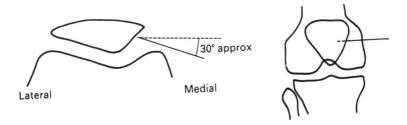

30° approx

Lateral

Medial

Fig. 11.1 Technique of knee arthrography.

is released from the plunger of the syringe it will be forced back into the syringe. This test is not infallible and occasionally air can be injected into soft tissue with little resistance. A test injection of a small volume of contrast medium can be made under fluoroscopic control to ensure the needle is correctly positioned and, if so, the contrast medium should be seen to flow rapidly away from the needle tip. If a satisfactory position is demonstrated, then the full volume of contrast medium and air may be injected.

5. The needle is then removed and the knee is manipulated to ensure even distribution of contrast medium within the joint; this is easily facilitated by asking the patient to walk around the room several times whilst bending the knee through as full a movement as is comfortable.

6. The patient is placed in the prone position with a pad or bolster under the thigh of the side to be examined. It is necessary to apply varus or valgus strain to the knee during the procedure and this is facilitated by applying a strap around the thigh and attaching this to the edge of the table top.

Films
1. Spot films:
   (a) The knee joint is divided into quadrants for the purpose of the examination — an anterior and posterior quadrant for each of the medial and lateral compartments. The X-ray beam is collimated to the compartment being examined.
   (b) Traction is applied to the joint and simultaneously valgus or varus strain is applied

either with a lead glove or, as mentioned before, with the aid of a strap applied to the thigh. A variable degree of flexion may also be required to bring the tibial plateau and meniscus into profile.

(c) Four views of each quadrant are taken, rotating the leg approximately 20° between each spot view. This will result in 8 views per meniscus.

2. Overcouch films: as for preliminary views.

3. In some instances when there is doubt it will be advisable to repeat the spot views. It is recognized that small meniscal tears may not be visible immediately and contrast may take time to adhere. Also meniscal cysts may be better seen on delayed films.

Aftercare The patient is warned that there may be some discomfort in the joint for 1–2 days after the procedure. It is also necessary to refrain from strenuous exercise during this time.

Complications

Due to the contrast medium
1. Allergic reactions.
2. Chemical synovitis.

Due to the technique
1. Pain.
2. Infection.
3. Capsular rupture.
4. Trauma to adjacent structures.

Hip Arthrography

Indications	1. Congenital dislocation of the hip. 2. Loose body. 3. Trauma. 4. Perthes' disease. 5. Proximal focal femoral deficiency. 6. Arthropathy. 7. Painful hip prosthesis.
Contraindications	Local sepsis.
Contrast medium	LOCM 240. 1. Child — 1–2 ml. 2. Adult — 3–5 ml (in loose prostheses the false capsule may take 15–20 mls).
Equipment	1. Fluoroscopy unit. 2. Overcouch tube. 3. Lumbar puncture needle (7.5 cm, 20 or 22G, short bevel).
Patient preparation	1. Nothing orally for 4 hours prior to the procedure. 2. Children under 10 years may require general anaesthesia.
Preliminary films	Hip: 1. AP. 2. Lateral. ADDITIONAL FILMS FOR CHILDREN: Frog lateral.
Technique	1. The patient lies supine on the X-ray table, the leg is extended, internally rotated and the position maintained with sandbags so that the entire length of the femoral neck is visualized. 2. The position of the femoral vessels is marked to avoid inadvertent puncture. 3. The skin is prepared in a standard aseptic manner. 4. A metal marker (sterile needle) or a point on the skin is marked to show the position of entry (Figure 11.2). The needle is then advanced vertically onto the femoral neck under fluoroscopic

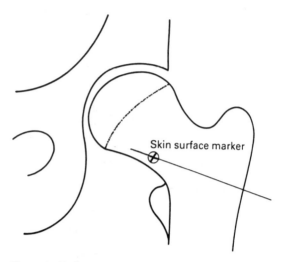

Fig. 11.2 Technique of hip arthrography.
x = site of entry into joint

control; the capsule may be thick and a definite 'give' felt when the needle enters the joint.

5. A test injection of contrast will demonstrate correct placement off the needle, the contrast will flow away from the needle tip. Any fluid in the joint should be aspirated at this stage and sent for analysis.

6. Approximately 3–5 ml (1–2 ml in children) of contrast medium is injected. The exact amount depends on the capacity of the joint capsule. If examining a prosthetic joint, larger volumes of contrast may be required (15–20 ml). By adding a radioactive tracer to the infusate ([99m] Tc-colloid) and subsequent imaging with a gamma camera, a more accurate assessment of loosening can be made, perhaps because the tracer is less viscous than the contrast medium and extends to a greater extent along the prosthesis.

7. After injection of the contrast medium the needle is removed and the joint is passively exercised to distribute the contrast medium evenly. Films are taken immediately.

Films

Adult
1. AP hip.
2. AP in full internal rotation.
3. AP in full external rotation.
4. Lateral.
5. Delayed films at 30 min if indicated.

Children
1. AP hip.
2. Frog lateral.
3. Abduction and internal rotation.
4. Maximum abduction.
5. Maximum adduction.
6. Push/pull views to demonstrate instability.

Prosthetic joint
1. AP prior to injection of contrast.
2. AP with limb immobilized after injection of contrast.
3. Subtraction film using either digital or photographic method. This technique facilitates interpretation, as the metal prosthesis and the barium impregnated cement are subtracted out of the final image.

Aftercare   If the procedure was carried out under general anaesthetic the patient may require admission overnight. The patient should be warned of possible discomfort for 1–2 days and told to avoid strenuous exertion and driving for this time.

Complications   See under knee arthrography (p. 308).

Double Contrast Shoulder Arthrography

Indications
1. Supraspinatus tears.
2. Loose body.
3. Recurrent dislocation.
4. Synovitis or capsulitis.

Contraindications
Local sepsis.

Contrast medium
1. LOCM 320.
2. Air. Approx. 8–10 ml.

Equipment
1. Fluoroscopy unit.
2. Overcouch tube.
3. Lumbar puncture needle (9 cm, 22G, short bevel).

Patient preparation
None.

Preliminary films
Shoulder:
1. AP in internal rotation.
2. AP in external rotation.
3. Axial.

Technique
1. The patient lies supine, with the arm of the side under investigation close to the body and the hand supinated. This is to rotate the long head of the biceps out of the path of the needle. The articular surface of the glenoid will face slightly forwards, which is important as it allows a vertically placed needle to enter the joint space without damaging the glenoid labrum.
2. The coracoid process is located by palpation. Using a sterile technique, the skin and soft tissues are anaesthetized at a point 1 cm inferior and 1 cm lateral to the coracoid process. Position is optimized by fluoroscopy.
3. A lumbar puncture needle (22G) or a 21G needle is inserted vertically down into the joint space (Figure 11.3). The vertical direction allows precise control of the medial–lateral course of the needle. The position of the needle should be checked by intermittent screening. When it meets the resistance of the articular surface of the humeral head

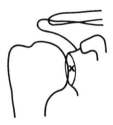

Fig. 11.3 Technique of double contrast shoulder arthrography.
x = site of entry into joint

it is withdrawn by 1–2 mm to free the tip.
4. The intra-articular position of the needle is then confirmed by the injection of a few drops of the contrast medium under fluoroscopic control.
5. The remainder of the contrast medium and sufficient air to distend the synovial sac (8–10 ml) is injected. Patients with an adhesive capsulitis may experience pain after much smaller amounts. If this is severe then injection should be stopped. Resistance to injection is common, unlike injection into the knee, and more force is often required.
6. The needle is removed and the joint is gently manipulated to distribute the contrast medium.

Films
1. AP in neutral — erect.
2. AP in external rotation — erect.
3. AP in internal rotation — erect.
4. Axial.

Additional films
1. Repeat steps 2 and 3 above with the tube angled caudad to bring the under surface of the acromion parallel to the beam.
2. AP in neutral with shoulder under load (5 kg) may help demonstrate supraspinatus tear.

Aftercare
The patient is warned of slight discomfort persisting for 1–2 days.

Complications
As for knee arthrography.

Further reading
Ghelman, B & Goldman, A.B. (1977) The double contrast shoulder arthrogram: evaluation of rotary cuff tears. *Radiology* **124**, 251–254.

CT Shoulder Arthrography

Indication As for double contrast arthrography but particularly useful in joint instability.

Technique
1. Contrast medium is injected as outlined in the steps for double contrast arthrography. Too much contrast will flood the joint and so a smaller volume is all that is required (2.5–3 ml).
2. If any delay is anticipated in transfer to the CT scanner, then dilution of the contrast medium can be reduced by the addition of 0.2 ml of adrenaline 1:1000 to the injection.
3. CT examination is performed with the patient supine and positioned slightly eccentrically within the scanner to ensure that the shoulder is well within the scan field.
4. The contralateral arm can be elevated above the head to minimize image artefacts.
5. Scanning should be undertaken during arrested respiration to minimize motion artefact.

Films
1. Contiguous slices (3–4 mm) are obtained from the acromiom to the axillary recess. Images should be targeted to the relevant shoulder with a magnification factor of 4.
2. Images should be viewed on both soft tissue and bone windows.
3. Additional information can occasionally be obtained by scanning prone. Direct sagittal scanning to better visualize the rotator cuff can also be employed, but it adds to time taken and the position may be difficult for the patient to maintain.

Further reading Davies, A.M. (1991) The current role of computed tomographic arthrography of the shoulder. *Clin. Radiol.* **44**, 369–375.

Elbow Arthrography

Indications
1. Loose body.
2. Ligament injury.
3. Capsular rupture.

Contraindications Local sepsis.

Contrast medium LOCM 240. 3–4 ml.

Equipment
1. Fluoroscopy unit.
2. Overcouch tube.

Patient preparation None.

Technique
Single contrast
1. The patient sits next to the table with his elbow flexed and resting on the table, the lateral aspect uppermost.
2. The radial head is located by palpation during gentle pronation and supination of the forearm. Using a sterile technique the skin and soft tissues are anaesthetized at a point just proximal to the radial head.
3. A 23G needle is then inserted vertically down into the joint space between the radial head and the capitellum (Figure 11.4).
4. An injection of a small volume of local anaesthetic will flow easily if the needle is correctly sited. This can be confirmed by the injection of a few drops of contrast medium under fluoroscopic control.

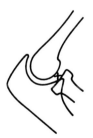

Fig. 11.4 Technique of elbow arthrography.
x = site of entry into joint

5. The remainder of the contrast medium is injected and the joint gently manipulated to distribute it evenly.

Double contrast

1. Position the patient as for single contrast technique and follow steps 1–4 above.
2. Inject 0.5 ml of contrast medium followed by 6–12 ml of air until the olecranon fossa is distended.

Films

1. AP.
2. Lateral.
3. Both 45° posterior obliques.
4. Delayed films at 30 min, if indicated.

Aftercare

The patient is warned that there may be discomfort for 1–2 days afterwards.

Complications

As for knee arthrography.

Wrist arthrography

RADIOCARPAL JOINT

Indications	1. Ligament injury. 2. Synovial swelling.
Contraindications	Local sepsis.
Contrast medium	LOCM 240. 2–4 ml.
Equipment	1. Overcouch tube. 2. Fluoroscopy unit.
Patient preparation	None.
Preliminary films	1. PA. 2. Lateral
Technique	1. The patient is seated next to the screening table with the forearm resting in a neutral prone position. The wrist should be supported over a wedge with about 10–15° of flexion.

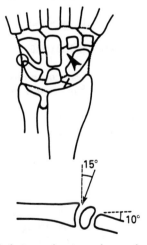

Fig. 11.5 Technique of wrist arthrography. Arrow and x = site of entry into radiocarpal joint. Arrowhead = site of entry into midcarpal joint.

2. Using a sterile technique, the skin and soft tissues are anaesthetized on the dorsal aspect of the wrist at a point just distal to the mid-point of the lower end of the radius (Figure 11.5).
3. A 23G needle is inserted into the joint by advancing it downwards and at an angle of about 15° proximally.
4. Contrast medium is injected under fluoroscopic control; if any leakage occurs into the midcarpal joint or distal radioulnar joints, then spot views should be taken. If this is not done, it is possible to miss small tears that later become obscured by the anterior and posterior extensions of the radiocarpal joint.

Films
1. PA.
2. PA with ulnar deviation.
3. PA with radial deviation.
4. Lateral.
5. 45° oblique.

MIDCARPAL JOINT

Indications   Ligamentous injury

Contraindications   Local sepsis.

Contrast medium   LOCM 240. 3 ml.

Equipment   Overcouch tube.
Fluoroscopy unit with video facility.

Preliminary films
1. PA.
2. Lateral.

Technique
1. The wrist is positioned as for radiocarpal injection but with ulnar deviation, as this widens the joint space.
2. The skin and soft tissues are anaesthetized at point over the mid-point of the scaphocapitate joint (Figure 11.5).
3. A 23G needle is inserted vertically into the joint space under fluoroscopic control.
4. Contrast is injected under fluoroscopic control, ideally with video-recording facility, until the

joint space is full. Without continuous monitoring it may not be possible to tell which of the ligaments separating the midcarpal from the radiocarpal joint are torn from the plain films alone.

Films
1. PA.
2. PA with ulnar deviation.
3. PA with radial deviation.
4. Lateral.
5. 45° oblique.

Aftercare The patient should be warned of possible discomfort for 1–2 days after the procedure.

Complications As for knee arthrography.

Further reading Robert, M., et al (1985) Midcarpal wrist arthrography for the detection of tears of the scapholunate and lunotriquetral ligaments. *Am. J. Roentg.* **144**, 107–108.

Ankle Arthrography

Indications
1. Ligament injury.
2. Loose body.
3. Joint rupture.
4. Osteochondral defect.

Contraindications   Local sepsis.

Contrast medium   LOCM 240. 6–8 ml.

Equipment   Overcouch tube.

Patient preparation   None.

Preliminary films
1. AP.
2. Lateral.

Technique
1. The patient lies supine with the ankle slightly plantar-flexed. An anterior approach is used.
2. Using a sterile technique, the skin is anaesthetized at a point 1 cm above and 1 cm lateral to the tip of the medial malleolus (Figure 11.6). Position is optimized by fluoroscopy.
3. A 21G needle is inserted and advanced in an AP direction into the joint space.

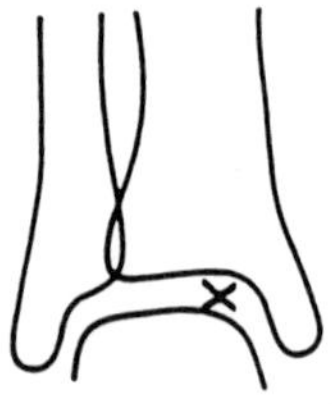

Fig. 11.6   Technique of ankle arthrography.
x = site of entry into joint

Films
1. AP.
2. Lateral.
3. 45° obliques.
4. Inversion and eversion stress films.

Additional films   AP and lateral tomography.

Aftercare   The patient should be warned of possible discomfort for 1–2 days following the procedure and to avoid strenuous activity and driving for this time.

Complications   As for knee arthrography.

CT Ankle Arthrography

Indication　Osteochondral defects.

Technique
1. Contrast medium is introduced into the joint as outlined in the steps above for standard single contrast arthrography. Low osmolar contrast has the advantage of slower dilution in the event of delay prior to scanning. Adrenaline, 0.1 ml of 1:1000, can be used to delay absorption further.
2. The patient is positioned in the scanner, supine with the knee flexed and the foot placed sole-flat on the couch.
3. The scanner gantry is then tilted to obtain, as close as is possible, true coronal sections through the ankle joint.

Films
1. Contiguous thin sections are acquired (3–4 mm) through the joint from anterior to posterior.
2. Direct axial sections may also be acquired if necessary.

Further reading　Davies, A.M., & Cassar-Pullicino, V.N. (1989) Demonstration of Osteochondritis dissecans of the talus by coronal computed tomography arthrography. *Br. J. Radiol.* **62**(744), 1050–1055.

Temporomandibular Joint Arthrography

Indications	Dysfunction, pain, clicking or failure of conservative management.
Contraindications	Local sepsis.
Contrast medium	LOCM 300. 2 ml.
Equipment	1. Fluoroscopy unit. 2. Overcouch tube.
Patient preparation	None.
Technique	Two methods are described.
Single contrast	1. The patient lies on his side, with a pad under the lower shoulder, and the head resting on the table. The degree of lateral flexion of the head is adjusted using fluoroscopy to obtain the optimum visual-

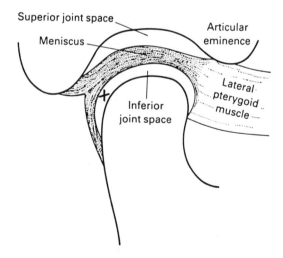

Fig. 11.7 Technique of temporomandibular joint arthrography.
x = site of entry into joint

ization of the temporomandibular joint under investigation.

2. Using a sterile technique, the overlying skin and soft tissues are anaesthetized.

3. With the mouth a little open, a 25G needle is advanced down onto the posterosuperior aspect of the condyle of the mandible (Figure 11.7). If satisfactorily sited, it will move forwards with the condyle as the mouth is opened.

4. A small volume (0.3–0.6 ml) is injected under fluoroscopic control. It should flow freely forward to the anterior aspect of the head of the condyle.

FILMS

1. Lateral oblique-mouth open.
2. Lateral oblique–mouth closed.
3. Video full range of temporomandibular joint movement.

Double contrast

1. Position the patient as for single contrast technique (see above).

2. Using a 25G needle, the lower joint is entered as described above. Approx. 0.5 ml of air is injected followed by 0.1 ml of contrast followed by a further 0.8 ml of air.

3. The needle is repositioned level with and 3 mm posterior to the upper tip of the condyle. The needle is advanced until it meets the articular eminence. It is then withdrawn slightly and 0.5 ml of air is injected followed by 0.15 ml of contrast and a further 1 ml of air. This should outline the superior joint compartment.

FILMS

AP and lateral tomography with the mouth closed.

Aftercare   The patient is warned of possible discomfort for 1–2 days after the procedure.

Complications   As for knee arthrography.

Further reading   Doyle, T. (1983) Arthrography of the temporomandibular joint: a simple technique. *Clin. Radiol.* **34**, 147–151.
Bell, K.A. et al (1983) Videofluoroscopy during arthro-

graphy of the temporomandibular joint. *Radiology* **147**, 879.

Westessen, P.-L. et al., (1980) Double contrast tomography of the temporomandibular joint. *Acta. Radiol. (Diagn.)* **21**, 777–782.

Tenography

Methods of imaging tendons
1. Tenography.
2. Ultrasound.
3. CT.
4. MRI.

General points
1. Tenography is used to detect abnormalities of tendons and their surrounding sheaths. With the advent of CT and MRI, the number of such procedures performed has declined.
2. Although MRI can show fluid within tendon sheaths, the resolution is not capable of detailing fine irregularity of tendons seen in minimal to moderate tenosynovitis or the scarring that develops in stenosing tenosynovitis.
3. Tenography can be used to identify with certainty the positioning of therapeutic injections of local anaesthetic and steroid.
4. Tenography can be used for any tendon that has an approachable sheath and one which has suitable anatomical surface landmarks. Commonly evaluated tendon sheaths around the ankle joint include peroneal, posterior tibial, extensor hallucis longus, anterior tibial, flexor digitorum longus and flexor hallucis longus. In the wrist and hand, the carpal tunnel and abductor pollicis longus can be evaluated in this way.
5. The technique is essentially similar for any tendon sheath.

Indications
1. Tenosynovitis:
   − acute
   − chronic stenosing.
2. Capsular or tendon sheath tears.
3. Traumatic rupture.
4. Extrinsic compression.
5. Tendon displacement.
6. Therapeutic placement of steroid.

Contraindication Local sepsis.

Contrast medium LOCM 240. Volume depends on the tendon to be evaluated.

Equipment	1. Fluoroscopy unit.
	2. Overcouch tube.

Technique
1. Before injection, the origin, course and insertion of the tendon should be familiarized.
2. By moving the joint passively the tendon of interest can be palpated. The point of insertion should be marked.
3. Using an aseptic technique the skin and soft tissue is anaesthetized with local infiltration with lignocaine 1%.
4. A 23 or 25G needle is advanced into the tendon sheath until firm resistance is met from the tendon. The needle is slowly withdrawn, exerting gentle pressure to a syringe containing local anaesthetic. When this flows easily the needle is within the sheath. This is then confirmed by the injection of 1 ml of contrast under fluoroscopic control; contrast will be seen to flow away from the needle.
5. Sufficient contrast material is then injected to fill the sheath to its distal reflection.
6. Fluoroscopy during injection is advisable to identify filling defects or lobulations.

Films
1. Spot films during fluoroscopy.
2. AP.
3. Lateral.
4. Both 45° obliques.

ADDITIONAL FILMS
1. Spot films after full range of movement of the tendon under evaluation.
2. AP or lateral with skin marker to identify point of maximal tenderness.

Aftercare Patient should be warned of discomfort lasting for 24–48 hours.

Complications As for arthrography.

Further reading Baker, K.S., Gilula, L.A. (1990) The current role of tenography and bursography. *Am. J. Roentg.* **154**, 129–133.

Ultrasound of the Paediatric Hip

Indications
1. Developmental hip dysplasia.
2. Hip effusion.
3. Slipped femoral capital epiphysis.

Equipment
5–7.5 MHz linear transducer.

Technique
Developmental hip dysplasia

With ultrasonography the unossified elements of the hip — femoral head, greater trochanter, labrum, triradiate cartilage — as well as the bony acetabular roof, can be identified in the first 6 months of life[1]. After 9–12 months the degree of ossification precludes adequate imaging by ultrasound and plain film radiography becomes superior. There are two main methods — static and dynamic, and both may be used during one examination.

STATIC (GRAF) METHOD
This assesses the morphology and geometry of the acetabulum. Although independent of the position of the infant, it is recommended that the infant be placed in the decubitus position. A single longitudinal image is obtained with the transducer placed over the greater trochanter and held at right angles to all the anatomical planes. The following landmarks are identified, and in the following sequence: chondro-osseous boundary between femoral shaft and head, joint capsule, labrum, cartilaginous roof, superior bony rim of acetabulum. Although most images can be 'eyeballed', two angles can be measured from the image and form the basis for the Graf classification[2].

DYNAMIC METHOD
This assesses the stability of the hip when stressed. The hip is studied in the coronal and axial planes with the infant supine. With the hip flexed and adducted, the femur is pushed and pulled with a piston-like action[3].

Hip joint effusion

Approximately 50% of children with acute hip pain have intra-articular fluid[4] and the sensitivity of ultrasound for detecting effusion approaches 100%.

With the child supine, the hip is scanned anteriorly with the transducer parallel to the femoral neck. Bulging of the anterior portion of the joint capsule can be readily identified[5]. The normal distance between the bony femoral neck and the joint capsule is always less than 3 mm, and the difference between the affected and unaffected sides should not be greater than 2 mm.

Slipped femoral capital epiphysis

Although plain radiographs constitute the usual means of diagnosis, a mild posterior slip can be identified in the acute situation by longitudinal scanning along the femoral neck.

References

1. Youzefzadeh, D. & Ramilo J.L. (1987) Normal hip in children: correlation of U.S. with anatomic and cryomicrotome sections. *Radiology* 165, 647–655.
2. Graf, R. (1987) *Guide to Sonography of the Infant Hip*. New York: Thième Medical Publishers.
3. Clark, N.M.P., Harcke, T.H., McHugh, P. et al (1985) Real time ultrasound in the diagnosis of congenital dislocation and dysplasia of the hip. *J. Bone Joint Surg.* 67B, 406–412.
4. Dörr, U., Zieger, M. & Hanke, H. (1988) Ultrasonography of the painful hip. Prospective studies in 204 patients. *Pediatr. Radiol.* 19, 36–40.
5. Miralles, M., Gonzalea, G., Pulpeiro, J.R. et al (1989) Sonography of the painful hip in children: 500 consecutive cases. *Am. J. Roentg.* 152, 579–582.

Radionuclide Bone Scan

Indications
1. Staging of cancer and response to therapy, especially breast, prostatic and bronchial carcinoma.
2. Assessment of primary bone tumours.
3. Bone infections.
4. Metabolic bone disease.
5. Bone pain.
6. Painful hip and knee prosthesis.
7. Avascular necrosis and bone infarction.
8. Trauma not obvious on X-ray.
9. Arthritis.
10. Assessment of non-accidental injury.

Contraindications None.

Radiopharmaceuticals ^{99m} *Tc-methylene diphosphonate (MDP) or other* ^{99m} *Tc-labelled diphosphonate.* 500 MBq typical, 600 MBq max.

These compounds are phosphate analogues which are stable *in vivo* and rapidly excreted by the kidneys, so giving a good contrast between bone and soft tissue.

Equipment
1. Gamma camera, preferably with whole body imaging facility.
2. Low-energy general purpose or high-resolution collimator.
3. Tomographic capability with high-resolution collimator where precise localization of lesions is required.

Patient preparation The patient must be well hydrated.

Technique
1. ^{99m} Tc-diphosphonate is injected i.v. When infection is suspected or blood flow to bone or primary bone tumour is to be assessed, a bolus injection is given with the patient in position on the camera. A three-phase study is then performed with arterial, blood-pool and delayed static imaging.
2. The patient should be encouraged to drink plenty and empty the bladder frequently.
3. The bladder is emptied immediately prior to imaging.

4. Delayed static imaging is performed 2–4 hours after injection.

Images

Standard With digital cameras, high-resolution images are acquired with a pixel size of 1–2 mm.

1. The whole skeleton. The number of views will depend upon the field of view of the camera and whether a whole-body imaging facility is available. A point to consider is that whole-body images will have lower resolution than spot views over parts of the skeleton where the camera is some distance from the patient (unless a body-contour tracking facility is available), since resolution falls off with distance. Spot views should be overlapping.
2. Anterior oblique views of the thorax are useful to separate sternum and spine uptake.
3. For examination of the posterior ribs, scapula or shoulder, an extra posterior thorax view with arms above the head should be taken to move the scapula away from the ribs.
4. For imaging small bones and joints, magnified views should be taken, with a pinhole collimator if necessary.
5. Tomography can be useful for lesion localization, e.g. in vertebrae and joints, and to detect avascular necrosis[1].

Three-phase

1. Arterial phase: 1–2 s frames of the area of interest for 1 min post-injection.
2. Blood pool: 3-min image of the same area 5 min post-injection.
3. Delayed: views 2–4 hours post-injection, as for standard imaging.

Analysis

1. For the arterial phase, time–activity curves are created for regions of interest symmetrical about the mid-line.
2. For tomography, reconstruction of transaxial, coronal, sagittal and possibly oblique slices to demonstrate the lesion.

Additional technique   Additional information about renal function may be obtained with dynamic imaging during the first 20–30 min post-injection, e.g. in prostatic carcinoma[2].

Aftercare   Normal radiation safety precautions (see Chapter 1).

Complications   None.

References
1. Murray, I.P.C., Dixon, J. (1989) The role of single photon emission computed tomography in bone scintigraphy. *Skeletal Radiol.* **18**, 493–505.
2. Narayan, P., Lillian, D., Hellstrom, W., Hedgcock, M., Jajodia, P.B. & Tanagho, E.A. (1988) The benefits of combining early radionuclide renal scintigraphy with routine bone scans in patients with prostate cancer. *J. Urol.* **140**, 1448–1451.

Further reading
Fogelman, I. (ed.) (1987) *Bone Scanning in Clinical Practice.* London: Springer-Verlag.
Freeman, L.M. & Blaufox, M.D. (eds) (1988) Nuclear orthopedics. *Semin. Nucl. Med.* **18**(2).
Lamki, L.M. (1985) Bone scintigraphy: current trends and future prospects. *J. Nucl. Med.* **26**, 312–314.
Smith, F.W. The skeletal system. In: Sharp, P.F., Gemmell, H.G. & Smith, F.W. (eds) (1989) *Practical Nuclear Medicine*, pp. 245–264. Oxford: Oxford University Press.

12 Central Nervous System

Methods of imaging the brain

1. Plain films.
2. Tomography — especially the pituitary fossa and internal auditory meati.
3. Angiography.
4. CT.
5. MRI.
6. Radionuclide imaging
   - conventional brain scan
   - regional cerebral blood flow scan
   - positron emission tomography (PET).
7. Ultrasound.

Further reading

Bernard, M.S., Hourihan, M.D. & Adams, H. (1991) Computed tomography of the brain: does contrast enhancement really help? *Clin. Radiol.* **44**, 161–164.

Methods of imaging acoustic neuromas

Gadolinium-enhanced MRI is the definitive test and could be considered to be the only imaging investigation necessary[1]. However, it is a limited resource and only 1 in 100 patients who present with symptoms suggestive of an acoustic neuroma will ultimately be shown to have one. Investigation is, therefore, a two-stage process of screening followed by definitive imaging[2,3].

SCREENING
Using a combination of three techniques the majority of acoustic neuromas can be identified.
1. *Evoked response audiometry* — a normal result virtually excludes acoustic neuroma but there is a high false-positive rate.
2. *Caloric response.*
3. *Conventional tomography* — an acoustic neuroma is highly likely if there is a discrepancy of >1 mm between the sizes of the internal auditory meati.

DEFINITIVE IMAGING

1. *MRI – all* acoustic neuromas show enhancement with i.v. gadolinium and this technique is the method of choice. It has replaced CT air meatography[4], although the latter is still more sensitive than unenhanced MRI[5].

2. *CT* – with contrast enhancement and imaged with soft tissue and bone windows. There are false negatives with small and/or intracanalicular tumours.

3. *CT air meatography* – is associated with a significant morbidity[6].

References

1. Anon. (1988) Imaging patients with acoustic neuroma. *Lancet* 3, 1294.

2. Terkildsen, K. & Thomsen, J. Diagnostic screening for acoustic neuromas. *Clin. Otolaryngol.* 8, 295–296.

3. Clifton, A.G., Phelps, P.D. & Lloyd, G.A.S. (1991) The investigation of acoustic neuroma. *Clin Radiol.* 44, 232–235.

4. Phelps, P.D. & Lloyd, G.A.S. (1982) High resolution air CT meatography: the demonstration of normal and abnormal structures in the cerebellopontine cistern and the internal auditory meatus. *Br. J. Radiol.* 55, 19–22.

5. Haughton, V.M., Rimm, A.A., Sobocinski, K.A. et al (1986) A blinded clinical comparison of MR imaging and CT in neuroradiology. *Radiology* 160, 751–755.

6. Greenberger, R., Khangure, M.S. & Chakera, T.M.H. (1987) The morbidity of CT air meatography: a follow-up of 84 patients. *Clin Radiol* 38, 535–536.

Methods of imaging the spine

1. Plain films.
2. Tomography.
3. Myelography/radiculography.
4. Discography.
5. Facet arthrography.
6. Epidurography.
7. Lumbar epidural venography.
8. Arteriography.
9. CT ± enhancement with intrathecal or i.v. contrast medium.
10. Radionuclide imaging.
11. Magnetic resonance, imaging ± i.v. gadolinium enhancement.
12. Ultrasound
    – oblique measurements

— intraoperative
— the paediatric spine.

Further reading   Cacayorin, E.D. & Kieffer, S.A. (1982) Applications and limitations of computed tomography of the spine. *Radiol. Clin N. Am.* **20**, 185–206.

DiChiro, G. & Wener, L. (1973) Angiography of the spinal cord: a review of contempory techniques and applications. *J. Neurosurg.* **39**, 1–29.

Emery, I. & Hamilton, G. (1980) Epidurography using metrizamide. An out-patient examination *Clin. Radiol.* **31**, 643–649.

Han, J.S., Benson, J.E. & Yoon, Y.S. (1984) Magnetic resonance imaging in the spinal column and craniovertebral junction. *Radiol. Clin. N. Am.* **22**, 805–827.

McCormick, C.C. (1978) Radiology in low back pain and sciatica. An analysis of the relative efficacy of spinal venography, discography and epidurography in patients with a negative or equivocal myelogram. *Clin. Radiol.* **29**, 393–406.

Park, W.M. (1980) The place of radiology in the investigation of low back pain. *Clin. Rheum. Dis.* **6**, 93–132.

Porter, R.W., Wicks, M. & Otterwell, D. (1978) Measurement of the spinal canal by diagnostic ultrasound. *J. Bone Joint Surg.* **60B**, 481–484.

Rubin, J.M., DiPietro, M.A., Chandler, W.F. & Venes, J.L. (1988) Spinal ultrasonography. Intraoperative and pediatric applications. *Radiol. Clin. N. Am.* **26**, 1–27.

Ultrasound of the infant brain

Indications Any suspected intracranial pathology.

Contraindications None, but a small or closed anterior fontanelle will severely limit the success of the technique.

Equipment 5 MHz sector transducer. Occasionally a 3.5 MHz transducer may be needed for larger brains and a 7.5 or 10 MHz transducer may be necessary to visualize superficial structures.

Patient preparation None. A restless child may be consoled with a dummy or examined while cuddled in the arms of a carer.

Methods
1. Via the anterior fontanelle.
2. Through the squamosal portion of the temporal bone to visualize extracerebral collections and the region of the circle of Willis and to obtain Doppler signals of the middle cerebral arteries.
3. Via the posterior fontanelle, for the posterior fossa.

The method via the anterior fontanelle will be described.

Technique
Coronal A basic six coronal and six sagittal images are obtained and supplemented with other images of specific areas of interest. The base of the skull must be perfectly symmetrical on coronal scans. The first image is obtained with the transducer angled forward and subsequent images obtained by angling progressively more posteriorly. The anatomical landmarks that define each view are:
1. The orbital roofs and cribriform plate (these combine to produce a 'steer's head' appearance); anterior interhemispheric fissure; frontal lobes.
2. Greater wings, lesser wings and body of sphenoid (these produce a 'mask' appearance); the cingulate sulcus; frontal horns of lateral ventricles
3. 'Pentagon' view: five-sided star formed by the internal carotid, middle cerebral and anterior cere-

bral arteries (these may be observed to pulsate and may be interrogated with Doppler); frontal horns of lateral ventricles; cavum septum pellucidum; basal ganglia.

4. Bilateral C-shaped echoes from the parahippocampal gyri; thalami.

5. Trigones of lateral ventricles containing choroid plexus; echogenic inverted V from the tentorium cerebelli; cerebellum.

6. Occipital horns of lateral ventricles; parietal and occipital cortex; cerebellum.

For the sagittal images, the reference plane should be a mid-line image with the third ventricle, cavum septum pellucidum (if present) and fourth ventricle all on the same image. The more lateral parasagittal images are obtained with the transducer angled laterally and slightly oblique because the occipital horn of the lateral ventricle is more lateral than the frontal horn.

Sagittal
1. Two views of the mid-line.
2. Parasagittal scan of the left lateral ventricle. This is angled approximately 15° from the mid-line.
3. Steep parasagittal scan, approximately 30° from the mid-line, of the left frontal, temporal and parietal cortex.
4. Parasagittal scan of the right lateral ventricle.
5. Steep parasagittal scan of the right frontal, temporal and parietal cortex.

Further reading
Cremin, B.J., Chilton, S.J. & Peacock, W.J. (1983) Anatomical landmarks in anterior fontanelle ultrasonography. *Br. J. Radiol.* **56**, 517–526.

Conventional Radionuclide Brain Scan (Blood–Brain Barrier Imaging)

Indications
1. Cerebral tumours.
2. Subdural haematoma.
3. Assessment of carotid and cerebral artery blood flow.
4. Cerebrovascular disease.
5. Infection.
6. Confirmation of brain death.

Contraindications   None.

Radiopharmaceuticals
1. ^{99m}Tc-*glucoheptonate*. 500 MBq max. for static imaging only, 800 MBq max. for dynamic imaging.
   Crosses the damaged blood–brain barrier and demonstrates areas of increased vascularity. Higher lesion-to-background ratio than pertechnetate because of faster plasma clearance.
2. ^{99m}Tc-*DTPA*. 500 MBq max. for static imaging only, 800 MBq max. for dynamic imaging.
   Similar efficacy to glucoheptonate.
3. ^{99m}Tc-*pertechnetate*. 500 MBq max. for static imaging only, 800 MBq max. for dynamic imaging.
   Crosses the damaged blood–brain barrier, but accumulates in the choroid plexus, thyroid and salivary glands, so requires prior blocking with potassium perchlorate. Considered inferior to the above agents[1].

Equipment
1. Gamma camera.
2. Low-energy general purpose collimator.
3. Imaging computer.

Patient preparation   Pertechnetate only: blockade with 200–400 mg potassium perchlorate orally 30–90 min before study or 50–100 mg sodium perchlorate i.v. at the time of radiopharmaceutical injection.

Technique   The study consists of a dynamic or vascular phase followed by static imaging.
1. The patient lies supine with the camera centred over head and neck to include the carotid arteries.

If information about intracranial arterial flow alone is required, the camera is positioned over the vertex of the skull.

2. A rapid i.v. injection of radiopharmaceutical in a small volume is given, starting computer acquisition at the same time.
3. Dynamic images are acquired for 1 min following injection to assess flow in the major arteries.
4. Static views 1–2 hours after injection.
5. Delayed images at 3–5 hours can improve the sensitivity.

Images
1. *Dynamic.* Anterior, 60 × 1-s frames on computer. Hard copy: 2-s images from first arrival of bolus generated from computer images, or 2–6 s analogue images for 1 min post-injection.
2. *Static.* Patient sitting if capable. 300–500 kilocounts per view:
   (a) anterior, forehead and nose in contact with camera
   (b) posterior, head well flexed to separate posterior fossa from nasal mucosa
   (c) left and right lateral
   (d) a vertex view may be taken to improve demonstration of lesions high in the cerebral hemispheres.

Analysis
Dynamic. Time–activity curves are produced from regions over the carotid arteries and cerebral hemispheres.

Aftercare
Normal radiation safety precautions (see Chapter 1).

Complications
None.

Reference
1. Banzo, J.I., Banzo, J., Abós, M. D., Prats E., Morales, F. & Teijeiro, J. (1982) ^{99m}Tc-DTPA and ^{99m}Tc-GH cerebral imaging: a comparative analysis. *Nucl. Med. Commun.* **3**, 304–308.

Further reading
Nisbet, A.P., Ratcliffe, G.E., Ellam, S.V., Rankin, S.C. & Maisey, M.N. (1983) Clinical indications for optimal use of the radionuclide brain scan. *Br. J. Radiol.* **56**, 377–381.

Smith, F.W. (1989) The central nervous system. In: Sharp, P.F., Gemmell, H.G. & Smith, F.W. (eds) *Practical Nuclear Medicine*, pp. 109–135. Oxford: Oxford University Press.

Regional Cerebral Blood Flow Imaging

Indications
1. Localization of epileptic foci.
2. Cerebrovascular disease.
3. Diagnosis of dementia including Alzheimer's disease.
4. Differential diagnosis of depression and depressive dementia.
5. Diagnosis of Huntington's disease.
6. Assessment of effects of treatment regimes.
7. Diagnosis and serial assessment of AIDS dementia complex.
8. Confirmation of brain death.

Contraindications   None.

Radiopharmaceutical   *^{99m}Tc-D,L-hexamethylpropyleneamineoxime (HMPAO)*[1]. 500 MBq max.

HMPAO is a lipophilic complex that crosses the blood–brain barrier and localizes in proportion to cerebral blood flow. It has moderate cerebral extraction on the first pass, with minimal redistribution (about 86% remains in the brain at 24 hours).

Other radiopharmaceuticals ^{123}I-N-isopropyl-p-iodoamphetamine (IMP)[2].
^{123}I-N.N.N'-trimethyl-N'(2-hydroxyl-3-methyl-5-iodo-benzyl)-1,3-propanediamine (HIPDM)[2].
200 MBq typical.

These are lipophilic amines with maximum brain uptake in proportion to blood flow at 20–30 min (IMP) or 10–15 min (HIPDM), with good extraction on first pass. Redistribution occurs after about 60 min, so imaging should be completed within this time. Inferior image quality to HMPAO with standard injected dose, and availability is limited.

Equipment
1. Tomographic gamma camera.
2. Tomography bed with head extension.
3. Low-energy high-resolution collimator (or more specialized slant-hole or fan-beam collimator).

Patient preparation   Since cerebral blood flow is continuously varying with motor activity, sensory stimulation, emotional arousal, etc., it is important to standardize the conditions under which the HMPAO is administered, especially if serial studies are to be undertaken in the same individual. Familiarization with the procedure to reduce anxiety and injection in a relaxing environment through a previously positioned i.v. cannula should be considered.

Technique
1. If blood flow in the carotid and major cerebral arteries is of interest, the patient lies supine with the camera anterior. If information about intracranial arterial blood flow alone is required, the camera is positioned over the vertex of the skull.
2. ^{99m}Tc-HMPAO is administred i.v. (rapidly for dynamic imaging).
3. Immediate dynamic imaging for 1 min following injection may be carried out to assess flow in the major arteries.
4. Tomographic imaging is performed any time from 5 min after injection with the patient supine. Ensure that the head is not rotated and care is taken to obtain the smallest orbit possible – a 12 cm radius orbit should be feasible on most heads, with the shoulders moved down as far as possible.

Images
1. *Dynamic*. Anterior, 60 × 1 s frames on computer. Hard copy: 2 s images from first arrival of bolus generated from computer images, or 2–6 s analogue images for 1 min post-injection.
2. *Tomographic*. The acquisition protocol will depend upon the system available. Suitable parameters for a modern single-headed gamma camera might be:
   (a) 360° circular or elliptical orbit
   (b) 60–120 projections or continuous rotation over a 20–30 min acquisition
   (c) Combination of matrix size and zoom to give a pixel size of 3–4 mm.

Analysis
1. *Dynamic*. Time–activity curves are produced from regions over the carotid arteries and cerebral hemispheres.
2. *Tomographic*. Transverse, coronal and sagittal slices parallel and orthogonal to the orbitomeatal

plane with a thickness of approximately 8 mm are reconstructed. Quantitative analysis of tomographic images is an area of increasing interest[3], but is not yet in routine use.

Aftercare Radiation dose may be reduced by administration of a mild laxative on the day after the study and maintenance of good hydration to promote urine output.

Complications None.

References
1. Kung, H.F. (1990) New technetium 99m-labeled brain perfusion imaging agents. *Semin. Nucl. Med.* **20**, 150–158.
2. Moretti, J.L., Cinotti, L., Cesaro, P. et al (1987) Amines for brain tomoscintigraphy. *Nucl. Med. Commun.* **8**, 581–595.
3. Lamoureux, G., Dupont, R.M., Ashburn, W.L. & Halpern, S.E. (1990) "CORT-EX": a program for quantitative analysis of brain SPECT data. *J. Nucl. Med.* **31**, 1862–1871.

Further reading
Costa, D.C. & Ell, P.J. (1991) *Clinician's Guide to Nuclear Medicine: Brain Blood Flow in Neurology and Psychiatry*. Edinburgh: Churchill Livingstone.

Freeman, L.M. & Blaufox, M.D. (eds) (1990) SPECT imaging of the brain: part I. *Semin. Nucl. Med.* **20**(4).

Freeman, L.M. & Blaufox, M.D. (eds) (1991) SPECT imaging of the brain: part II. *Semin. Nucl. Med.* **21**(1).

Holman, B.L. & Devous, M.D. (1992) Functional brain SPECT: the emergence of a powerful clinical method. *J. Nucl. Med.* **33**, 1888–1904.

Imaging Approach to Back Pain and Sciatica

With the ever increasing horizon and spectrum of costly complex imaging procedures, it is imperative that the radiologist plays a pivotol role in directing the investigative algorithm to assist the clinical requirement. Each diagnostic imaging procedure has different degrees of sensitivity and specificity when applied to a particular diagnostic problem. The combination of imaging techniques can be used in a complementary way to enhance diagnostic accuracy. The appropriate use of the available methods of investigating the spine is essential, requiring a sensible sequence and timing of the procedures to ensure cost-effectiveness, maximal diagnostic accuracy, and minimum discomfort to the patient.

The philosophy underlying the management of low back pain and sciatica encompasses the following fundamental points:
1. Radiological investigation is an essential prerequisite for surgery.
2. Radiological findings must be compatible with the clinical picture before surgery is entertained, offered and undertaken.
3. The main aim of both the surgeon and radiologist is to help the patient avoid surgery.
4. If that is not possible, they have one chance to get the diagnosis right and 1 month to do it in[1,2].

The need for radiological investigation of the lumbosacral spine is based on the results of a thorough clinical examination. A useful and basic preliminary step which will avoid unnecessary investigations, is to determine whether the predominant symptom is back pain or leg pain. Leg pain extending to the foot is indicative of nerve root compression and imaging needs to be directed towards excluding lesions such as a disc prolapse. This is most commonly seen at the L4/5 or L5/S1 levels (90–95%), and the non-invasive techniques, CT and MRI, should be employed as the primary modes of imaging. If the predominant symptom is back pain with or without proximal lower limb radiation, then it is more likely that invasive techniques will be required in the form of discography and facet joint arthrography. Unfortunately, the presence of degenerative disc and facet disease demonstrated by a plain film, CT and MRI, bears no direct correlation with the incidence of clinical symptomatology. The annulus fibrosus of the intervertebral disc and the facet joints are richly innervated, and only direct injection can assess them as a potential pain source.

Plain radiography

Routine plain radiographic evaluation at the initial assessment of a patient with acute low back pain, often does not provide clinically useful information. As 85% of such patients return to work within 2 months of conservative therapy, the potential for non-contributory plain film requests is high. Attempts to reduce the amount of unnecessary radiation should be directed at minimizing the number of patients and not the number of films per patient. Despite the known limitations of plain films, it is essential that a full series of routine radiographs of the lumbar spine are obtained before any other investigation is requested. Any or all of the features of degenerative disc disease can be found in both the symptomatic and asymptomatic individuals and in this respect, plain films offer very little information. The role of plain radiographs can be summarized in the following points:

1. They exclude conditions that can mimic mechanical or discogenic pain, e.g. infection, spondylolysis, ankylosing spondylitis, and bone tumours. ^{99m}Tc scintigraphy, CT and MRI are, however, more sensitive.
2. They serve as a technical aid to assess and localize the vertebral column and spinal canal prior to myelography, CT cnd MRI.
3. They disclose the presence of congenital lumbosacral anomalies, e.g. lumbarization or sacralization, to avoid mistakes in interpreting the correct level of the abnormalities before surgery.
4. The non-invasive techniques for the spine enhance the contrast of bone and soft tissues. The superior spatial and contrast resolution of CT and MRI is undoubted, but correlation with plain film appearances is essential to avoid mistakes in interpretation. Plain films should be available before

investigations are performed, and radiological appearances of the lumbar spine correlated with the CT and MRI findings at the time of reporting.

CT and MRI   The advent of CT and MRI has resulted in a marked reduction in the popularity of invasive techniques such as epidurography and lumbar epidural venography. There is no doubt that both CT, and preferably MRI if available, should replace myelography as the first mode of investigating suspected disc prolapse. Axial imaging by CT or MRI is the best determinant of neural compression. Plain CT is excellent in the delineation of disc contour, bony outlines, and root compression, while CT myelography can enhance the information of neural compression by local vertebral disease. Sagittal imaging by reconstructed CT images or MRI is useful to assess vertebral alignment, neural foraminae and disc status. These techniques visualize directly the cause of neural compression, unlike myelography in which distortions of the intrathecal contrast medium infers the presence of extradural disease. It is for this reason that CT and MRI are essential in the exclusion of the 'far-out' or lateral disc prolapses not diagnosed by myelography[3]. In the absence of any realistic alternative and in the presence of clinical conservatism, myelography is still popular. However, even in the presence of CT and MRI scanners, it still has a role to play when the non-invasive methods fail to provide the necessary information. Myelography excludes the unexpected tumour at the level of the conus medullaris when a CT from L3-S1 is normal, and it also allows a dynamic assessment of the spinal canal in instances of spinal stenosis and instability. MRI clearly has significant advantages compared to CT in the assessment of the lumbar spine. Apart from the absence of ionizing radiation, it directly images the two components of the disc and the intrinsic status of the cord, producing a myelographic effect of the cerebrospinal fluid (CSF) on the T2 sequences. However, in view of the different contrast characteristics of tissues assessed by CT and MRI, the axial CT quite often has an advantage over MR axial imaging because the contrast between bone and disc is greater, the bone detail is better, and the contributions of bone and soft tissue components in lumbar canal stenosis, better assessed.

Since the classical paper describing lumbar disc herniation by Mixter and Barr in 1934, great strides have been made in its diagnosis and management. Apart from a diagnosis of this condition, modern radiological imaging has a role defining the therapeutic options by differentiating the 'contained' disc from the 'sequestrated' disc with free migratory disc fragments. This distinction is crucial in the consideration of conservative versus surgical therapy and percutaneous from open surgical techniques.

The problems of the 'post-laminectomy' or 'failed back surgery syndrome' are well known. Accurate preoperative assessment can go a long way to prevent the causes due to 'wrong diagnosis', 'wrong operation' and 'wrong levels'. The investigation of the postoperative lumbar spine is difficult. The distinction of a residual or recurrent disc prolapse at the operated level from epidural fibrosis is fundamental in the consideration of further surgery. Intravenous enhancement by large volumes of contrast medium at CT and Gd-DTPA at MRI allows the accurate differentiation to be made.

Arachnoiditis is a cause of postoperative symptoms and its features are well known on myelography, CT myelography and, more recently, MRI. Its true incidence is probably not known, and the exact role of preoperative Myodil myelography in its causation is not yet fully defined. There is no doubt that when MRI techniques become more refined true incidence can be determined more accurately.

Conclusions   MRI has revolutionized the imaging of spinal disease. Its superior soft tissue contrast enables the distinction of the nucleus pulposus from the annulus fibrosus of the healthy disc and enables the early diagnosis of degenerative changes. Initial reports comparing MRI appearances with discography showed good correlation of morphological alteration in the nucleus pulposus. Subsequent studies have shown that MRI is at present not as accurate in the diagnosis and delineation of annular disease. Instead of a reduction in the popularity of discography, MRI has stimulated a resurgence of interest and application. Primarily this is directed to using MRI as a predictor of the causative levels contributing to the back pain. To date, no such correlation has been proven and discography still plays a significant role in investigating the patient with discogenic pain prior to surgical fusion.

The ultimate aim must be the ideal of investigating the spine non-invasively. However, it is well known that up to 35% of asymptomatic individuals before 40 years of age have significant intervertebral disc disease of at least one level on MRI images. Correlation with clinical symptomatology is essential before any relevance is attached to their presence and surgery undertaken. Invasive 'needle work' techniques still play a significant role in their assessment, and it seems unlikely that they can be completely dispensed with.

References

1. Nachemson, A.C. (1985) Advances in low back pain. *Clin. Orthopaed. Rel. Res.* **200**, 266–278.
2. Butt, W.P. (1989) Radiology for back pain. *Clin. Radiol.* **40**, 6–10.
3. Novetsky, G.L., Berlin, L., Epstein, A.J. et al (1982) The extra foraminal herniated disc: detection by computed tomography. *Am. J. Neuroradiol.* **3**, 653–655.

Further reading

Antti-Poika, I. Soini, J., Tallroth, K. Yrjonen, T. & Konttinen Y.T. (1990) Clinical relevance of discography combined with CT scanning: a study of 100 patients. *J. Bone Joint Surg.* **72B**, 480–485.

Boden, S., Davis, D.O., Dina, T.S. et al (1990) Abnormal magnetic resonance scans of the lumbar spine in asymptomatic subjects. *J. Bone Joint Surg.* **72A**, 403–408.

Braun, I.F., Hoffman, J.C. Jr, Davis, P.C. et al (1985) Contrast enhancement in CT differentiation between recurrent disc herniation and post-operative scan. *Am. J. Roentg.* **145**, 785–790.

Butler, P. (1991) Editorial. The current status of myelography *Clin. Radiol.* **44**, 1–2.

Colhoun, E., McCall, I.W., Williams, L, & Cassar-Pullicino, V.N. (1988) Provocation discography as a guide to planning operations on the spine. *J. Bone Joint Surg.* **70B**, 267–271.

Du Boulay, G.H., Hawkes, S. Lee, C.C. et al (1990) Comparing the cost of spinal MR with conventional myelography and radiculography. *Neuroradiology* **32**, 124–136.

Eisenstein, S.M., Parry, C.R. (1987) The lumber facet arthrosis syndrome. *J. Bone Joint Surg.* **69B**, 3–7.

Gibson, M., Buckley, J., Mawhinney, R., Mulholland, R.C. & Worthington, B.S. (1986) Magnetic resonance imaging and discography in the diagnosis of disc degeneration. *J. Bone Joint Surg.* **68B**, 369–373.

Heuftle, M.G., Modic, M.T., Ross, J.S. et al (1988) Lumbar spine: post-operative MR imaging with gadolinium-DTPA. *Radiology* **167**, 817–824.

Horton, W.C. & Daftari, T.K. (1992) Which disc as visualised by magnetic resonance imaging is actually a source of pain? A correlation between magnetic resonance imaging and discography. *Spine* **17(6)**, 164–171.

Johnson, C.E. & Sze, G. (1990) Benign lumbar arachnoiditis: MR imaging with gadopentate dimeglumine. *Am. J. Roentg.* **155**, 873–880.

Osti, O.L. & Fraser, R.D. (1992) MRI and discography of annular tears and intervertebral disc degeneration. *J. Bone Joint Surg.* **74B**, 431–435.

Powell, M.C., Szypryt, P. Wilson, M. et al (1986) Prevalence of lumbar disc degeneration observed by magnetic resonance in symptomless women. *Lancet* **2**, 1366–1367.

Simmons, J.W., Emery, S.F., McMillin, J.N. et al (1990) Awake discography. A comparison study with magnetic resonance imaging. *Spine* **16(6)**, 216–221.

Szypryt, E.P., Twining, P., Wilde, G.P. et al (1988) Diagnosis of lumber disc protrusion: a comparison between magnetic resonance imaging and radiculography. *J. Bone Joint Surg.* **70**, 717–722.

Walsh, T.R., Weinstein, J., Spratt, K.F. et al (1990) Lumbar discography. A controlled prospective study of normal volunteers to determine the false positive rate. *J. Bone Joint Surg.* **72A**, 1081–1088.

Zucherman, J., Derby, R., Hsu, K. et al (1988) Normal magnetic resonance imaging with abnormal discography. *Spine* **13**, 1355–1359.

Contrast Media For
Myelography/Radiculography

Historical perspective

Historically the contrast media that have been used for myelography are:

Gas (CO_2, air). An unsatisfactory contrast medium because of the poor contrast obtainable. Tomography was necessary for adequate visualization of the cord and the nerve roots were not seen.

Lipiodol. Introduced in 1921, this was too viscous and too toxic, producing arachnoiditis.

Abrodil (sodium iodomethanesulphonate). Introduced by Lidstrom and Arnell in 1931 this was the first water-soluble contrast medium to be used in the subarachnoid space but it was also very toxic. A preliminary spinal anaesthetic was necessary to relieve the pain produced by the contrast medium.

Myodil, Pantopaque (ethyl esters of ethyl iodophenylundecyclic acids) was used since 1944. Although less viscous and less toxic than Lipiodol, Myodil has now been replaced by safer water-soluble contrast media.

Conray 280 (meglumine iotholamate). Too toxic, producing arachnoiditis and leptomeningitis.

Dimer X (meglumine iocarmate). This was, basically, two iothalamate molecules linked together. Although of lower toxicity than Conray 280, it still produced leptomeningitis in a large number of patients. Severe muscle spasms resulting in fractures were well described, as was epilepsy. Its use was limited to the lumbar subarachnoid space. Both Conray 280 and Dimer X have been withdrawn from use in the subarachnoid space.

Amipaque (metrizamide). Available since 1977, this was the first non-ionic, low-osmolar water-soluble contrast medium. Although almost devoid of the risks of leptomeningitis and arachnoiditis, it does have neurotoxic effects — transient confusion, hallucinations and disturbed hearing, vision or speech. It is also expensive and, because it is packaged as a freeze-dried solute which has to be dissolved in very dilute sodium bicarbonate to the required concentration, it is time-consuming to use. A concentration of 170 mg I ml^{-1} is isotonic with CSF and a solution between 240 and 300 mg ml^{-1} is usually preferred. A total dose of 3000 mg I should not be injected intrathecally in a single examination. Although still available, it has been replaced by non-ionic monomeric water-soluble contrast media, iopamidol and iohexol, and more recently by non-ionic dimers such as iotrolan. These contrast media are both cheaper and safer than metrizamide.

Iopamidol (Niopam) became available for intrathecal use in the UK in late 1982. It was the first of the second generation of non-ionic water soluble contrast agents. Unlike metrizamide it is stable and autoclavable in solution, and is available in concentrations from 200 to 370 mg I ml^{-1}.

Iohexol (Omnipaque) was available for myelography in the UK by 1983. Like metrizamide and iopamidol it is a non-ionic amide. Electroencephalographic abnormalities have been observed in 34% of patients after myelography, but the findings are unreliable in predicting which patients may develop convulsions. The use of electroencephalographic studies and measurements of visual evoked responses as indicators of neurotoxicity have shown that, when present, a demonstrable difference always favoured iohexol as less toxic.

Iotrolan (Isovist). This water-soluble non-ionic dimer with low neurotoxicity for intrathecal use was licensed in the UK in 1990. The data from the completed UK trial are not yet published, but preliminary reports from Europe suggest a better tolerance with low chemotoxicity compared with iohexol and iopamidol, with a reduction in the incidence, severity and duration of side-effects.

Historically, all forms of myelography were performed as inpatient procedures. The inherent safety of non-ionic media has made outpatient lumbar radiculography a safe procedure, provided there is informed consent, careful patient selection, adequate advice and easy access to medical help. There is no statistically significant difference in the incidence and severity of side-effects between outpatient and inpatient controls. In a comparative study on outpatient lumbar radiculography utilizing iopamidol and iohexol, there were no statistically significant differences in the incidence and severity of post-procedure side-effects within 24 hours. A higher incidence of delayed side-effects (within 7 days; headache, nausea, dizziness) was found in the iopamidol group of outpatients. More recently, outpatient cervical myelography using iohexol administered via a lateral C1/2 puncture or the lumbar route has also been shown to be safe and cost-effective.

Lateral Cervical C1/2 Puncture

Indications
1. Examination limited to the cervical region.
2. Demonstration of the upper level of a spinal block.
3. When lumbar puncture has failed. A 'dry tap' may occur in the presence of large tumours within the canal, spinal stenosis, e.g. achondroplasia, or because of severe degenerative changes and spinal deformity which prevents the successful passage of a needle into the spinal canal.

Contraindications
1. Suspected mass lesion in the upper cervical canal including cerebellar tonsillar herniation.
2. When the whole spinal canal must be examined. Less dilution of contrast meclium occurs with 'run-up' examination via a lumbar puncture.
3. Suspected lumbar spinal dysraphism. The lumbar canal is often very large and marked dilution will occur when contrast medium is injected from above.
4. Spinal deformity which leads to loss of the C1/2 interspace, e.g. congenital fusion, rheumatoid arthritis.

Equipment
Tilting fluoroscopy table, preferably with biplane facility.

Patient preparation
Due to the epileptogenic potential of intrathecal contrast media and the possible spill into the posterior cranial fossa, phenobarbitone sodium (200 mg) or diazepam 10 mg i.m. are administered 30 min before and 4 hours after cervical myelography.

Technique
1. The patient lies prone with arms at the sides and chin resting on a soft pad so that the neck is in a neutral position or in slight extension. Hyperextension is undesirable as it promotes patient discomfort and reduces the C1/2 interlaminar distance. It can further compromise a narrow canal and produce symptomatic cord compression. The patient must be comfortable and able to breathe and swallow easily. If the examination is being undertaken to examine the thoracic region, the patient can lie supine and the table be tilted

slightly feet-down so that the contrast medium can run downwards to the lesion.

2. The area around the mastoid process is shaved and hair restrained with a cap.

3. Using lateral fluoroscopy the C1/2 space is identified. The beam should be centred at this level to minimize errors due to parallax. Head and neck adjustments may be needed to ensure a perfect lateral position. The aim is to puncture the subarachnoid space between the laminae of C1 and C2, at the junction of the middle and posterior thirds of the spinal canal, behind the spinal cord.

4. Using aseptic technique the skin is anaesthetized with 1% lignocaine. A 22G spinal needle with stilette is introduced at right-angles to the spine and parallel to the table top. Lateral fluoroscopy is used to adjust the direction of the needle, and ensure the maintenance of a perfect lateral position as the needle is advanced. A nurse placed at the head of the table to steady the patient's head is essential. AP fluoroscopy may be required to confirm that the needle tip has not traversed the mid-line.

5. The sensation of the needle penetrating the dura is similar to that experienced during a lumbar puncture and the patient not infrequently complains of some discomfort at this stage. Another sign that indicates that the needle tip is close to the dura is the observation of venous blood droplets at the needle hub as the epidural space is crossed. N.B. With the tenting effect on the dura, the needle may appear to cross the mid-line before CSF is encountered. *Unlike* in lumbar spinal punctures, the needle should *not* be advanced 1–2 mm once puncture has been successful. Severe acute neck or radicular pain indicates that the needle is incorrectly sited.

6. Following removal of the stilette, CSF should drip from the end of the needle. The needle position can be checked by screening in the AP plane.

7. Under fluoroscopy a small amount of contrast medium is injected to ensure correct needle tip placement. This will flow away from the needle tip and gravitate downwards to layer behind the vertebral bodies. A further 3 ml are injected to

ensure the absence of an obstructing lesion which would promote spill into the head.
8. The required amount of contrast medium is injected under intermittent fluoroscopy in the AP projection.

Aftercare
1. Although many centres request the patient to remain sitting or semi-recumbent for about 6 hours, the incidence of side-effects is not increased by allowing the patient to remain ambulant.
2. High fluid intake.

Further reading
Amundsen, P. & Skalpe, I.O. (1975) Cervical myelography with a water soluble contrast medium (metrizamide). A preliminary clinical report with special reference to clinical aspects. *Neuroradiology* 8, 209–212.

Lamb, J.T. (1981) Cervical myelography by lateral C1-2 puncture. In: Grainger, R.G. & Lamb, J.T. (eds) *Myelographic Techniques with Metrizamide*, pp. 59–73. Birmingham: Nyegaard (UK).

Orrison, W.W., Eldevik, O.P. & Sackett, J.F. (1983) Lateral C1-2 puncture for cervical myelography Part III — historical, anatomical and technical considerations. *Radiology* 146, 401–408.

Robertson, H.J. & Smith, R.D. (1990) Cervical myelography survey of modes of practice and major complications. *Radiology* 174, 79–83.

Teasdale, E. & MacPherson, P. (1983) Incidence of side effects following direct puncture cervical myelography. Bed rest versus normal mobility. *Neuroradiology* 25, 85–86.

Cisternal Puncture

Indications As for lateral cervical puncture

Technique 1. The area from the external occipital protuberance to the mid-cervical region is shaved.
2. The patient is placed in the lateral decubitus position with his head supported so that the cervical spine is horizontal. The neck is flexed.
3. The spinous process of C2 is palpated with a finger (this is the highest palpable spinous process) and, with aseptic technique, the skin and subcutaneous tissues 1.5 cm cephalad to it are infiltrated with local anaesthetic.
4. A 20G spinal needle with stilette is introduced into the anaesthetic puncture point and directed towards the nasion, keeping the needle in the midline. Increased resistance is felt at about 3 cm as the needle penetrates the atlanto-occipital membrane, followed by a diminution as the needle point pops into the cisterna magna. The stilette is remove and CSF should drip from the end of the needle. If no CSF appears (even with slight suction) the tip of the needle may be in the epidural space and should be advanced a further 0.5 cm.
5. If the needle strikes bone (probably the occiput), it should be partially withdrawn and reintroduced, angling it slightly more caudally.
6. Contrast medium should be injected via a short tube connection and under fluoroscopic control to ensure that the needle bevel is entirely within the cistern.

Aftercare As for lateral cervical puncture.

Complications 1. Puncture of the cord, which presents clinically as transient paraesthesiae or pain radiating down the body or a limb.
2. Subarachnoid haemorrhage due to puncture of the posterior inferior cerebellar artery or its branches.

Myelography/Radiculography with Water-soluble Contrast Media

The introduction of radio-opaque contrast medium into the spinal subarachnoid space allows the identification of the spinal cord (myelography) and its nerve roots (radiculography).

Indications　Any suspected intraspinal or nerve root abnormality.

Any region of the spine may be examined, but when the entire length of the spinal canal is to be examined dilution may occur, with subsequent impairment of image quality.

Contraindications
1. Papilloedema.
2. Cerebral aneurysms and AV malformations.
3. Recent lumbar puncture. A small amount of CSF often leaks into the subdural or extradural space after a lumbar puncture; and if a second lumbar puncture is performed within a week of the first, it is this pool of CSF that may be tapped instead of the subarachnoid space. If the need for myelography is urgent, a lateral cervical or cisternal puncture can be made.
4. Previous adverse reaction to intrathecal injection of the same contrast medium. A previous adverse reaction to i.v. contrast medium is not associated with an increased incidence of contrast medium reaction to myelography.

Contrast medium
1. Omnipaque.
2. Niopam.
3. Iotrolan.

The volume and concentration of contrast medium will depend on the site of injection, the region under examination, the clinical problem under investigation and the size of the subarachnoid space (see Table 12.1). For example, a patient with spinal stenosis would need less contrast medium than a patient of the same size with a large meningocoele.

Equipment
1. Fluoroscopy unit with spot film device.
2. Tilting table (90–90° tilt). A simpler table with less

Table 12.1 Water-soluble contrast medium dosage in myelography.

Region under examination	Lumbar puncture		Cisternal/lateral cervical puncture	
	Iodine concentration (mg ml^{-1})	Volume (ml)	Iodine concentration (mg ml^{-1})	Volume (ml)
Lumbar	200	10–15		
	240	10		
	300	≤ 10		
Thoracic	240	10–12		
	300	7–10		
Cervical	300	7–10	240 or 200	5

The maximum dose of 300 mg I should not be exceeded.

tilt is suitable for radiculography only.
3. Overcouch tube (for horizontal beam laterals).
4. Spinal needle with stylet (22G).

Patient Preparation Avoid dehydration.

Preliminary films AP and lateral projections of the regions to be studied.

It is critical that assessment of the plain radiographs is made to exclude anomalies such as sacralization/lumbarization of vertebrae, before the interpretation of any surgically correctable abnormality demonstrated on the radiculogram. This will avoid any misunderstanding and ensure that the operation takes place at the correct disc level.

Technique The site of injection of contrast medium can be:
1. Via lumbar puncture—L2/3 or L3/4. L2/3 is preferred if there is a suspected lumbar disc lesion, as most of these lesions occur below that level.
2. Via lateral C1/2 puncture.
3. Via cisternal puncture.

Lumbar puncture is the technique commonly used and will be described here. The indications for lateral cervical and cisternal puncture are given in the relevant sections.

Lumbar region

Technique
1. Lumbar puncture is easiest to perform with the patient sitting. With the patient leaning forward, legs over the far side of the table and arms crossed on a pillow across the knees, the spinous processes are separated and the spinal theca is distended because of the effect of gravity. Alternatively, the patient may be placed in the prone or lateral decubitus position. Fluoroscopy ensures correct needle placement and enables the volume of contrast medium to be adjusted to the capacity of the spinal canal under examination. In the latter two instances, the table is tilted slightly feet-down to facilitate the outflow of CSF and pooling of contrast medium in the lumbar subarachnoid space.
2. The lumbar puncture is performed with aseptic technique. The needle should be no greater than 22G, to reduce CSF leakage after it has been withdrawn. Once fluid is obtained the needle is advanced a further 2 mm to ensure that all the bevel is within the subarachnoid space. If flow ceases, rotation of the needle will probably re-establish it. A small volume of CSF is usually sent for laboratory examination but the value of this is in doubt[1]. The contrast medium is injected slowly.

FILMS
With the patient prone in the erect or semi-erect position:
1. Frontal.
2. 15–30° prone obliques. The patient is positioned with fluoroscopy to show the nerve roots as they pass beneath the pedicles.
3. Lateral in neutral to include L5/S1 junction.
4. Laterals in flexion and extension — to show the dynamics of a posterior disc protrusion, spinal instability and dynamic spinal stenosis.
5. Routine AP and lateral views of the conus medullaris and lower thoracic cord are mandatory to exclude unsuspected intraspinal tumours which can mimic a disc prolapse. These are obtained by running the contrast column up into the lower thoracic spine with the patient in the lateral decubitus position. The supine position allows optimal visualization of the conus medullaris.

ADDITIONAL FILMS
1. Shoot through lateral. If a meningocoele is present, its full extent will be demonstrated when contrast medium enters it in the supine position.
2. Lateral decubitus with 15° obliquity to show degenerate nerve roots.
3. Erect lateral.
4. Post-radiculogram CT.

Thoracic region
Technique
1. If this is the primary region of interest the injection is best made with the patient prone or lying on his side, with the head of the table lowered and the patient's head elevated to prevent contrast medium from running up into the head.
2. If an obstruction to flow is expected, about half the volume of contrast medium is injected and the needle left in position. When the obstruction has been demonstrated, the remainder of the contrast medium is injected under pressure and this may cause the contrast medium to flow around the lesion and demonstrate its superior extent[2]. If there is no obstruction, the full volume is injected and the patient placed supine.

FILMS
Table horizontal
1. AP.
2. Lateral.

As soon as these films are seen to be satisfactory the table is tilted head up to return the contrast medium to the lumbar region.

3. Post-myelogram CT.

Cervical region
Technique
1. This is best examined by lateral cervical or cisternal puncture, but good results are obtainable by screening up the contrast column introduced by lumbar puncture.
2. The lumbar puncture is made with the patient in the prone or decubitus, slightly head-up position so that the contrast medium pools in the lumbar canal. Following the injection of contrast medium, the patient is turned prone, with his neck extended and chin on a pad to prevent contrast medium

from flowing into the head. The table is tilted 40° head-down and contrast medium runs rapidly, as a bolus, into the cervical canal.
3. Once contrast medium has reached the cervical region the table is returned to the horizontal and the degree of neck extension reduced.

FILMS
1. AP.
2. Lateral.
3. Obliques.

ADDITIONAL FILMS
1. AP with craniocaudal angulation – will demonstrate the upper cervical region when the neck is extended.
2. Swimmer's view – to show the lower cervical region. This is a lateral projection with one arm beside the body and the other alongside the head.
3. Lateral with the patient supine – to demonstrate the cerebellar tonsils.
4. Post-myelogram CT.

CT myelography (CTM)

In the lumbar spine, the CTM should be delayed 2–4 hours to reduce the density by dilution of the contrast medium. Turning the patient a few times prior to CT ensures even distribution and reduces layering effects. In evaluating the spinal cord a delay is not as critical unless syringomyelia is being entertained, when a 24 hour lapse is optional to show the syrinx. The superior sensitivity of CT to contrast difference allows detection of very dilute contrast medium, e.g. beyond a spinal block. It defines the extent and avoids the need for a C1/2 puncture. The full value of CTM is observed when CT follows a conventional myelographic procedure. The practice of obtaining CTM as a separate procedure using small amounts (3–5 ml) of dilute water-soluble contrast medium (160–170 mg per 100 ml) exposes the patient to the same risks of a lumbar puncture and should not be practised as it does not obviate the future necessity of a myelogram.

Paediatric myelography

A few points need to be borne in mind when carrying out myelography in the paediatric age-group.
1. General anaesthetic is mandatory for all children

aged 6 or younger and for most children up to the age of 12.

2. Lumbar puncture in cases of spinal dysraphism carries the risk of damaging a low-lying cord due to tethering. The thecal sac is usually wide in these conditions and the needle needs to be placed laterally in the thecal sac. In addition, as low a puncture as possible will aid in minimizing the risk. Even when the spinal cord is inadvertently punctured, injury is uncommon, or masked by the neurologic deficit that is present.

3. The frequent association of cerebellar tonsillar herniation precludes lateral C1/2 puncture.

Aftercare

1. Hospitalize overnight.

2. The patient is allowed to remain ambulant if he wishes. The incidence and severity of side-effects are similar for those confined to bed and those allowed to remain ambulant[3].

3. Encourage high fluid intake.

4. Phenobarbitone sodium (see lateral cervical puncture).

Complications
Due to the anaesthetic

1. Headache (30–40%)

2. Nausea and vomiting (20–30%)

both more frequent in females and with increasing dose and extent of subarachnoid space examined.

3. Transient increase in lumbar or sciatic pain in patients with sciatica (10%). Possibly due to direct irritation of nerve roots.

4. Convulsions — rare. The incidence is reduced by limiting the flow of contrast medium intracranially and by not exceeding the maximum recommended dose. The incidence of seizures with metrizamide was increased by the concurrent administration of phenothiazines and tricyclics. Treatment is with diazepam 10 mg i.v, followed by phenobarbitone 200 mg i.m. as prophylaxis against further convulsions.

5. Transient confusion, hallucinations, disturbed hearing, vision or speech were very common after metrizamide myelography[4], but are much less frequent with the new contrast media. Treatment is supportive.

Due to puncture technique

1. Hypotension. This is a particular problem if the lumbar puncture is performed in the sitting position. The examination should be continued in the prone or decubitus position.
2. Headache, nausea and vomiting. Both technique and contrast medium make a contribution to these symptoms.
3. Subdural injection of contrast medium. This occurs when the whole of the needle bevel is not within the subarachnoid space. Contrast medium initially remains loculated near the end of the needle rather, but can track freely to simulate intrathecal flow. When in doubt, stop injecting and obtain AP and lateral views with the needle in situ. Resist the temptation of interpreting such an examination.
4. Extradural injection of contrast medium outlines the nerve roots well beyond the exit foraminae.
5. Intramedullary injection of contrast medium. This is a complication of lateral cervical puncture and is recognized as a slit-like collection of contrast medium in the spinal canal. Small collections are without clinical significance.
6. Haemorrhage. A small amount of blood in the CSF is not significant, but if there is heavy blood staining, thought to be iatrogenic, then the examination should be deferred.

During lateral cervical puncture it is possible, though uncommon, to puncture the vertebral or posterior inferior cerebellar arteries. The vertebral arteries overlie the posterior one-third of the spinal canal in less than 1% of patients[5].

References

1. Kuuliala, I.K. & Göransson, H.J. (1987) Diagnostic contribution of routine cerebrospinal fluid analysis during myelography *Clin. Radiol* **38**, 169–170.
2. Kendall, B.E. & Valentine, A.R. (1981) Myelographic study of the obstructed spinal theca with water-soluble contrast medium. *Br. J. Radiol.* **54**, 408–412.
3. Macpherson, P. & Teasdale, E. (1984) Radiculography with non-ionic contrast medium: routine bed rest is unnecessary. *Clin. Radiol.* **35**, 287–288.
4. Richert, S., Sartor, K. & Holl, B. (1979) Subclinical organic pyschosyndromes on intrathecal injection of metrizamide for lumbar myelography. *Neuroradiology* **18**, 177–184.

5. Cox, T.C.S., Stevens, J.M. & Jendall, B.E. (1981) Vascular anatomy in the suboccipital region and lateral cervical puncture. *Br. J. Radiol.* **54**, 572–575.

Further reading   Bien, S., Schumacher, M., Berger, W. & Wenzel-Hora, B.I. (1989) Iotrolan, a nonionic dimeric contrast medium in myelography. In: Taenzer, V. & Wende, S. (eds.) *Recent Developments in Nonionic Contrast Media*, pp. 58–60. Stuttgart: Georg Thieme Verlag.

Davies, A.M., Evans, N. & Chandy, J. (1989) Out-patient lumbar radiculography: comparison of iopamidol and iohexol and a literature review. *Br. J. Radiol.* **62**, 716–723.

Davies, A.M., Fitzgerald, R. & Evans, N. (1989) Out-patient lumbar radiculography with iohexol. *Clin. Radiol.* **40**, 413–415.

Dublin, A.B., McGahan, J.P. & Reid, M.H. (1983) The value of computed tomographic metrizamide myelography in the neuro-radiological evaluation of the spine. *Radiology* **146**, 79–86.

Grainger, R.G. (1977) Technique of lumbar myelography with metrizamide. *Acta. Radiol.* **355**, 31–37.

Grainger, R.G., Kendall, B.E. & Wylie, I.G. (1976) Lumbar myelography with metrizamide – a new non-ionic contrast medium. *Br. J. Radiol.* **49**, 996–1003.

Kendall, B. & Stevens, J. (1984) Cervical myelography with iohexol. *Br. J. Radiol.* **57**, 785–787.

Kendall, B., Schneidau, A., Stevens, J. & Harrison, M. (1983) Clinical trial of iohexol for lumbar myelography. *Br. J. Radiol.* **56**, 539–542.

Ringel, K., Klotz, E., Wenzel-Hora, B.I. (1989) Iotrolan versus Iopamidol: a controlled, multicenter, double-blind study of lumbar and direct cervical myelography. In: Taenzer, V. & Wende, S. (eds) *Recent Developments in Nonionic Contrast Media*. pp. 153–157. Stuttgart: Georg Thieme Verlag.

Rolfe, E.B. & Maguire, P.D. (1980) The incidence of headache following various techniques of metrizamide myelography. *Br. J. Radiol.* **53**, 840–844.

Teasdale, E. & Macpherson, P. (1984) Guidelines for cervical myelography: lumbar versus cervical puncture technique. *Br. J. Radiol.* **57**, 789–793.

Wang, H., Kumar, A.J., Zinreich, S.J. et al (1991) Iohexol cervical myelography in adult out-patients. *Spine* **16**(12), 1356–1358.

Arachnoiditis and Myelographic Contrast Media

Chronic adhesive spinal arachnoiditis is a chronic, progressive, inflammatory response of the pia-arachnoid membrane, considered to be a significant cause of the 'failed back surgery' syndrome. Fibroblastic proliferation results in collagen deposition between the nerve roots and the pia-arachnoid, promoting adhesions between nerve roots within the subarachnoid space. The combination of marked pia-arachnoid proliferation with the dense collagen deposition leads to complete encapsulation of the nerve roots which become ischaemic, compressed, and atrophic. These secondary changes in neural structures are probably responsible for the neurological disability. Although arachnoiditis is well defined, with characteristic radiological appearances, there is no clear consensus on the clinical features of arachnoiditis.

Numerous aetiological factors have been implicated including myelography, spinal stenosis, disc herniation, intraspinal tumours and spinal surgery. The most frequently reported irritants associated with arachnoiditis were mainly the slowly absorbable oily contrast media, iophendylates (Myodil) and ionic substances such as meglumine iothalamate (Conray 280) and meglumine iocarminate (Dimer X). The combination of intrathecal corticosteroid with Dimer X produced a florid arachnoiditis. Furthermore, the combination of oily contrast medium with blood in the subarachnoid space potentiates the inflammatory reaction, as does laminectomy following myelography. Arachnoiditis does not occur with non-ionic contrast media now used for myelography at the doses recommended in clinical practice.

Recent medicolegal interest has focused on the extent to which Myodil used in lumbar myelography could be responsible for chronic arachnoiditis. A wide range of incidence is found in the reported literature, but the true incidence of *symptomatic* lumbar arachnoiditis due *solely* to the presence of intrathecal

Myodil is unknown. Indeed a retrospective study of 98 patients in whom Myodil was introduced remote from the lumbar spine (by ventriculography and cisternography) revealed no cases of symptomatic chronic lumbar arachnoiditis[1]. This study was based on clinical findings only, without inclusion of any radiological investigations. What seems more likely is that the inadvertent trauma on the micro-vasculature of the arachnoid during surgery is an important potentiating factor[2]. There is every likelihood that preoperatively the spinal conditions of spinal stenosis and disc herniation by virtue of the compressive effect on the theca cause arachnoiditis by a similar mechanism. In re-operations on the lumbar spine concomitant epidural fibrosis was seen around the sac associated with a thickened dura. These findings were most marked at the previously operated site and the proliferative dural changes were marked on the side of the discectomy extending above and below the operated interspace[3]. In one study of 54 patients with chronic arachnoiditis, 43 (80%) gave a history of myelography and spinal surgery, 6 (11%) myelography but no surgery, 3 (6%) surgery without myelography, and 2 (4%) neither[4].

In 1991 this problem prompted the British Society of Neuroradiology and the Council of the Royal College of Radiologists[5] to make a combined statement on Myodil. In summary, the guidelines are as follows:
1. Myodil was the correct contrast medium of choice for radiculography and full myelography between 1944 and 1972. Due to the known inadequacies of clinical examination in precise localization of a lesion, myelography was necessary.
2. Myodil was still the medium of choice for run-up myelography, and still acceptable for radiculography during the Conray/Dimer X era.
3. Metrizamide became widely accepted as a myelographic contrast medium in the early 1980s. Its introduction did not automatically signal the redundancy of Myodil. Despite its advantages, a decision still had to be made balancing the quality of the images against the potential severity of the immediate complications. Myodil was largely abandoned, not because of considerations of tox-

icity (metrizamide was more toxic), but because of better images with metrizamide.

4. It was a common and acceptable practice in the UK not to aspirate the small amounts of injected Myodil. Aspiration failed to prevent the development of arachnoiditis and, if it necessitated a second lumbar puncture, increased the risks of arachnoiditis.

5. 'Informed consent' did not apply in the Myodil era and more so when reports indicated only a 1% incidence of post-Myodil arachnoiditis.

Although myelography is the major modality for the diagnosis of arachnoiditis, MRI will probably become the primary imaging modality for the diagnosis, and in assessing the response of inhibitors of fibroblastic activity and collagen synthesis. It is only by applying this non-invasive technique to asymptomatic and symptomatic patients who have had Myodil myelography will the true incidence be established. At present it has a reported range of 1–70%.

References

1. Hughes, D.G. & Isherwood, I. (1992) How frequent is chronic lumbar arachnoiditis following intrathecal myodil? *Br. J. Radiol.* **65**, 758–760.

2. Quencer, R.M., Tenner, M. & Rothman, L. (1977) The post-operative myelogram: radiographic evaluation of arachnoiditis and dural/arachnoid tears. *Radiology* **123**, 667–679.

3. Jorgensen, J., Hansen, P.H., Steenskov, V. & Ovensen, N. (1975) A clinical and radiology study of chronic lower spinal arachnoiditis. *Neuroradiology* **9**, 139–144.

4. Mooij, J.J.A. (1980) Spinal arachnoiditis: disease or coincidence? *Acta Neurochirug.* **53**, 151–160.

5. The Royal College of Radiologists. 'Statement on Myodil'. December 1991.

Further reading

Grahame, P., Clark, B., Watson, M., Polkey, C. (1991) Toward a rational therapeutic strategy for arachnoiditis: a possible role for D-penicillamine. *Spine* **16(2)**, 172–176.

Kendall, B.E., Stevens, J.M. & Thomas, D. (1991) Arachnoiditis. *Curr. Imaging* **3(2)**, 113–118.

Rowland Hill, C.A., Hunter, J.V., Moseley, I.F. & Kendall, B.E. (1992) Does Myodil introduced for ventriculography lead to symptomatic lumbar arachnoiditis? *Br. J. Radiol.* **65**, 1105–1107.

Lumbar Discography

Aims
1. To outline the intranuclear disc morphology by contrast medium as well as to show the presence and direction of annular damage.
2. To provoke and reproduce the patient's symptomatology due to disc disease and to assess its response to anaesthetic injection.

Indications
1. Symptomatic disc degeneration without radicular signs.
2. Traumatic annular tears and ruptures.
3. Suspected disc prolapse in a negative or equivocal radiculogram, especially at the L5/S1 disc level.
4. Post-discectomy syndromes.
5. Acute traumatic intraosseous disc herniation.
6. Confirmation of a normal disc above or below a proposed surgical fusion.
7. Assessment of disc(s) above or below a mechanically altered segment, e.g. spondylolisthesis, transitional vertebrae, post-surgical fusion, etc.
8. Biopsy.

Contraindications
1. None absolute.
2. Any local or distant sepsis will add to the risk of infective discitis.

Contrast medium
Non-ionic contrast media (Iopamidol, Iohexol) abolish the risks associated with intrathecal injection or communication from a disc prolapse. N.B. Sodium salts are directly irritant and produce different pain sensations, confusing the interpretation and significance of the provoked pain complex. A normal disc will usually allow up to 1.0 ml to be injected. More contrast medium may be injected without overt disc damage.

Equipment
1. Fluoroscopy unit with spot film facility.

An overcouch tube besides providing a better image and radiographic result is also more practical giving more room for the operator and diminishes the risk of de-sterilization. The significant increased radiation dose must borne in mind.

2. A second image intensifier with its own TV monitor for accurate biplane needle positioning. A portable C-arm is sufficient.
3. Discography needles — a set of two needles are used for each level:
   (a) outer needle, 21G, 12.5 cm
   (b) inner needle, 26G, 15.8 cm.

Patient preparation

No specific instructions are necessary. The procedure is done under local anaesthesia. Any premedication and analgesia may alter the patient's subjective response to discography, diminishing its efficacy and usefulness. Diazepam may, however, occasionally be required in particularly anxious patients. Broad spectrum antibiotic cover (e.g. cephalosporins) are given immediately before the examination to minimize the risk of infection.

Preliminary films

1. AP.
2. Lateral.

Technique

1. There are two possible needle approaches:
   (a) The posterior approach, which is also transdural — this transgresses the spinal canal, and is sometimes used at the L5/S1 level when the lateral approach is technically difficult, owing to high iliac crests, bony interalar fusions, etc.
   (b) The lateral extradural approach, which avoids puncture of the dura and the susceptible part of the posterior annulus — this is the preferred approach and can be carried out with the patient in the prone or left lateral decubitus position.
2. The number and sequence of disc examinations is decided prior to commencement, based on clinical requirements.
3. The procedure and its aim are explained to the patient. It is important that the patient be asked to describe what pain he experiences and that he should *not* be told that he may get his symptomatic pain. This reduces the chance of a programmed response.
4. Patient positioning — the left lateral decubitus position is preferred, with the patient's head

rested on a pillow and a pad placed in the lumbar angle to maintain a straight spine. Spinal flexion is useful, especially in the L5/S1 examination.

5. Using a full aseptic technique, the level of commencement is determined utilizing fluoroscopy, and the skin is anaesthetized, usually a hand's breadth from the spinous processes.

6. The outer 21G needle is then directed towards the posterior aspect of the disc under intermittent fluoroscopic control, at an angle of 45–60° to the vertical. An additional caudal tilt may be necessary for the L5/S1 level.

7. This needle should reach but not traverse the annulus fibrosus. This point is recognized by a distinct feeling of resistance when the outer fibres are encountered. The 26G needle is then introduced through the 21G needle and its tip in the nucleus pulposus confirmed in two planes with the aid of the image intensifiers prior to contrast medium injection.

8. Contrast medium is injected steadily using a 1 ml syringe. This is done under intermittent fluoroscopic control, while the pain response, the disc volume and its radiographic morphology are assessed. The resistance to flow will gradually increase in a normal disc during the 0.5–1.0 ml stage, and a back-flow may occur.

9. The normal discographic patterns are:
   (a) a unilocular or 'cottonball' appearance
   (b) a bilocular or 'hamburger in a bun' appearance.

   Abnormal patterns include:
   (a) internal annular disruption with concentric rings of contrast
   (b) posterior or anterior annular tears
   (c) degeneration — contrast medium extends throughout the disc in both AP and lateral directions.

10. Patient interrogation — normal discs are asymptomatic. Some abnormal discs are asymptomatic. In the symptomatic abnormal discs, the exact pattern, distribution, and similarity to the usual symptomatology are assessed and recorded. At each symptomatic level a variable

amount of 0.5% Marcaine (bupivacaine hydrochloride) is injected and its efficacy at producing relief recorded prior to withdrawing the needles. (If contrast medium leaks into the epidural space, Marcaine injected may anaesthetize other levels and lead to inaccuracies in pain reproduction.)

11. The outer and inner needles are simultaneously withdrawn and the next level is examined, repeating the above steps.

Films
1. Spot lateral films are taken of each discogram, with the needle in situ.
2. When all the levels are examined, AP and lateral flexion/extension views are carried out. Standing films are also useful in a number of instances.
3. CT can be useful to define the disc abnormalities conclusively.

Aftercare
Analgesics may be required.

The examination is performed on an inpatient basis for the patient's comfort. An overnight stay after the examination depends on the level of low back discomfort.

Technical problems and complications
Apart from local backache, the after-effects are minimal.

Annular injection due to faulty needle placement jeopardizes the examination.

Recognized potential but rare sequelae include:
1. Discitis. Pain with or without pyrexia heralds this problem in a few days. Narrowing of the disc space with a variable degree of end-plate sclerosis is seen after a few weeks. All cases are probably due to low-grade infection.
2. A needle inserted too deep or anterior could penetrate a major vessel, causing a retroperitoneal haemorrhage. (Furthermore, if the bowel is penetrated and the needle withdrawn and then introduced into the disc centre, inoculation with infective organisms will produce an infective discitis).
3. A needle placed too superficial or posterior may transgress the dural sac, entering the subarachnoid

space. In this context, the complications seen following a posterior transdural approach can be expected, especially headache.

Further reading   Calhoun, W., McCall, I.W., Williams, W. & Cassar-Pullicino, V.N. (1988) Provocation discography as a guide to planning operations on the spine. *J. Bone Joint Surg.* (Br) **70B**, 267–71.

Henson, J., McCall, I.W. & O'Brien, J.P. (1993) Disc damage above a spondylolisthesis. *Br. J. Radiol.* (in press).

McCall, I.W., Park, W.M., O'Brien, J.P. & Seal, P.V. (1985) Acute traumatic intra-osseous disc herniation. *Spine* **10(2)**, 134–137.

McCulloch, J.A. & Waddell, G. (1978) Lateral lumbar discography. *Br. J. Radiol.* **51**, 498–502.

Intradiscal Therapy

For the herniated nucleus pulposus in the lumbar spine.

In 1934 Mixter and Barr[1] first showed that herniation of the lumbar disc is a cause of low back pain and sciatic pain. Since then disc surgery has evolved with recent employment of microsurgical techniques to minimize the trauma and invasiveness. Percutaneously guided intradiscal techniques have also been employed as an alternative to open surgery in patients in whom conservative treatment has failed.

Patient selection for intradiscal therapy

To produce success rates in the order of 70–80%, criteria for patient selection are essential:
1. MRI or CT scan documentation of a contained, non-sequestrated disc herniation.
2. Radicular pain is predominant symptom.
3. Failed conservative treatment – 3 months.
4. Retention of good disc height, no evidence of subarticular or foraminal stenosis.
5. No previous surgery at disc level.
6. Informed consent.

Intradiscal steroids

On the assumption that a chemical inflammatory response forms the basis of pain generated in the degenerate intervertebral disc, intradiscal steroids should alter inflammation of nuclear aetiology. However, the results vary from favourable to insignificant, and are never dramatic. Intradiscal administration can be used at the same time as discography.

Chemonucleolysis

Chymopapain, a proteolytic enzyme derived from papaya latex, catalyses rapid hydrolysis of the non-collagenous polypeptides that maintain the structure in the chondromuco protein of the nucleus pulposus. This destroys the water-binding capacity of the nucleus pulposus and therefore reduces the pressures that it can exert. The technique of utilizing this enzyme property in the treatment of patients with herniation of the intervertebral disc is called chemonucleolysis.

Technically the procedure of correct needle placement in the centre of the nucleus pulposus is carried out as outlined above. However, the patient is sedated by an anaesthetist and full premedication is administered. A general anaesthetic is contraindicated. Severe anaphylactic reactions have occurred, with an incidence of between 0.1% and 0.5%, usually occurring within 5 min of the injection. The drug is extremely toxic when injected intrathecally. The transdural approach is absolutely contraindicated. Discography done immediately before the chymopapain injection confirms proper placement of the needle tip in the nucleus pulposus and has the advantage of demonstrating any communication with the subarachnoid space or intervertebral venous channels, which would clearly contraindicate the chymopapain injection. Unfortunately, despite its value, it is important to remember that in nearly all of the cases of serious neurological adverse complications, discography was performed as part of the chymopapain procedure. If discography is employed, only a small amount of contrast medium is used to minimize both the risk of enzyme leakage due to elevation of intradisc pressure and the alleged inhibitory action on the chymopapain. Each disc should be treated with a single injection and, at the present time, the enzyme should not be used in a patient who has had previous chemonucleolysis.

The pressure/volume relationship in the closed hydraulic space of the intervertebral disc lends itself to therapeutic manipulation in that a small change in disc volume results in a large change of intradiscal pressure. Percutaneous nucleotomy and percutaneous laser disc decompression as treatment for the non-sequestered disc herniation are designed to reduce the intradiscal pressure which, in the presence of an intact annulus, relieves nerve root compression.

Percutaneous discectomy

This was introduced by Hijikata et al[2] in 1975. The 'nucleotome' introduced by Onik et al[3] in 1985 consists of a trochar with a side-window, a cutting device and suction capability. The trochar is introduced percutaneously under fluoroscopic guidance into the centre of the disc, suction is applied, and the nuclear material which sequentially protrudes into the window is sliced and aspirated. The procedure is performed utilizing local anaesthetic and can be done on an outpatient basis.

Percutaneous laser disc decompression

Introduced in 1986, this new advance in the treatment of the herniated disc uses lasers to vaporize a small portion of nucleus pulposus thereby decompressing the disc. Studies to ascertain the optimal laser wavelength for disc vaporization are being undertaken. Although incomplete, they suggest that the Holmium–YAG lasers should prove most suitable.

References

1. Mixter, W.J. & Barr, J.S. (1934) Rupture of the intervertebral disc with involvement of the spinal canal. *N. Eng. J. Med.* **211**, 210.
2. Hijikata, S., Yamiagishi, M., Nakayama, T. et al (1975) Percutaneous discectomy: a new treatment method for lumbar disc herniation. *Todem Hosp.* **5**, 5–13.
3. Onik, G., Helms, C.A., Cinsberg, L. et al (1985) Percutaneous lateral discectomy using a new aspiration mode: procine and cadaver model. *Radiology* **155**, 251–252.

Further reading

Choy, D.S.J., Ascher, P.W., Saddekni, S. et al (1992) Percutaneous laser disc decompression: a new therapeutic modality. *Spine* **17(8)**, 949–956.

Ebata, M. & Takahashi, Y. (1966) Proteolytic specificity of Chymopapain: hydrolysis of the fraction B of oxidized insulin. *Biochim. Biophys. Acta* **118**, 201–203.

Hendry, N.G. (1958) The hydration of the nucleus pulposus and its relation to intervertebral disc derangement. *J. Bone Joint Surg.* **40B**, 132–144.

Onik, G., Maroon, J., Helms, C. et al (1987) Automated percutaneous discectomy: Initial patient experience. *Radiology* **162**, 129–132.

Simmons, J.W., McMillin, J.N., Emery, S.F., Kimmich, J.J. (1992) Intra-discal steroids: a prospective double blind clinical trial. *Spine* **17(6S)**, 172–175.

Stern, J.J. (1969) Biochemistry of Chymopapain. *Clin. Orthop. Rel. Res.* **67**, 42–46.

Facet Joint Arthrography

This is performed for diagnostic and therapeutic purposes, primarily at the lumbar level. Intraarticular injection is the only means available to assess the facet joints as a source of back pain.

Indications
1. 'Facet' syndrome: due to degenerative disease. The facet joint capsule is richly innervated by the dorsal ramus of the lumbar spinal nerves which supplies at least two facet joints.
2. Nerve root compression by synovial cyst.
3. Spondylolysis.
4. Inflammatory spondyloarthropathy.

Equipment
1. Standard table with single plane fluoroscopy ideally with rotating table top.
2. 22G spinal needle.

Contrast medium
Non-ionic contrast medium 0.1–0.2 ml.

Technique
1. Outpatient procedure which involves the simultaneous injection of both joints at each level for diagnostic purposes, done on consecutive days from L3–S1 levels.
2. The joint space is profiled by slowly rotating the patient from a prone position into a prone oblique orientation with the relevant side raised. The degree of rotation varies from level to level, and it is not uncommon to find asymmetric facet joint orientation at the same level.
3. Sterile technique.
4. The spinal needle is inserted and advanced perpendicularly to the facet joint, under fluoroscopic control. Caudal needle angulation is sometimes needed if the iliac crest overlies the L5/S1 facet joints.
5. In the majority of cases a noticeable 'give' indicates that the capsule is penetrated. The needle tip almost immediately abuts onto the facet joint cartilage because of the curved nature of the joint.
6. Contrast medium injection confirms correct needle placement by demonstrating immediate opacification of a superior and inferior recess.

7. Plain spot films are taken to document intra-articular location. The arthrographic appearances are rarely of any diagnostic consequence. In cases of spondylolysis, injection of one facet joint above the defect in the pars inter-articularis may demonstrate it, and in turn outline the facet joint below it.

8. For diagnostic purposes up to 1 ml of 0.5% bupivacaine hyrochloride (Marcaine) is injected in the facet joint and the response over the ensuing 24 hour period documented. When a therapeutic injection is indicated, 0.5 ml of 0.5% Marcaine with 0.5 ml of long-acting corticosteroid containing 20 mg of methylprednisolone (Depo-Medrone) is injected after arthrography.

9. During the injection of contrast material, local anaesthetic and corticosteroid, any pain reproduction is documented. More often than not this is unreliable in predicting therapeutic response, probably due to the multilevel innervation of each facet joint.

Further reading

Fairbank, J.C.T., Park, W.M., McCall, I.W. & O'Brien, J.P. (1981) Apophyseal injection of local anaesthetic as a diagnostic aid in primary low back syndromes. *Spine* 6, 598–605.

Maldague, B., Mathurin, P. & Malghem, J. (1981) Facet joint arthrography in lumbar spondylolysis. *Radiology* 140, 29–36.

McCall, I.W., Park, W.M. & O'Brien, J.P. (1979) Induced pain referral from posterior lumbar elements in normal subjects. *Spine* 4, 441–446.

Mooney, V. & Robertson, J. (1976) The facet syndrome. *Clin. Orthopaed.* 115, 149–156.

Percutaneous Vertebral Biopsy

The percutaneous approach to obtaining a representative sample of tissue for diagnosis prior to therapy is both easy and safe, avoiding the morbidity associated with open surgery. It enjoys a success rate of close to 90%. Accurate lesion localization prior to and during the procedure is of paramount importance and a CT scan is obtained routinely.

Indications

In the presence of a proven vertebral abnormality where knowledge of the nature of the lesion is necessary to effect appropriate therapy.

Commonest pathologies encountered are infection and neoplasia.

Contraindications

Absolute

1. Abnormal and uncorrected bleeding or clotting time are absolute contraindications, including a low platelet count of < 50 000.

Relative

2. Lesions suspected of being highly vascular, e.g. aneurysmal bone cyst, renal metastasis. It is always wise to perform an ultrasound examination of the kidneys before a biopsy of a destructive bone lesion. Use a fine-needle aspiration instead of a trephine needle for these cases.
3. A more accessible lesion in the appendicular skeleton. It is always wise to obtain a radionuclide bone scan to demonstrate such a lesion.

Equipment

1. A vertebral lesion seen on plain radiographs is best biopsied under fluoroscopic control. Bi-plane screening is essential with spot film facility.
2. Small lesions, especially those located in the posterior neural arch, are best done under CT control.
3. *Biopsy needle*: Numerous types are available. The commonest types used are the Jamshidi and Ackerman sets. A trephine needle with an internal diameter of 2 mm or more is ideal, minimizing histological distortion and reducing sampling error without increasing the complication rate.

Advantages of Jamshidi needle:
(a) non-serrated cutting edge avoids tearing of surrounding soft tissues
(b) tapered tip reduces crushing of the specimen
(c) practical handle.

Disadvantages:
(a) lacks a protective cannula
(b) lacks a central guide wire.

The Ackerman needle is 12G and provides specimens 1.6 mm calibre.

4. Sterile equipment and trolley.

Medication　Sedation, analgesia and, where necessary, general anaesthesia are required, preferably administered and monitored by an anaesthetist.

Technique
1. The patient is placed in the lateral decubitus position and restrained by Velcro bands. The approach is governed by the location of the lesion and risks to major structures.
2. Preliminary fluoroscopy checks the correct level and ensures a true lateral position.
3. Skin entry point from the mid-line varies, and is about 8 cm for the lumbar region and 5 cm in the thoracic region.
4. The aim of the procedure is to enter the vertebral body in the posterior third of its lateral dimension. When done under local anaesthesia, the preliminary positioning of a 21G spinal needle allows infiltration of the soft tissues and periosteum.
5. The needle is advanced at between 30 and 45° to the sagittal plane in the thoracic and lumbar spine, respectively.
6. When the biopsy needle impinges correctly on the cortex of the vertebral body its position is confirmed in both AP and lateral planes. The trocar is then pushed through the cortex and withdrawn.
7. Using alternate clockwise and anticlockwise rotation the cannula is advanced under fluoroscopic control for about 1 cm.
8. By twisting the needle firmly several times in the same direction the specimen is severed.

9. At least two cores of bone are obtained by withdrawing the needle back to the cortex, angulating and re-entering the vertebral body.
10. The needle is then withdrawn while simultaneous suction is applied by a syringe attached to the hub.
11. The trocar is re-inserted through the cutting end and specimens pushed out onto a gauze swob. Always include blood clot as part of the specimen.

In suspected infection

1. The end-plate and not the disc is biopsied. Most of these cases are due to an osteomyelitis involving the disc space.
2. Every attempt should be made to aspirate a paravertebral abscess demonstrated before the procedure.
3. Appropriate specimen bottles for aerobic, anaerobic and tuberculous cultures are included.

Aftercare

1. Overnight stay with routine nursing observation.
2. Chest X-ray is obtained routinely immediately after the procedure and before discharge following thoracic vertebral biopsy.
3. Analgesia if needed.

Complications

(Rare — 0.2%)
1. Bleeding — usually transient and stops spontaneously.
2. Haematoma — treated conservatively.
3. Nerve root damage
   (a) more likely to happen if procedure is done under general anaesthesia
   (b) usually transient.
4. Cord injuries — transient or permanent.
5. Pneumothorax — most do well with conservative management.
6. Tumour spread along needle — only 3 cases reported.

Further reading

Shaltot, A., Michell, P.A., Betts, J.A., Darby, A.J. & Gishen, P. (1982) Jamshidi Needle biopsy of bone lesions. *Clin. Radiol.* **33**, 193–196.
Stoker, D.J. & Kissin, C.M. (1985) Percutaneous vertebral biopsy: a review of 135 cases. *Clin. Radiol.* **36**, 569–577.

13 Lacrimal System

Dacryocystography

Indications   Epiphora — to demonstrate the site and degree of obstruction.

Contraindications   None.

Contrast medium   Lipiodol. 0.5–2.0 ml per side.

Equipment
1. Skull unit (using macroradiography technique).
2. Silver dilator and cannula, or 18G blunt needle with polythene catheter (the catheter technique has the advantage that the examination can be performed on both sides simultaneously, and films can be taken during the injection).

Patient preparation   None.

Preliminary films   Skull:
1. Occipitomental.
2. Lateral (centred to the inferior orbital margin).

Technique
1. The lacrimal sac is massaged to express its contents prior to injection of the contrast medium. The lower eyelid is everted to locate the lower cannaliculus at the medial end of the lid. The lower cannaliculus is dilated and the cannula or catheter is inserted. The lower lid should be drawn laterally during insertion to straighten the bend in the cannaliculus, and so avoid perforation by the cannula.
2. The contrast medium is injected, and radiographs are taken immediately afterwards (or during the injection if a catheter is used).

Films   The preliminary views are repeated.

Aftercare   None.

Complications   Perforation of the cannaliculus.

Further reading   Campbell, W. (1964) Radiology of the lacrimal system. *Br. J. Radiol.* **37**, 1–26.
Bunce, A.H. (1972) Macrodacryocystography. *Radiography* **38**, 335–338.

14 Salivary Glands

Methods of imaging the salivary glands

1. Plain films.
2. Sialography.
3. CT ± enhancement by sialographic or i.v. contrast medium.
4. Ultrasound.
5. MRI.
6. Radionuclide imaging (sialoscintigraphy)
   - ^{99cm}Tc-pertechnetate (40 MBq max.) i.v. followed by dynamic imaging during uptake and oral stimulation of saliva secretion
   - incidental visualization also occurs with:
     - ^{123}I- or ^{131}I-iodide
     - ^{123}I- or ^{131}I-MIBG
     - ^{67}Ga-citrate, especially in radiation sialitis and sarcoidosis
   - unstable or poor ^{99m}Tc radiopharmaceutical preparations resulting in significant amounts of free pertechnetate.

Further reading

Bryan, R.N., Miller, R.H., Ferreyro, R.I. & Sessions, R.B. (1982) Computed tomography of the major salivary glands. *Am. J. Roentg.* **139**, 547–554.

Kassel, E.E. (1982) CT sialography, Part I: Introduction, technique, anatomy and variants. Part II: Parotid masses. *J. Otolaryngol.* **11** (12), 1–24.

Neiman, H.L. Philips, J.F., Darrell A.J. & Brown, T.L. (1976) Ultrasound of the parotid gland *J. Clin. Ultrasound* 1976 **4**, 11–13.

Pilbrow, W.J., Brownless, S.M., Cawood, J.I., Dynes, A., Hughes, J.D. & Stockdale, H.R. (1990) Salivary gland scintigraphy — a suitable substitute for sialography? *Br. J. Radiol.* **63**, 190–196.

Rabinov, K., Kell, T. & Gordon, P.H. (1984) CT of the salivary glands. *Radiol. Clin. N. Am.* **22**, 145–159.

Stone, D.N., Mancuso, A.A., Rice, D. & Hanafee, W.N. (1981) Parotid CT sialography. *Radiology* **138**, 393–397.

Whyte, A.M. & Byrne, J.V. (1987) A comparison of computed tomography and ultrasound in the assessment of parotid masses. *Clin. Radiol.* **38**, 339–343.

Wittich, G.R., Scheible, W.F. & Hajek, P.C. (1985) Ultrasonography of the salivary glands. *Radiol. Clin. N. Am.* **23**, 29-37.

Yasumoto, M., Shibuyu, H. Suzuki, S. et al (1992) Computed tomography and ultrasonography in submandibular tumours. *Clin. Radiol.* **46**, 114-120.

Sialography

Indications
1. Pain
2. Swelling

Contraindications
Acute infection or inflammation.

Contrast medium
1. HOCM or LOCM 240–300.
2. Lipiodol Ultra Fluid.

Neither contrast medium has a clear advantage over the other.

Equipment
1. Skull unit (using macroradiography technique).
2. Silver lachrymal dilator.
3. Silver cannula or 18G blunt needle and polythene catheter.

Patient preparation
Any radio-opaque artefacts are removed (e.g false teeth).

Preliminary films
Parotid gland
1. AP with the head rotated 5% away from the side under investigation. Centre to the mid-line of the lower lip.
2. Lateral, centred to the angle of the mandible.
3. Lateral oblique, centred to the angle of the mandible, and with the tube angled 20% cephalad.

Submandibular gland
1. Inferosuperior using an occlusal film. This is a useful view to show calculi.
2. Lateral, with the floor of the mouth depressed by a wooden spatula.
3. Lateral oblique, centred 1 cm anterior to the angle of the mandible, and with the tube angled 20% cephalad.

Technique
1. The orifice of the parotid duct is adjacent to the crown of the second upper molar, and that of the submandibular duct is at the base of the frenulum of the tongue. If they are not visible, a sialogogue (e.g. citric acid) is placed in the mouth to promote secretion from the gland, and so render the orifice visible.

2. The orifice of the duct is dilated with the silver wire probe and the cannula or polythene catheter is introduced into the duct. The catheter can be held in place by the patient gently biting on it.
3. Up to 2 ml of contrast medium is injected. The injection is terminated immediately any pain is experienced. The duct must not be overfilled.
4. If the cannula method is used, films are taken immediately after the injection. The catheter method has the advantage that films can be taken during the injection, with the catheter in situ, and that both sides can be examined simultaneously.

Films
1. *Immediate* – the same views as for the preliminary films are repeated. The occlusal film for the submandibular gland may be omitted, as this is only to demonstrate calculi.
2. *Post-secretory* – the same views are repeated 5 min after the administration of a sialogogue. The purpose of this is to demonstrate sialectasis.

Aftercare   None.

Complications
1. Pain.
2. Damage to the duct orifice.
3. Rupture of the ducts.
4. Infection.

Further reading

Adnam, E.J., Wilson, S.A., Corcoran, M.O. & Hobsley, M. (1983) The value of parotid sialography. *Br. J. Surg.* **70**, 108–110.

Bladey, J.V. & Hocker, A.F. (1983) Sialography, its technique and application in the roentgen study of neoplasms of the parotid gland. *Surg. Gynecol. Obstet.* **67**, 777–787.

Nicholson, D.A. (1990) Contrast media in sialography: a comparison of lipiodol, ultra fluid and urografin 290. *Clin. Radiol.* **42**, 423–426.

Stacey-Clear, A., Evans, R., Kissin, M.W., Kark, A.E. & Wilkins, R. (1985) Sialography does not alter the management of parotid space-occupying lesions. *Clin. Radiol.* **36**, 389–390.

Verhoeven, J.W. (1984) Choice of contrast medium in sialography. *Oral Surg.* **57**, 323–336.

15 Thyroid and Parathyroids

Methods of imaging the thyroid gland
1. Plain film.
2. Ultrasonography.
3. Radionuclide imaging.
4. CT.
5. MRI.

Ultrasound of the Thyroid

Indications
1. Palpable thyroid mass.
2. Suspected thyroid tumour.
3. 'Cold spot' on radionuclide imaging.
4. Suspected retrosternal extension of thyroid.
5. Guided aspiration or biopsy.

Contraindications None.

Patient preparation None.

Equipment 5–10 MHz transducer. Linear array for optimum imaging.

Technique Patient supine with the neck extended. Longitudinal and transverse scans of both lobes of the thyroid. The isthmus is imaged in a transverse scan as it crosses anterior to the trachea. If there is retrosternal extension, angling downwards and scanning during swallowing may enable the lowest extent of the thyroid to be visualized.

Further reading Solbiati, L., Cioffi, V. & Ballarati, E. (1992) Ultrasonography of the neck. *Radiol. Clin. N. Am.* **30**, 941–954.

Radionuclide Thyroid Imaging

Indications
1. Investigation of thyroid nodules.
2. Investigation of the origin of thyrotoxicosis.
3. Diagnosis and post-intervention assessment of thyroid cancer.
4. Suspected ectopic thyroid.
5. Assessment of goitre.

Contraindications   None.

Radiopharmaceuticals
1. ^{99m}Tc-*pertechnetate*. 60 MBq typical, 80 MBq max.
   Pertechnetate ions are trapped in the thyroid by an active transport mechanism, but are not organified. Cheap and readily available. Inferior to ^{123}I, but is considered an acceptable alternative.
2. ^{123}I-*sodium iodide*. 20 MBq max.
   Iodide ions are trapped by the thyroid in the same way as pertechnetate, but are also organified, allowing overall assessment of thyroid function. The agent of choice, but ^{123}I is a cyclotron product and is therefore currently expensive with limited availability.

Equipment
1. Gamma camera.
2. Pinhole, converging or high resolution parallel hole collimator.

Patient preparation   None, but uptake may be modified by antithyroid drugs.

Technique
^{99m}Tc-*pertechnetate*
1. I.V. injection of pertechnetate.
2. After 15 min, immediately before imaging, the patient is given a drink of water to wash away pertechnetate secreted into saliva.
3. The patient lies supine with the neck slightly extended and the camera anterior. For a pinhole collimator, the pinhole should be positioned to give the maximum magnification for the camera field of view (usually 7–10 cm from the neck).
4. The patient should be asked not to swallow during imaging.

5. An image is acquired with markers on the suprasternal notch, clavicles, edges of neck and any palpable nodules.
6. Start imaging 15–20 min post-injection when the target-to-background ratio is maximum.

^{123}I-sodium iodide The technique is similar to that for pertechnetate except:
1. Sodium iodide may be given orally.
2. Imaging is performed 3–4 hours later.
3. A drink of water is not necessary, since ^{123}I is not secreted into saliva in any significant quantity.

Images 200 kilocounts or 15 min maximum:
1. Anterior.
2. Left and right anterior oblique views as required, especially for assessment of multinodular disease.

Analysis The percentage thyroid uptake may be estimated by comparing the background-subtracted attenuation-corrected organ counts with the full syringe counts measured under standard conditions before injection.

Additional techniques Whole-body ^{131}I imaging is often performed after thyroidectomy and/or ablation for thyroid cancer to locate sites of metastasis[1].

Aftercare None.

Complications None.

Reference 1. Maisey, M.N. & Fogelman, I. (1991) Thyroid disease. In: Maisey, M.N., Britton, K.E. & Gilday, D.L. (eds) *Clinical Nuclear Medicine*, pp. 198–234, 2nd edn. London: Chapman & Hall.

Further reading Biersack, H.J. & Hotze, A. (1991) The clinician and the thyroid. *Eur. J. Nucl. Med.* **18**, 761–778.
Clarke, S.E.M. (1988) Radionuclide imaging in thyroid cancer. *Nucl. Med. Commun.* **9**, 79–84.
Tindall, H., Griffiths, A.P. & Penn, N.D. (1987) Is the current use of thyroid scintigraphy rational? *Postgrad. Med. J.* **63**, 869–871.
Fogelman, I. & Maisey, M.N. (eds) (1988) *An Atlas of Clinical Nuclear Medicine*, pp. 160–216. London: Martin Dunitz.

Radionuclide Parathyroid Imaging

Indications
1. Investigation of suspected hyperparathyroidism.
2. Preoperative localization of parathyroid adenomas and hyperplastic glands.

Contraindications   None.

Radiopharmaceuticals
1. *99mTc-pertechnetate* (80 MBq max.) and *201Tl-thallous chloride* (80 MBq max.).

   Both ^{99m}Tc and ^{201}Tl are trapped by the thyroid, but only ^{201}Tl accumulates in hyperactive parathyroid tissue. With computer subtraction of ^{99m}Tc from ^{201}Tl images, abnormal accumulation of ^{201}Tl may be seen[1]. In patients in whom ^{99m}Tc thyroid uptake is suppressed, e.g. with use of iodine-containing skin preparations, oral ^{123}I administered several hours before ^{201}Tl may be considered[2].

2. *99mTc-methoxyisobutylisonitrile (MIBI or sestamibi)* has recently been used for parathyroid imaging with encouraging results[3,4]. ^{99m}Tc-sestamibi accumulates in both thyroid and hyperactive parathyroid tissue, but washes out of normal thyroid tissue faster, so delayed images (2–3 hours) should highlight abnormal parathyroid activity. Early images (10–15 min) show the thyroid and may be used for anatomical reference. ^{99m}Tc has better imaging characteristics than ^{201}Tl and results in a greatly reduced radiation dose. Although not yet widely used, if early promise is borne out, ^{99m}Tc-sestamibi may become the parathyroid imaging agent of choice[5].

Equipment
1. Gamma camera with dual isotope capability for ^{99m}Tc/^{201}Tl.
2. Collimator choice depends upon system characteristics, but a general order of preference might be[6]:
   (a) high-resolution converging
   (b) pinhole
   (c) high-resolution parallel hole.
3. Imaging computer.

Patient preparation   None, but uptake may be modified by antithyroid drugs.

Technique   A variety of imaging protocols have been used[6-9], in particular dividing into those where ^{99m}Tc and those where ^{201}Tl is injected first, although no consistent difference in diagnostic efficacy between the two techniques has been found. A typical protocol is described:

1. 75 MBq ^{99m}Tc-pertechnetate is administered i.v.
2. The camera is set for dual isotope imaging (if available) with 20% energy windows about 140 keV for ^{99m}Tc and 70 keV for ^{201}Tl.
3. After 15 min the patient is given a drink of water immediately before imaging, to wash away pertechnetate secreted into saliva.
4. The patient lies supine with the neck slightly extended.
5. The camera is positioned anteriorly with the thyroid towards the top of the image and the upper mediastinum in view.
6. The patient should be asked not to swallow or move during imaging. Head immobilizing devices may be useful. Movement is more critical if dual isotope imaging is not available[8].
7. 15–20 min post-injection, a 5 min 128 × 128 or 64 × 64 image is acquired in both energy windows on computer (or consecutive 5 min views in each window if no dual isotope facility is available).
8. Without moving the patient, 75 MBq ^{201}Tl-thallous chloride is injected i.v.
9. 1–2 min dynamic images are acquired for 20–30 min on the same matrix size as above, using dual isotope mode if available.

Analysis   1. Motion correction is performed if necessary.
2. Correct ^{201}Tl images for scatter from ^{99m}Tc by subtracting ^{201}Tl energy window image in initial frame (i.e. before ^{201}Tl injection).
3. If the lesion is not obvious from comparison of summed ^{201}Tl and ^{99m}Tc images, perform subtraction of normalized ^{99m}Tc images (or initial ^{99m}Tc image if single isotope acquisition) from the corresponding ^{201}Tl images.

Aftercare   None.

Complications   None.

References

1. Young, A.E., Gaunt, J.I., Croft, D.N. et al (1983) Location of parathyroid adenomas by thallium-201 and technetium-99m subtraction scanning. *BMJ* **286**, 1384–1386.
2. Picard, D., D'Amour, P., Carrier, L., Chartrand, R. & Poisson, R. (1987) Localization of abnormal parathyroid gland(s) using thallium-201/iodine-123 subtraction scintigraphy in patients with primary hyperparathyroidism. *Clin. Nucl. Med.* **12**, 60–64.
3. O'Doherty, M.J., Kettle, A.G., Wells, P., Collins, R.E.C. & Coakley, A.J. (1992) Parathyroid imaging with technetium-99m-sestamibi: preoperative localisation and tissue uptake studies. *J. Nucl. Med.* **33**, 313–318.
4. Taillefer, R., Boucher, Y., Potvin, C. & Lambert, R. (1992) Detection and localization of parathyroid adenomas in patients with hyperparathyroidism using a single radionuclide imaging procedure with technetium-99m-sestamibi (double-phase study). *J. Nucl. Med.* **33**, 1801–1807.
5. Potchen, E.J. (1992) Parathyroid imaging — current status and future prospects. *J. Nucl. Med.* **33**, 1807–1809.
6. Brownless, S.M. & Gimlette, T.M.D. (1989) Comparison of techniques for thallium-201-technetium-99m parathyroid imaging. *Br. J. Radiol.* **62**, 532–535.
7. Coakley, A.J. & Wells, C.P. (1991) Parathyroid scanning. In: Maisey, M.N., Britton, K.E. & Gilday, D.L. (eds) *Clinical Nuclear Medicine*, pp. 254–270, 2nd edn. London: Chapman & Hall.
8. Sandrock, D., Dunham, R.G. & Neumann, R.D. (1990) Simultaneous dual energy acquisition for ^{201}Tl/^{99}Tc^{m} parathyroid subtraction scintigraphy: physical and physiological considerations. *Nucl. Med. Commun.* **11**, 503–510.
9. Sandrock, D., Merino, M.J., Norton, J.A. & Neumann, R.D. (1990) Parathyroid imaging by Tc/Tl scintigraphy. *Eur. J. Nucl. Med.* **16**, 607–613.

Further reading

Goris, M.L., Basso, L.V. & Keeling, C. (1991) Parathyroid imaging. *J. Nucl. Med.* **32**, 887–889.

Samanta, A., Wilson, B., Iqbal, J., Burden, A.C., Walls, J. & Cosgriff, P. (1990) A clinical audit of thallium —

technetium subtraction parathyroid scans. *Postgrad. Med. J.* **66**, 441–445.

Gooding, G.A.W., Okerlund, M.D., Stark, D.D. & Clark, O.H. (1986) Parathyroid imaging: comparison of double-tracer (Tl-201, Tc-99m) scintigraphy and high-resolution US. *Radiology* **161**, 57–64.

Appendix I Water-soluble Contrast Media

Proprietary name	Chemical name	Iodine concentration (mg ml^{-1})
Conray series		
Conray 280	meglumine iothalamate	280
Conray 325	sodium iothalamate	325
Conray 420	sodium iothalamate	420
Hypaque series		
Hypaque 25	sodium diatrizoate	150
Hypaque 45	sodium diatrizoate	270
Urografin series		
Urografin 150	meglumine diatrizoate / sodium diatrizoate	146
Urografin 290	meglumine diatrizoate / sodium diatrizoate	292
Urografin 310M	meglumine diatrizoate	306
Urografin 325	meglumine diatrizoate / sodium diatrizoate	325
Urografin 370	meglumine diatrizoate / sodium diatrizoate	370
Uromiro series		
Uromiro 300	meglumine iodamide	300
Uromiro 340	meglumine iodamide / sodium iodamide	340
Uromiro 380	meglumine iodamide / sodium iodamide	380
Uromiro 420	meglumine iodamide / sodium iodamide	420

395

Proprietary name	Chemical name		Iodine concentration (mg ml^{-1})
Isopaque			
Cysto 100	sodium metrizoate calcium metrizoate magnesium metrizoate meglumine metrizoate	}	100
Amin 200	meglumine metrizoate calcium metrizoate	}	200
Cerebral 280	meglumine metrizoate calcium metrizoate	}	280
350	sodium metrizoate calcium metrizoate magnesium metrizoate meglumine metrizoate	}	350
Coronar 370	sodium metrizoate meglumine metrizoate calcium metrizoate	}	370
Hexabrix			
Hexabrix 320	meglumine ioxaglate sodium ioxaglate	}	320
Niopam			
Niopam 150	iopamidol		150
Niopam 200	iopamidol		200
Niopam 300	iopamidol		300
Niopam 340	iopamidol		340
Niopam 370	iopamidol		370
Omnipaque			
Omnipaque 140	iohexol		140
Omnipaque 180	iohexol		180
Omnipaque 240	iohexol		240
Omnipaque 300	iohexol		300
Omnipaque 350	iohexol		350
Ultravist			
Ultravist 150	iopramide		150
Ultravist 240	iopramide		240
Ultravist 300	iopramide		300
Ultravist 370	iopramide		370
Isovist			
Isovist 240	iotrolan		240
Isovist 300	iotrolan		300

Appendix II Emergency Equipment for the X-ray Department

Equipment   Oxygen — piped or in a cylinder
Suction and catheters
Face mask — adult and paediatric sizes
Airway — adult and paediatric sizes
Laryngoscope
Endotracheal tubes
Ventilation bag
Needles and syringes
I.V. giving set
Scalpel, blade and French's needle
Stethoscope and sphygmomanometer

Drug	Route	Adult dose	Paediatric dose
Adrenaline 1:1000	s.c.	0.5 ml	0–1 yr: 0.01 ml kg^{-1} 1 yr: 0.12 ml 7 yr: 0.25 ml
Aminophylline 250 mg in 10 ml	i.v.	250 mg over 5 min	4 mg kg^{-1} over 10 min
Atropine 600 μg in 1 ml	i.v.	600 mg	0–1 yr: 15 mg kg^{-1} 1 yr: 150 mg 7 yr: 300 mg
Sodium bicarbonate 8.4%, 200 ml	i.v.		
Calcium gluconate 10%, 10 ml	i.v., slowly	10 ml	30 mg kg^{-1} 10% solution diluted to 2.5%
Chlorpheniramine 10 mg in 1 ml	i.v. diluted with blood over 1 min	10 mg	0–1 yr: 0.25 mg kg^{-1} 1 yr: 2.5 mg 7 yr: 5 mg
Dextrose 5%, 500 ml	i.v.		
Dextrose 50% w.v.	i.v.	50 ml	1 ml kg^{-1}
Diazepam 10 mg in 2 ml	i.v.	10–20 mg at a rate of 0.5 ml per 30 s. Repeat after 30 min if necessary	200–300 μg kg^{-1}
Dopamine 800 mg in 5 ml to be diluted in 500 ml N saline or 5% dextrose	i.v. infusion	2–5 μg kg^{-1} min^{-1} initially increase if necessary	
Frusemide 10 mg ml^{-1} 2 ml, 5 ml and 25 ml ampoules	i.v.	20–50 mg (diuretic effect proportional to dose)	0.5–1.5 mg kg^{-1}
Hydrocortisone 100 mg	i.v. slowly	100–500 mg	4 mg kg^{-1}
Lignocaine 100 mg in 10 ml	i.v.	100 mg over a few mins	
N saline 500 ml	i.v.		
Naloxone 400 μg in 1 ml	i.v.	0.8–2 mg	10 μg kg^{-1}
Protamine sulphate 10 mg ml^{-1}	i.v. slowly	1 mg for each 100 U of heparin up to 50 mg. If more than 15 min has elapsed since heparin was given, then give less, as heparin is rapidly excreted.	
Water for injection			

Appendix III   Treatment of Emergencies

The flow charts on the following pages outline the steps to be taken during the most frequently occurring emergencies in the X-ray department. Drug dosages are given in Appendix II.

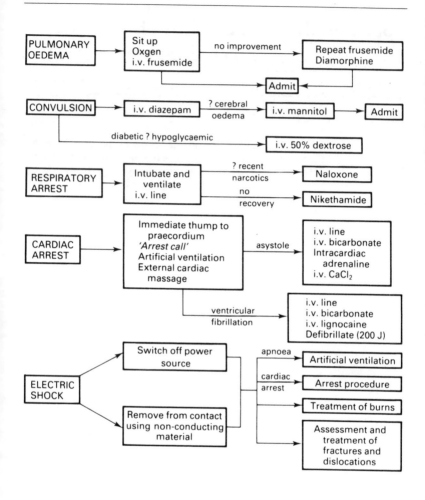

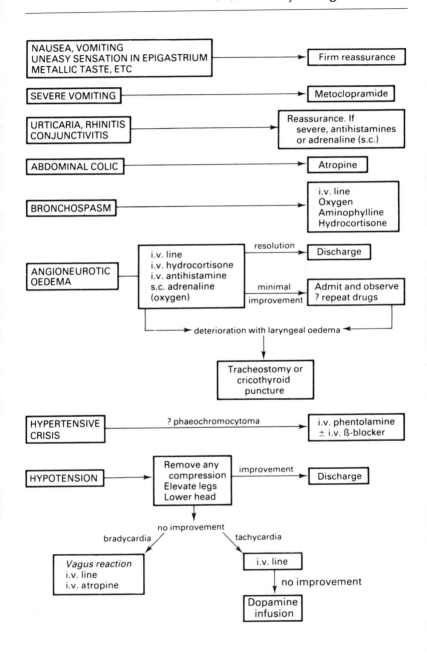

Appendix IV Average Effective Dose Equivalents for some Common Examinations

Examination	Effective dose equivalent*	Equivalent no. of chest X-rays*	Equivalent period of natural background radiation*	Probability of radiation effect occurring ($\times 10^{-6}$) (fatal somatic)	
	(mSv)			Male	Female
Chest (PA)	0.02	1	3 days	0.27	0.47
Skull	0.1	5	2 weeks	1.7	1.7
Cervical spine	0.1	5	2 weeks		
Thoracic spine	1.0	50	6 months	7.0	11
Lumbar spine	2.4	120	14 months	25	26
Hip (1 only)	0.3	15	2 months		
Pelvis	1.0	50	6 months	3.9	3.9
Abdomen	1.5	75	9 months	9.4	9.5
Extremity (e.g. hand, foot)	<0.01	<0.5	<1.5 days		
Barium:					
Meal	5.0	250	2.5 years	26	31
Small bowel	6.0	300	3 years		
Large bowel	9.0	450	4.5 years	37	38
IV Urography	4.6	6.5	2.5 years	26	37
CT					
Head	2.0	100	1 year	62	69
Chest	8.0	400	4 years	330	370
Abdomen	8.0	400	4 years	330	370

*These figures are based on National Radiation Protection Board calculations for average doses in the UK. Recent changes in the weighting factors used to calculate effective dose equivalents will mean that the above figures will need recalculation. Figures are expected to vary by less than 20%.

Appendix V   Safety in MRI

Potential hazards associated with magnetic resonance imaging which may affect patients and staff are due to:
1. Magnetic fields
   (a) static field
   (b) gradient field
   (c) radiofrequency field.
2. Auditory effects of noise.
3. Inert gas quench.
4. Claustrophobia.
5. Intravenous contrast agents (see Chapter 2).

Effects due to magnetic fields The effects due to magnetic fields are largely dependent on the field strengths used, and as a result guidelines have been issued by the various regulatory authorities that advise on the maximum to be used (Table 1).

Table 1   Guidelines on exposure in MRI.

	USA FDA guidelines	UK NRPB guidelines
Max. static field (Tesla)	2.0	whole body: 2.5 part body: 4.0
whole-body specific absorption rate (W kg^{-1}); (see text)	0.4	$t^* > 30$ min: 1 $15 < t < 30$: $30/t$ $t < 15$ min: 2
Temperature rise		
Whole body (°C)	1	0.5
Skull	38	38
trunk	39	39
limb	40	40

$^*t =$ time of exposure.

Static field BIOLOGICAL EFFECTS

Despite extensive research, no deleterious physiological effects have been found. There have been reports of minor changes, such as alteration in electrocardiogram (T wave elevation) presumed to be due to eddy currents induced in circulating electrolytes. This change is purely temporary and disappears on removal from the field. Alterations in length of cardiac cycle, changes in red cell morphology, alterations in haemostasis, increased nerve cell excitability, alterations in growth patterns and activity, alteration in behaviour in rats, changes in blood-brain barrier permeability have all been reported but do not appear to be significant in vivo. Reports of chromosomal aberrations in lymphocyte culture, and also increased malformations in chick and frog embryo development, have been made but are not considered to be a significant danger in mammalian development, and teratogenesis in humans is thought unlikely at the field strengths used in clinical MRI.

NON-BIOLOGICAL EFFECTS

There are two main areas of concern.

1. Ferromagnetic materials may undergo rotational or translational movement as a result of the field.

   Rotational movement occurs as a result of an elongated object trying to align with the field. This may result in displacement of the object, and this applies to certain types of surgical clip. Not all materials implanted are ferromagnetic and many are only weakly so. Each type should be checked individually for any such risk. In many cases, post-operative fibrosis (greater than 6 weeks) is strong enough to anchor the material so that no danger of displacement exists.

   Translational movement occurs when loose ferromagnetic objects are attracted to the field. Objects such as paperclips or hairgrips may reach considerable speeds and could potentially cause severe damage to patient or equipment. This is the so called missile effect.

2. Electrical devices such as cardiac pacemakers may be affected by the static field strengths as low as 5

Gauss. Most modern pacemakers have a sensing mechanism that can be bypassed by a magnetically operated relay and this relay can be triggered by fields as low as 5 Gauss. Relay closure can be expected in virtually all pacemakers placed in the bore of the magnet.

Gradient field

BIOLOGICAL EFFECTS

Sudden changes in field strength during acquisition may induce voltages in the body. The strength of these is dependent on the rate of change of the field, the cross sectional area and the conductivity of the tissue. Possible effects include direct stimulation of nerve or muscle. Magnetophosphenes are visual flashes perceived by the subject. They are produced by direct stimulation of the optic pathways and are the most likely effects to occur since the threshold is much lower than for other direct nerve or muscle depolarization.

NON-BIOLOGICAL EFFECTS

Rapidly varying fields can induce currents in conductors. Metal objects may heat up rapidly and cause tissue damage. Instances of partial and full thickness burns, arising when conducting loops (e.g. ECG electrodes or surface imaging coils) have come into contact with skin, are well recorded.

Radiofrequency fields

Energy is absorbed by the stimulation of protons and is largely dissipated as heat. Radiofrequency (RF) energy also induces voltages similar to the time-varying field. These voltages are oscillating, and currents thus produced are not capable of inducing depolarization but are capable of producing heat through resistive losses. Energy deposited in this way is calculated in terms of the specific absorption rate (SAR) measured in Watts per kilogram ($W\,kg^{-1}$). Total body temperature rises do occur but are insignificant ($0.3°C$). Of more concern are the temperature rises in tissue close to surface coils. Temperature rises of several degrees Celsius have been measured in the skin of the scrotum and the cornea. No adverse effects on spermatogenesis has yet been found within the defined power limits used.

Noise During imaging, noise arises from vibration in the gradient coils and other parts of the scanner due to the varying magnetic fields. The amplitude of this noise does depend on such physical characteristics as the strength of the magnetic fields, pulse sequence and the design.

Noise levels may reach as much as 95 dB for long periods of time. This level is greater than agreed noise limits in industry. Temporary or even permanent hearing loss has been reported.

Where noise levels are excessive the use of earplugs or headphones is advised.

Inert gas quench Where superconducting magnets are used the coolant gases, liquid helium or nitrogen, can vaporize should the temperature inadvertently rise. This could potentially lead to asphyxiation or exposure to extreme cold and result in frostbite. To prevent this, a well-ventilated room with some form of oxygen monitor to raise alarm should be installed.

Psychological effects Some patients find the interior of the scanner a very disconcerting environment and report claustrophobic and even acute anxiety symptoms. This may occur in as many as 10% of patients. Approximately 1% of investigations may have to be curtailed as a result.

To decrease the number of scans aborted, the counselling, explanation to and reassurance of patients by well-trained staff should be routine.

Intravenous contrast See Chapter 2.

RECOMMENDATIONS FOR SAFETY

Controlled and restricted access Access to the scanning suite should be limited. Areas should be designated as controlled (10 Gauss line) and restricted (5 Gauss line). No patient with a pacemaker should be allowed to enter the restricted area. Any person who enters this area should be made aware of the hazards and in particular the 'missile effect'. Any person entering the controlled area should remove all loose ferromagnetic materials such as paperclips and pens, and it is advisable that any magnetic tape or credit cards do not come near the magnet. Other considerations include the use of specially adapted cleaning equipment such as long extensions to vacuum cleaners. Fire extinguishers must be constructed from non-ferromagnetic materials. Anaesthetic equipment must be specially adapted in the same way.

Table 2 Some common metallic implants.

Type	Deflection[*]	Max. field strength tested (Tesla)
Aneurysm and heamostatic clips		
Drake DR20	yes	1.5
Downs multipositional	yes	1.44
Autosuture GIA	no	1.5
Hemoclip tantalum	no	1.5
Heart valves[†]		
Starr Edwards 1260	yes	2.35
Bjork–Shiley	no	1.5
Intravascular devices		
Gianturco coil	yes	1.5
Greenfield filter		
Steel	yes	1.5
Titanium	no	1.5
Orthopaedic implants[‡]		
Charnley THR	no	
AO plates	no	
Dental materials		
Amalgam	no	
Wire	yes (probably safe)	
Miscellaneous		
CSF shunt	no	
Bullet	yes	
AMS 800 artificial sphincter	no	
IUD, Copper 7	no	
Copper T	no	

[*]Deflection refers to rotational movement as a result of the primary field.
[†]Many heart valves are safe because the deflection force is insignificant when compared with the mechanical forces already present. The exception are some valves pre-1964 in origin.
[‡]Most orthopaedic implants are safe.

Implants As mentioned above, persons with pacemakers must not enter the controlled area. All other persons must be screened to ensure there is no danger from implanted ferromagnetic objects such as aneurysm clips. Where an object is not known to be 'magnet safe', then the person should not be scanned. Lists of safe and unsafe implants are available and some common examples are included in Table 2.

Occupational screening is also advisable to assess the risk of shrapnel; intraocular foreign bodies in metal workers have been known to migrate and cause further damage.

Pregnancy Although no conclusive evidence of teratogenesis exists in humans, scanning should be avoided, particularly during the first trimester, unless alternative diagnostic procedures would involve the exposure of the foetus to ionising radiation. Pregnant staff are advised to remain outside the controlled area (10 Gauss line) and to avoid exposure to gradient or RF fields.

References
1. Kanal, E. et al (1990) Safety considerations in MR imaging. *Radiology* **176**, 593–606.
2. Jehensen, P. et al (1988) Change in human cardiac rythm induced by a 2T static imaging field. *Radiology* **166**, 227–230.
3. Brummett, R.E. et al (1988) Potential hearing loss resulting from MR imaging. *Radiology* **169**, 539–540.
4. Quirk, M.E. et al (1989) Anxiety in patients undergoing MR imaging. *Radiology* **170**, 463–466.
5. Carrington, B.M., (1991) Biosafety. In: Hricak, H. and Carrington, B.M. (eds) *MRI of the Pelvis* pp. 37–42. London: Martin Dunitz.

Appendix VI   MRI Signal Intensity

Substance	T1-weighted	T2-weighted
Water	dark grey	light grey or white
Fat	white	light grey
Muscle	grey	grey
Air	black	black
Cortical bone	black	black
Fatty bone marrow	white	light grey
Liver	grey	grey
Spleen	grey	grey
Flowing blood*	black	black
Brain		
White matter	light grey	grey
Grey matter	grey	v. light grey
CSF in ventricle	dark grey	light grey or white
CSF 'fast' flow	dark grey or black	dark grey or black

*Depends on signal sequence and velocity of flow.

Appendix VII   Artefacts in MRI

Chemical shift

Protons in fat and water have different resonant frequencies. Signal arising from protons in fat will be interpreted as arriving from a different point along the frequency encoded read-out axis relative to signal from water. This difference will depend on the strength of the main magnetic field and will be more apparent at higher field strengths. Shift artefact will also be greater when the field gradient is less.

Motion

All motion—cardiac, CSF pulsation, gastrointestinal, respiratory and that due to blood vessel pulsation—causes artefact. This increases noise, edge blurring and streaking. Respiratory and cardiac artefact can be minimized by gating or compensation, but this adds significantly to the scan time. Peristalsis can be minimized by using relaxants such as glucagon. Blood flow produces signal loss as protons in arterial blood are moving rapidly and phase mismatches occur. Ghosting can occur, particularly noticeable in axial sections, in which faint images of blood vessels are seen at points distant from their true location in the phase encoded readout axis. Saturation radiofrequency (RF) pulses applied to tissue outside the region of interest can help reduce motion artefact.

Ferromagnetic

Ferromagnetic objects alter the T1 and T2 decay characteristics of the local magnetic environment and usually result in a signal void around the object. Nonferromagnetic metals can induce similar though less marked artefact due to induced eddy currents.

Radiofrequency

RF noise degrades MR images. Patient generated noise can occur due to eddy currents from thermal movement of ions. System-generated noise from coils or amplifiers may produce specific patterns such as herringbone artefact. Extrinsic RF may produce linear streaking and can arise from any malfunctioning electrical device, e.g. light bulb or leaking RF door seals.

Aliasing If the field of view is smaller than the area of tissue excited, structures that are peripheral to the field of view will wrap around the image and be seen on the opposite edge.

Partial volume averaging This is analogous to similar artefact occurring in CT. The signal intensity of any particular voxel is determined by the average signal intensity within it. Artefact due to partial volume averaging increases with the section thickness.

Further reading Artefacts in MR imaging. In: Edelmann R.R. & Hesselink J.R. (eds) (1990) *Clinical Magnetic Resonance Imaging*, Ch. 3. Philadelphia: WB Saunders.

Bellon, E.M. *et al.* (1986) MR artefact; a review. *J. Radiol.* **147**, 1271–1281.

Ludeke, K.M., Roschmann, A. & Tischler, R. (1985) Susceptibility artefacts in MR imaging. *Magn. Reson. Imaging* **3**, 327–343.

Index